NANDA Approved Diagnostic Labels Grouped by Human Response Pattern

EXCHANGING (Pattern 1)

Airway clearance, ineffective
Aspiration, risk for
Body temperature, risk for altered
Breathing pattern, ineffective
Cardiac output, decreased
Constipation
Constipation, colonic
Constipation, perceived
Diarrhea
Disuse syndrome, risk for
Dysreflexia
Fluid volume deficit
Fluid volume deficit, risk for
Fluid volume excess
Gas exchange, impaired
Hyperthermia
Hypothermia
Incontinence, bowel
Incontinence, functional (urinary)
Incontinence, reflex (urinary)
Incontinence, stress (urinary)
Incontinence, total (urinary)
Incontinence, urge (urinary)
Infection, risk for
Injury, risk for
Nutrition, altered: less than body
  requirements
Nutrition, altered: more than body
  requirements
Nutrition, altered: potential for more
  than body requirements
Oral mucous membrane, altered
Poisoning, risk for
Protection, altered
Skin integrity, impaired
Skin integrity, risk for impaired
Suffocation, risk for
Thermoregulation, ineffective
Tissue integrity, impaired
Tissue perfusion, altered (specify):
  cardiopulmonary, cerebral,
  gastrointestinal, peripheral, renal
Trauma, risk for
Urinary elimination, altered
Urinary retention
Ventilation, inability to sustain
  spontaneous
Ventilatory weaning response
  (dysfunctional)

COMMUNICATING (Pattern 2)

Communication, impaired verbal

RELATING (Pattern 3)

Caregiver role strain
Caregiver role strain, risk for
Family processes, altered
Parental role conflict
Parenting, altered
Parenting, risk for altered
Role performance, altered
Sexual dysfunction
Sexuality patterns, altered
Social interaction, impaired
Social isolation

VALUING (Pattern 4)

Spiritual distress (distress of the human
  spirit)

CHOOSING (Pattern 5)

Adjustment, impaired
Coping, defensive
Coping (family), ineffective: Compro-
  mised
Coping (family), ineffective: Disabling
Coping (family), potential for growth
Coping (individual), ineffective
Decisional conflict (specify)
Denial, ineffective
Health-seeking behaviors (specify)
Management of therapeutic regimen,
  ineffective
Noncompliance (specify)
Therapeutic regime
  ineffective man

MOVING (Patter

Activity intolerance
Activity intolerance,
Bathing/hygiene, Sel   deficit
  (specify level)
Breastfeeding, effective (potential for
  enhanced)
Breastfeeding, ineffective
Breastfeeding, interrupted
Diversional activity deficit

Dressing/grooming, Self-care deficit
  (specify level)
Fatigue
Feeding, self-care deficit (specify level)
Growth and development, altered
Health maintenance, altered
Home maintenance management,
  impaired
Infant feeding pattern, ineffective
Mobility, impaired physical
Peripheral neurovascular dysfunction,
  risk for
Relocation stress syndrome
Sleep pattern disturbance
Swallowing, impaired
Toileting, self-care deficit (specify level)

PERCEIVING (Pattern 7)

Body image disturbance
Hopelessness
Personal identify disturbance
Powerlessness
Self-esteem, chronic low
Self-esteem disturbance
Self-esteem, situational low
Sensory/perceptual alterations (specify):
  tactile, visual, auditory, gustatory,
  kinesthetic, olfactory
Unilateral neglect

KNOWING (Pattern 8)

Knowledge deficit (specify)
Thought processes, altered

attern 9)

  cipatory
  unctional
  ..., chronic
Post-trauma response
Rape-trauma syndrome
Rape-trauma syndrome: compound
  reaction
Rape-trauma syndrome: silent reaction
Self-mutilation, risk for
Violence, risk for: self-directed or
  directed at others

Used by permission, North American Nursing Diagnosis Association. *Nursing Diagnoses: Definitions and Classification, 1995–1996*. Philadelphia: NANDA.

NANDA Approved Diagnostic Labels (1995–1996) Grouped by Roy's Adaptational Model (1992)

PHYSIOLOGICAL MODE*

1. Exercise/Rest (Activity)
Disuse syndrome, risk for
Fatigue
Injury, risk for
Mobility, impaired physical
Self-care deficit, bathing/hygiene (specify level)
Sleep-pattern disturbance

2. Nutrition
Breastfeeding, effective (potential for enhanced)
Breastfeeding, ineffective
Breastfeeding, interrupted
Infant feeding pattern, ineffective
Infection, risk for
Nutrition, altered: less than body requirements
Nutrition, altered: more than body requirements
Nutrition, altered: potential for more than body requirements
Poisoning, risk for
Self-care deficit, feeding (specify level)
Swallowing, impaired

3. Elimination
Constipation
Constipation, colonic
Constipation, perceived
Diarrhea
Incontinence, bowel
Incontinence, functional (urinary)
Incontinence, reflex (urinary)
Incontinence, stress (urinary)
Incontinence, total (urinary)
Incontinence, urge (urinary)
Self-care deficit, toileting (specify level)
Urinary elimination, altered
Urinary retention

4. Fluids and Electrolytes
Fluid volume deficit
Fluid volume deficit, risk for
Fluid volume excess

5. Oxygenation/Circulation
Airway clearance, ineffective
Aspiration, risk for
Cardiac output, decreased
Gas exchange, impaired
Suffocation, risk for
Tissue perfusion, altered (specify): cardiopulmonary, cerebral, gastrointestinal, peripheral, renal
Ventilation, inability to sustain spontaneous
Ventilatory weaning response (dysfunctional)

6. Endocrine Function/Temperature Regulation
Body temperature, risk for altered
Hyperthermia
Hypothermia
Protection, altered
Thermoregulation, ineffective

7. Skin (and Tissue) Integrity
Oral mucous membrane, altered
Peripheral neurovascular dysfunction, risk for
Skin integrity, impaired
Skin integrity, risk for impaired
Tissue integrity, impaired

8. Senses
Pain
Pain, chronic
Sensory/perceptual alterations (specify): auditory, gustatory, kinesthetic, olfactory, tactile, visual
Trauma, risk for

9. Neurological Function
Dysreflexia
Peripheral neurovascular dysfunction, risk for
Unilateral neglect

SELF-CONCEPT MODE*
Anxiety
Body image disturbance
Coping, defensive
Decisional conflict (specify)
Denial, ineffective
Fear
Grieving, anticipatory
Grieving, dysfunctional
Health maintenance, altered
Health-seeking behaviors (specify)
Hopelessness
Noncompliance (specify)
Personal identity disturbance
Post-trauma response
Powerlessness
Rape-trauma syndrome
Rape-trauma syndrome: compound reaction
Rape-trauma syndrome: silent reaction
Self-care deficit, dressing/grooming (specify level)
Self-esteem, chronic low
Self-esteem, disturbance
Self-esteem, situational low
Self-mutilation, risk for
Spiritual distress (distress of the human spirit)
Thought processes, altered
Violence, risk for: self-directed

ROLE FUNCTION MODE*
Adjustment, impaired
Caregiver role strain
Caregiver role strain, risk for
Communication, impaired verbal (individual)
Diversional activity deficit
Home maintenance management, impaired
Knowledge deficit (specify)
Management of therapeutic regimen, ineffective
Parental role conflict
Parenting, altered
Parenting, risk for altered
Relocation stress syndrome
Role performance, altered
Therapeutic regimen, ineffective management of

INTERDEPENDENCE MODE*
Activity intolerance
Activity intolerance, risk for
Coping (family), ineffective: Compromised
Coping (family), ineffective: Disabling
Coping (family), potential for growth
Family processes, altered
Sexual dysfunction
Sexuality patterns, altered
Social interaction, impaired
Social isolation
Violence, risk for: directed at others

*The diagnosis Altered Growth and Development can occur in any of the modes.

NURSING PROCESS
A CRITICAL THINKING APPROACH
Second Edition

Judith M. Wilkinson, MA, MS, RNC

Johnson County Community College
Overland Park, Kansas

jwilkins@johnco.cc.ks.us.
(913) 469-8500 ext 3138

ADDISON-WESLEY NURSING

A Division of the Benjamin/Cummings Publishing Company, Inc.

Menlo Park, California
Reading, Massachusetts • New York • Don Mills, Ontario • Wokingham, U.K.
Amsterdam • Bonn • Paris • Milan • Madrid • Sydney • Singapore
Tokyo • Seoul • Taipei • Mexico City • San Juan, Puerto Rico

Executive Editor: Patricia L. Cleary
Acquisitions Editor: Erin Mulligan
Project Editor: Grace Wong
Managing Editor: Wendy Earl
Production Supervisor: Sharon Montooth
Text Designer: Irene Imfeld
Cover Designer: Yvo Riezebos
Copy Editor: John Hammett

Proofreader: Greg Teague
Indexer: Janet Perlman
Compositor: Fog Press
Prepress Supplier: R. R. Donnelley and Sons
Senior Manufacturing Coordinator: Merry Free Osborn
Text Printer and Binder: R. R. Donnelley and Sons
Cover Printer: Color Dot Litho

Library of Congress Cataloging-in-Publication Data

Wilkinson, Judith M., 1939–
    Nursing process: a critcal thinking approach / Judith M. Wilkinson. -- 2nd ed.
        p.   cm.
    Rev. ed. of: Nursing Process in action. c1992.
    Includes bibliographical references and index.
    ISBN 0-8053-9366-8
    1. Nursing.   2. Critical thinking.   I. Wilkinson, Judith M., 1946–. Nursing process in action.
II. Title.
    [DNLM: 1. Nursing Process.   2. Decision Making.   3. Patient Care Planning.   WY 100
W686n 1996]
RT41.W57   1996
610.73--dc20
DNLM/DLC
for Library of Congress   95-37177
                                                                                                          CIP

Care has been taken to confirm the accuracy of information presented in this book. The authors, editors, and the publisher, however, cannot accept any responsibility for errors or omissions or for the consequences from application of the information in this book and make no warranty, express or implied, with respect to its contents.

The authors and publisher have exerted every effort to ensure that drug selections and dosages set forth in this text are in accord with current recommendation and practice at time of publication. However, in view of ongoing research, changes in government regulations, and the constant flow of information relating to drug therapy and drug reactions, the reader is urged to check the package inserts of all drugs for any change in indications of dosage and for added warnings and precautions. This is particularly important when the recommended agent is a new and/or infrequently employed drug.

The quilt pictured on the cover, Circular Thinking, was designed by Melissa Hozinger, Arlington, WA.

ISBN 0-8053-9366-8
    4 5 6 7 8 9 10-DOW-99

Addison-Wesley Nursing
A Division of The Benjamin/Cummings Publishing Company, Inc.
2725 Sand Hill Road
Menlo Park, California 94025

The nursing process is the foundation for professional practice. It is within the framework of the entire nursing process that the professional applies the unique combination of knowledge, skills, and caring that constitute the art and science of nursing. Therefore, the purpose of this book is to promote professional practice through effective use of nursing process. To that end, the text integrates into the discussion of each nursing process step, consideration of:

- professional standards of care
- ethical issues
- wellness concepts
- nursing frameworks
- culture and spirituality

This is a serious text, with in-depth treatment of concepts, despite the fact that students find it easy, even enjoyable, to use.

Nurses need a conceptual understanding of nursing process as well as the practical ability to plan and implement nursing care. This text balances conceptual and practical aspects (e.g., Chapter 4 explains the diagnostic process, and Chapter 5 explains how to write a diagnostic statement; Chapter 6 discusses planning, and Chapter 9 is a detailed explanation of how to create a working care plan for a real patient).

Nursing diagnosis is an important part of the nursing process, but its emphasis in this book does not minimize the importance of the rest of the process. Nursing diagnosis is expanded more than other steps for the following reasons:

1. It is important in helping to define the domain of nursing.
2. I believe that students should be introduced to the diagnostic *process* before attempting to write diagnostic statements.
3. The complexity of the diagnostic process requires in-depth explanation and practice to enable students to grasp the concepts.
4. Students often have difficulty writing good diagnostic statements.
5. Ample opportunities for application and practice may make this step less intimidating for students.
6. Once a good nursing diagnosis is made, the rest of the nursing process falls into place with relative ease.

The Nursing Diagnosis Guide in the back of this text includes suggestions for using problematic diagnostic labels.

Ethics: In order to increase student awareness of ethical issues embedded in the practice of nursing, each chapter includes ethical considerations and principles pertinent to the nursing process step being presented (e.g., maintaining confidentiality of client data in the assessment step).

Collaborative Practice and Workplace Redesign: The text acknowledges the changing face of nursing and healthcare by emphasizing collaborative practice and expanding the references to work delegation by nurses. Case management and critical pathways receive extensive treatment as well.

Critical Thinking: I maintain that critical thinking should be promoted in the educational process from kindergarten through graduate school, and that it is especially important for nurses—perhaps in different degrees and for different uses, but at all levels. The nursing process provides an excellent vehicle for encouraging critical thinking; therefore, a chapter on critical thinking is included. In addition, the nursing process exercises are designed to foster critical thinking, and special critical thinking exercises are provided in each chapter to teach specific critical thinking skills. The critical thinking exercises are excellent for class discussion or small-group projects.

Interactive Format: The nursing process (and critical thinking) cannot be mastered merely by memorizing facts and principles. In order to remember and apply the concepts, students need practice; they need to "work problems." This text provides many practice problems. The exercises are not just a "workbook"; they are application exercises, designed to promote high-level thinking skills. The answer keys provide the rationale for both correct and incorrect answers and frequently demonstrate the thinking process used to arrive at the answers. This detailed feedback provides opportunity for truly interactive learning, as well as the kind of student-instructor dialogue that is so important in learning nursing process. Students are easily frustrated by the many ambiguities and seeming contradictions that arise when applying nursing process. The answer key discussions are vital because they decrease this frustration and model the thinking inherent in the process.

Wellness: Wellness language and examples are used frequently in order to promote awareness of health promotion as a vital part of the domain of nursing practice. Most chapters include a section in which wellness concepts are related to the chapter material, and the exercises include wellness examples where appropriate.

Terminology: Regarding terminology, *client* is used to emphasize the following points:

1. Nurses have independent functions.

2. Nurses are increasingly accountable to clients instead of institutions.

3. Nursing services are provided to both well and ill people.

4. People are increasingly more active in managing their own health care.

5. Nursing is not setting-bound; for example, it is not done only in hospitals.

Most nursing, however, still occurs in hospitals, and with ill people who are in a dependent state. Furthermore, most nurses are paid by an employing health agency rather than directly by a client. In these situations, the term *patient* seems more accurate. Because either term can be appropriate, depending on the situation, both terms are used in this text.

A similar approach is used for words denoting gender. I freely acknowledge and welcome the presence of men in nursing and, further, realize that patients are both men and women. However, terms like *s/he* or *she/he* are awkward to read, and they are not used in this text. Both nurses and clients are randomly assigned gender and referred to as *he* or *she.*

I have deliberately spoken directly to the reader as "you" (instead of "the nurse" or "the student"). I hope this will empower and engage the reader personally and promote active involvement with the text.

Nursing Frameworks: Theory-based practice is encouraged by integrating the use of nursing models in explaining each phase of the nursing process. In order to maintain flexibility, no one model was chosen for this text. Instead, several nursing frameworks are summarized and used. For some courses, teachers may choose not to emphasize the use of nursing theories; for others a particular framework could be chosen and emphasized.

Culture and Spirituality: In order to promote wholistic care, the cultural and spiritual dimensions of each step of the nursing process are explored.

Family and Community: Family and community examples are used to reflect that nursing care is increasingly given in settings other than acute care.

Teaching/Learning Features: A glossary is not included because (1) this text includes only a very few terms that are suitable for inclusion in a glossary and (2) key terms in each chapter appear in bold print.

This text is versatile; it is suitable for nursing students as an introduction to nursing process, or for use in the continuing education of professionals who may need refresher information and practice. It is effective for students who have had nursing process early in the curriculum and who later have difficulty applying the nursing process in a clinical course. The text is organized to accommodate the instructor's professional judgment—that is, it can be used for students of different levels, depending on what the instructor chooses to assign or emphasize. For example, if the instructor believes the concept of possible problems is too difficult for beginning students, this portion of Chapter 4 could be omitted without damaging the continuity of the material. Some instructors may choose to present Chapter 5 before Chapter 4; others prefer to use Chapter 9 just before Chapter 6. Both approaches are workable.

This text can be used for independent study, but it is in no way limited to that approach. It can be used as a text to supplement lectures, either in a discrete course or when the nursing process is integrated in the curriculum.

This text makes clear that nursing process and a written care plan are not one and the same. For teachers who question the exclusive use of written care plans as a teaching tool, this text will be helpful. I have used these chapters as learning units to teach nursing process to students of various levels, as well as in continuing education for practicing nurses. Student response has been overwhelmingly positive. The time previously allotted to lecture is now used mainly to discuss student questions about their ideas for care of their patients. Even more exciting, fewer instructor comments are needed on the student care plans that are written, and fewer in-depth individual conferences are being held to help students with nursing process.

Reviewers

I am grateful to the following for their comments and suggestions provided in their reviews of the manuscript: Sara Arneson, RN, PhD, University of Virginia; Janene Jeffery, RN, MSN, Austin Community College; Weslee Ann McGovern, RN, MA, Herbert Lehman College; Lois Owen, RN, PhD, Cleveland State University; and Cheryl Perrin, The University of Southern Queensland.

Special Appreciation

My thanks to Grace Wong and Erin Mulligan, who guided me painlessly through this revision.

Getting the Most from Your Reading

The following suggestions should help you get maximum benefit from your study of this text.

1. Begin each chapter by reading the chapter objectives. These direct your reading.

2. Key terms are in bold print in the chapter text. Be sure you are able to recognize and define these terms.

3. Next, read the chapter content.

4. Do the critical thinking exercises. Discuss these with your instructor and/or your classmates to be sure you are on the right track. There are no answer keys for these, because that would defeat the purpose of the exercises; the emphasis is not on the *correct answer* but on correct use of the *skill*, or how you arrived at your answer. These skills can be acquired best in discussions with your peers, either individually or in class.

5. Work the application activities. The nursing process must be *applied*, not simply memorized. You will be applying the nursing process in the real world, not simply recalling facts about it, so begin learning to do that now. Work the exercises before you look at the answer keys, and refer back to the chapter text as you need to. Be sure you understand the rationale provided in the answer keys.

   If you have difficulty with the exercises, reread the chapter and try again. If you are still having trouble, ask your instructor to suggest additional exercises, audiovisual materials, or further readings.

CHAPTER 1

OVERVIEW OF NURSING PROCESS

OBJECTIVES

On completing this chapter, you should be able to do the following:
- State the relationship between nursing process and the standards of care set by professional nursing organizations (e.g., the American Nurses Association).
- Define *human responses* in the context of nursing.
- Define nursing process in terms of purpose, characteristics, and organization.
- Name and describe the five steps of the nursing process.
- Explain how nursing process steps are both sequential and overlapping.
- Describe the qualities a nurse needs in order to use the nursing process successfully.
- Explain how nursing process can benefit the client, the nurse, and the profession.
- Discuss how nursing process applies to both well and ill clients.
- Differentiate among decision making, creative thinking, and critical thinking.

INTRODUCTION

When you first begin studying it, the nursing process may seem somewhat complicated. Because nursing process texts (and teachers) talk about *ideas* and *processes,* students sometimes wonder what all this has to do with taking care of patients. As you will learn in this chapter and throughout the book, the **nursing process** is a special way of thinking that nurses use. It is also what nurses *do* when giving patient care. In other words, the nursing process is a thinking/doing *approach* that nurses use in their work. Keeping this general idea in mind will help you as you work through the more detailed explanation developed in the following sections. The five basic steps of the nursing process are shown in Figure 1–1.

DEFINING NURSING

The nursing process is an essential part of nursing, but it is only one aspect of nursing. An understanding of what nursing is will help you to understand the nursing process and place it in proper perspective. **Nursing** is a unique blend of art and science applied within the context of interpersonal relationships for the purpose of promoting wellness, preventing illness, and restoring health.

Nursing has been defined by professional organizations and individual nursing leaders. The first nurse theorist, Florence Nightingale (1969 [1859]), said that what nurses do "is to put the patient in the best condition for nature to act

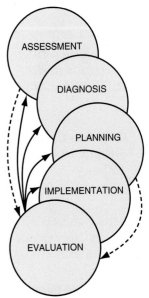

Figure 1–1. The five basic steps of the nursing process (Source: Kozier et al., *Fundamentals of Nursing,* 5th ed. Redwood City, CA: Addison-Wesley, 1995.)

upon him" (p. 133). More recently, the American Nurses Association (ANA), the professional organization for nurses, issued *Nursing: A Social Policy Statement* (1980), which defines nursing as "the diagnosis and treatment of human responses to actual or potential health problems" (p. 9).

Nursing Theory

A **theory** offers a way of looking at a discipline in clear, explicit terms that can be communicated to others. Nursing theories help to explain the unique place of nursing in the interdisciplinary team.

Table 1–1. Definitions of Nursing by Nurse Theorists

Theorist	Definition of Nursing
Hildegarde Peplau Interpersonal model (1952)	"A significant therapeutic interpersonal process which functions cooperatively with other human processes that make health possible for individuals" (p. 16). "A maturing force and educative instrument" (p. 8). A practice discipline.
Dorothy Johnson Behavioral System model (1961, 1980)	Nursing is concerned with behavior rather than biological functions. It is both art and science—a profession offering a distinctive service. Nursing is an external regulatory force that reduces stress and tension, helping individuals to achieve adaptation and system stability.
Martha Rogers Unitary Man model (1970, 1980)	Nursing is both art and science; a learned profession. It promotes achievement of maximum health potential by promoting "symphonic interaction between man and environment, to strengthen the coherence and integrity of the human field" (1970, p. 122). Nurses promote health, prevent illness, and care for and rehabilitate the sick and disabled (1970, p. vii).
Sister Callista Roy Adaptation model (1970, 1976, 1980)	Nursing is "a theoretical system of knowledge which prescribes a process of analysis and action related to care of the ill or potentially ill person" (1976, p. 31). Nurses promote adaptation of the client in the physiologic, self-concept, role-function, and interdependence modes by manipulating stimuli (or stressors).
Dorothea Orem Self-Care model (1971)	Nursing is a human service concerned with the need for continuous self-care action in order to sustain life and health or to recover from disease or injury. Nursing has both health and illness dimensions. Nurses help clients (mainly individuals) to achieve self-care agency and maintain an optimal state of health.
Betty Neuman Health-Care Systems model (1972, 1980)	The nurse helps the client to attain and maintain system equilibrium. Nursing is concerned with all variables that affect a person's response to stressors. The nurse attempts to help the client avoid or defend against stressors. Both client and nurse are active, but the nurse is more so.
Rosemarie Parse Human-Living-Health model (1974, 1981, 1987)	"Nursing is a human science profession concerned with the care of unitary man as he evolves from conception to death" (1974, p. 7). Nursing is a science and an art concerned with exploring personal meanings of lived experiences. The nurse guides clients in assuming responsibility for their health.

Nursing theories are based on the theorist's values and assumptions about health, the client, nursing, and the environment. Each theory describes these concepts and explains how they are related. There are almost as many definitions of nursing as there have been nurse leaders and theorists (see Table 1–1 for a few examples).

Although definitions of nursing vary, there is general agreement that even though nursing is concerned with health problems, it is not limited to concern with disease processes, and its phenomena of concern are different from those of medicine. Overall, nursing models describe nursing as an art and a science with its own evolving, scientific body of knowledge; as holistic, or concerned with the client's physical, psychosocial, and spiritual needs; as involving caring; as occurring in a variety of settings; and as concerned with health promotion, disease prevention, and care during illness. It is the blending of art (caring) and science (problem solving) within the person-to-person relationship that makes nursing special and unique.

Human Responses

According to the ANA definition of nursing, human responses are the phenomena of nursing concern. **Human responses** are biological, psychological, social, or spiritual reactions to an event or a stressor, such as a disease or injury. Nurses, viewing the client holistically, are interested in responses in all these dimensions. Nurses diagnose and treat the client's *responses* to diseases such as diabetes (e.g., lack of knowledge about diet, altered skin integrity, loss of self-esteem) rather than the disease itself.

> **Example:**   Consider the following possible responses to a heart attack:
>
> | | |
> |---|---|
> | Physical response | Pain |
> | Psychological response | Fear |
> | Sociological response | Returning to work before she is well |
> | Spiritual response | Praying |

There is an infinite variety of possible human responses. Note, too, that the stressors that cause health problems are not always diseases or microorganisms. They can be environmental (e.g., too much exposure to the sun produces a sunburn), interpersonal (e.g., the stress of adapting to parenthood when a new baby is born), or spiritual (e.g., guilt from falling away from one's religion may lead to depression).

Nursing, Medicine, and Collaborative Practice

The American Nurses Association definition emphasizes that nursing is different from medicine. Medicine is primarily concerned with diagnosing and treating disease; nursing is concerned with giving care during the cure. This is sometimes referred to as *curing versus caring*. Of course both nurses and physicians are capable of caring *about* patients. However, caring in this sense refers to the activities that nurses perform in *taking care of* patients; not the subjective feeling of caring *about* patients. That feeling may certainly be involved, but it does not necessarily differentiate nursing from medicine.

Nursing is a unique blend of art and science applied within the context of interpersonal relationships for the purpose of promoting wellness, preventing illness, and restoring health.

Medicine focuses on the pathophysiology of the disease and its physical effects on the person; nursing is concerned with the whole person, including psychosocial and spiritual responses to disease processes. Table 1–2 summarizes the differences between the concerns of nursing and medicine. In reality, all health team members work together to implement a plan of care. The nursing process enhances such collaboration.

Nursing in Wellness and Illness

Nursing is concerned with the whole person, well or ill. Nurses support ill people and help them to solve or reduce their health problems. They also help patients to adapt to and accept problems that cannot be treated, and help those who are terminally ill to achieve a peaceful death. For well people, nurses aim to prevent illness and promote wellness. This may involve a variety of activities, such as role-modeling a healthy lifestyle, being an advocate for community environmental changes, or teaching self-care strategies, decision-making, and problem-solving.

Example: Cara Wolinski is a nurse in a factory. Her health promotion efforts include supervising a daily exercise class for a group of employees. She also provides nutrition counseling for those who request it.

DEFINING NURSING PROCESS

Nursing process is a special way of thinking and acting. It is a systematic, problem-solving approach used to identify, prevent, and treat actual or potential health problems and promote wellness. It also provides the framework in which nurses use their knowledge and skills to express human caring. The nursing process can be more completely defined by explaining its relationship to the definition of nursing and its background, purpose, characteristics, and five-step organization.

Relationship to Nursing and Caring

Notice that the definition of the nursing process is similar to the definition of nursing. Nursing and the nursing process are interrelated, but nursing is more than just the nursing process. You may have an organized, systematic, deliberate

Nursing process
- ✓ is a special way of thinking and acting.
- ✓ is a systematic, problem-solving approach.
- ✓ is used to identify, prevent, and treat health problems and promote wellness.
- ✓ provides the framework in which nurses use their knowledge and skills to express human caring.

Table 1–2. Comparison of Nursing and Medical Concerns	
Medical Focus	**Nursing Focus**
1. Diagnose and treat disease	**1.** Diagnose and treat human responses
2. Cure disease	**2.** Care for patient
3. Biological, physical effects	**3.** Holistic—effects on whole person
4. Teach patients about the treatments for their diseases	**4.** Teach clients to do self-care and become more independent in daily activities

approach that is, nevertheless, mechanical and lacking in warmth and caring. You may also feel deeply for a patient, want to help, and yet not have the problem-solving skills that would enable you to do so. Although the nursing process is systematic and logical, its use does not negate the caring aspect of nursing. As you master the nursing process and it becomes second nature to you, it will actually facilitate your caring.

Nurses view caring in various ways, for example as comforting, involvement, kindness, nurturing, tenderness, and concern. Leininger (1978) states that care is the essence of nursing and that there can be no cure without caring. She emphasizes that there are cultural variations in the ways caring is expressed and that nurses should try to understand how clients of different cultures view care and work toward providing culture-specific care. Watson's nursing theory (1988, p. 75) describes nursing interventions (called carative factors) that are related to human care (Box 1–1 on page 6). Caring "sets up the conditions of trust that enable the [patient] to accept the help offered and to *feel* cared for" (Benner and Wrubel, 1989, pp. 1–4).

Background

Hall (1955) first described nursing as a *process*. Johnson (1959), Orlando (1961), and Wiedenbach (1963) were among the first to use the term *nursing process* to refer to a series of steps describing the process of nursing. Since then, it has evolved from a three-step process to a five-step process.

Using the nursing process as a basis, the American Nurses Association developed standards in 1973 for evaluating the quality of care that nurses deliver. The most recent ANA Standards of Care (1991) are shown in Box 1–2 below. A portion of the Canadian Nurses Association (CNA) publication *Definition of Nursing Practice: Standards for Nursing Practice* (1987) also includes standards that relate to the nursing process. The publication of the ANA standards provided the impetus for a number of states to revise their nurse practice acts to include assessment, diagnosis, planning, implementation, and evaluation as legitimate parts of the nursing role. Since then, the nursing process has been accepted by virtually all nurses as the basis of their practice.

The nursing process is now taught in nearly every school of nursing and included in most state nurse practice acts. The National Council Licensure Examination for registered nurses ("state board exams" or NCLEX) is organized around the nursing process. National accrediting bodies (e.g., the Joint Commission

Box 1–2. ANA Standards of Care	
I. Assessment	The nurse collects client health data.
II. Diagnosis	The nurse analyzes the assessment data in determining diagnoses.
III. Outcome Identification	The nurse identifies expected outcomes individualized to the client.
IV. Planning	The nurse develops a plan of care that prescribes interventions to attain expected outcomes.
V. Implementation	The nurse implements the interventions identified in the plan of care.
VI. Evaluation	The nurse evaluates the client's progress toward attainment of outcomes.

Source: American Nurses Association, *Standards of Clinical Nursing Practice* (1991). Kansas City, MO.: ANA. Used with permission.

Overview of Nursing Process

on Accreditation of Healthcare Organizations and the National League for Nursing) include use of the nursing process in their criteria for evaluating hospitals and schools of nursing.

Purpose

The purpose of the nursing process is to provide a framework within which nurses can identify clients' health status and assist them in meeting their health needs. The nursing process gives deliberate direction for planning, implementing, and evaluating effective, individualized nursing care. Often the vehicle for this is a written nursing or interdisciplinary care plan.

Characteristics

The following characteristics describe the nature of the nursing process and expand on its definition.

1. **Nursing process is *dynamic and cyclic*.** The word *process* suggests change. Nurses evaluate changing client responses to nursing interventions in order to make necessary revisions in the plan of care. Previously completed steps are constantly reexamined for accuracy and appropriateness. Because steps are interrelated, there is no absolute beginning or end.
2. **Nursing process is *client-centered*.** The plan of care is organized in terms of client problems rather than nursing goals. In the nurse-client relationship,

---

Box 1–1. Watson's Carative Factors: Interventions Related to Human Care

1. *Forming a humanistic-altruistic system of values:* Obtaining satisfaction through giving and extending the sense of self.
2. *Instilling faith and hope* through development of an effective nurse-client relationship.
3. *Cultivating sensitivity to one's self and others.* This includes the ability to recognize and express your own feelings.
4. *Developing a helping-trust (human care) relationship.* This involves effective communication, empathy, and nonpossessive warmth.
5. *Expressing positive and negative feelings* (e.g., feelings of sorrow, love, and pain), and accepting expression of those feelings from patients.
6. *Using a creative problem-solving caring process*—caring linked to the nursing process.
7. *Promoting transpersonal teaching and learning.* This factor differentiates caring from curing and shifts responsibility for wellness to the client.
8. *Providing a supportive, protective, or corrective environment.* This includes assessing the internal and external environment and the client's ability to cope with mental, physical, sociocultural, and spiritual changes; and making changes in the environment as needed.
9. *Helping with the gratification of human needs*—recognizing and attending to the physical, emotional, social, and spiritual needs of the client.
10. *Being sensitive to existential-phenomenologic-spiritual forces.* This means that you are alert to the mind-body-soul data of the immediate situation, allowing you to better understand the client's experience.

Adapted from Watson (1988). *Nursing: Human Science and Human Care. A Theory of Nursing.* National League for Nursing Publication No. 15-2236. New York: National League for Nursing.

the client's needs always take precedence. Clients are encouraged, to the extent they are able, to exercise control over their health and to make decisions about their care.

3. **Nursing process is *planned and goal-directed*.** Interventions are carefully considered and based on principles rather than tradition (e.g., "We've always done it that way"). The nursing orders are chosen for the purpose of achieving client goals.

4. **Nursing process is *universally applicable*.** It can be used with clients of any age, with any medical diagnosis, and at any point on the wellness-illness continuum. It is useful in any setting (e.g., schools, hospitals, clinics, home health, industries) and across specialties (e.g., hospice nursing, maternity nursing, surgical nursing).

5. **Nursing process is *problem-oriented*.** This means that care plans are organized according to patient problems. Of course the nursing process cannot eliminate every patient problem. (e.g., chronic health problems, such as the pain and immobility associated with arthritis). When problems cannot be eliminated, the nurse relieves them to the degree possible, supports the patient's strengths in coping with the problem, and helps patients to understand and find meaning in their situation.

6. **Nursing process is a *cognitive process*.** It involves the use of intellectual skills in problem solving and decision making. You will use critical thinking to apply nursing knowledge systematically and logically to client data, enabling you to determine its meaning and plan appropriate care. This characteristic is discussed further in Chapter 2.

Organization: The Steps of the Nursing Process

Nurses use the nursing process to process patient information and decide what to do. A series of five steps makes up the nursing process. The acronym *ADPIE* may help you remember their names.

Assessment—Getting the facts
In this step, the nurse collects, organizes, validates, and records data about a patient's health status. The nurse obtains data by examining patients, talking to them and their families, and reading charts and records. No conclusions about the data are drawn in this step.

Example: After Maura Greenberg's baby was born, the maternal-newborn nurse performed a comprehensive assessment. She recorded on the nursing history Ms. Greenberg's statements that she is often constipated, snacks frequently, doesn't drink much, and does not take laxatives.

Diagnosis—What is the problem? What factors are contributing to it?
In this step, the nurse (1) sorts, clusters, and analyzes the data in order to identify the patient's actual and potential health problems and strengths, (2) writes a precise statement of the problem and the factors contributing to the problem, and then (3) prioritizes the problems, providing the basis for the remaining steps of the process.

Example: The nurse wrote the following diagnosis on Ms. Greenberg's care plan: "Constipation related to insufficient intake of fiber and fluids."

Planning—What do you want to happen?
How can you make it happen?

In the planning step, the nurse works with the client to set goals (or outcomes); identify actions for preventing, correcting, or relieving health problems; and develop specific interventions for each nursing diagnosis. The product of the planning step is often a written nursing or interdisciplinary care plan. However, in some cases, planning is the mental process of choosing "what to do"; the nurse may act without a *written* plan (Wright, 1992).

Example: The nurse wrote the following on Ms. Greenberg's care plan:

Goal/Outcome	Nursing Orders
Will be able to name at least six high-fiber foods before dismissal on May 16.	**1.** Give the pamphlet "Fiber in Your Diet" to Ms. Greenberg.
	2. Help Ms. Greenberg fill out menu, identifying high-fiber foods.
	3. Explain the relationship of fiber and fluids to bowel elimination.

Implementation—Doing, delegating, and documenting

The nurse communicates the plan of care to other members of the health care team and carries out the interventions indicated on the care plan or delegates them to others. The final action in this phase is to record the care given and the client's responses on the appropriate documents (e.g., "nursing progress notes").

Example: The nurse took the pamphlet to Ms. Greenberg and talked with her about the importance of fiber and fluids and of preventing constipation in the postpartum period. She recorded these interventions in the nursing progress notes.

Evaluation—Did it work?

In this ongoing step the nurse determines the client's progress, using the goals of care as criteria. After implementing the nursing orders, the nurse identifies from the client's responses which orders were or were not helpful in achieving the goals. The nursing care plan is revised as needed. The nursing process is cyclic: the nurse must keep reexamining the previous steps of assessment, diagnosis, planning, and implementation to determine what is effective and what should be changed.

Example: Ms. Greenberg was dismissed from the hospital 24 hours after the birth of her infant. Because she had not yet had a bowel movement, the nurse advised her to continue her fluid-and-fiber regimen and to telephone her physician if she did not have a bowel movement within the next 48 hours.

Table 1–3 summarizes the five steps of the nursing process.

Table 1–3. Nursing Process Steps	
Step	**Activities**
Assessment	Collecting and organizing data
Diagnosis	Identifying client strengths and problems
Planning	Setting goals and choosing nursing actions
Implementation	Carrying out the plan of action
Evaluation	Determining if the plan was effective

Defining Nursing Process

Sequential Steps

The steps are sequential in that each step depends on the activities of the preceding steps. For example, you must have correct data (from the assessment step) in order to make the correct nursing diagnosis (in the diagnosis step). As another example, the goals you set (in the planning step) are used (during the evaluation step) to evaluate the effect of the nursing interventions.

However, the steps do not always occur in the ADPIE order; that is, you will not always perform one step completely before proceeding to the next. For example, a nurse does not always gather a complete set of data about a patient before taking action. In an emergency situation, for instance, you would quickly think of an action (planning) and implement it immediately (implementation) before doing any formal data collection or planning. Of course you would have made some observations (assessment) in order to realize that action was necessary, but the entire initial assessment step might not have been completed, and you may not have consciously formulated a problem statement. After taking action, you would evaluate whether the emergency was over and then return to a more thorough collection and analysis of data.

Example: The teacher brought Carlene Collins to the school nurse's office. Carlene was crying and complaining of severe abdominal pain (data). She seemed extremely anxious. Before doing a complete assessment, the nurse first acted (implementation) to calm Carlene. After evaluating that Carlene was calm enough to answer questions (evaluation), the nurse proceeded with the interview and physical examination (assessment).

Overlapping Steps

The steps of the nursing process are described separately in order to help you understand them. However, in practice they overlap a great deal. For example, even though the first encounter with a client nearly always begins with some form of data collection, assessment is actually an ongoing process. While you are bathing a client (implementation), you may at the same time be observing the condition of the skin over his bony prominences (assessment). If you observe some redness (assessment), you may conclude that the skin integrity goals are not being met (evaluation).

RELATIONSHIP TO THE PROBLEM-SOLVING PROCESS

The nursing process is similar to the method used in solving any kind of problem. In a **problem-solving process**, the first step is to identify the problem. The problem is then analyzed and carefully defined, and the problem statement serves as a guide for setting criteria by which to evaluate possible solutions. Data relating specifically to the problem is collected, and some solutions are generated. After considering the consequences of each, the preferred solution is put into effect, and the results are evaluated.

> ***Example:*** Suppose you are on your way to an important job interview when your car breaks down. Your analysis of the situation is that your most important and most immediate need is not to repair the car but to get a job. You have specified the exact nature of your problem: Possible loss of a job opportunity caused by being late to the interview. You have the following data: (1) it is too far to walk, and (2) no one is at home to come get you. You make a quick plan. Your goal is to get there on time. You decide to walk to the nearest telephone and call a taxi for yourself and a tow truck for the car. The outcome of your plan is a fabulous job and a new car—you evaluate that the plan was successful.

When using the nursing process, the problem is not usually so obvious. The nurse often begins with comprehensive data collection and uses the data to identify the problem(s). The problem-solving process is slightly different, in that the problem is identified before extensive data is collected and the only information gathered is that which pertains to the problem.

QUALITIES NEEDED FOR SUCCESSFUL USE OF NURSING PROCESS

The effectiveness of the nursing process depends on the nurse. The following qualities and attitudes of the nurse contribute to successful use of the nursing process. They are all qualities that you can improve through awareness, effort, and practice.

Intellectual (Cognitive) Skills

Nurses need to be able to think both logically and creatively. Intellectual skills used in the nursing process are creative thinking, critical thinking, problem solving, and decision making.

Decision making is the process of choosing the best action to take—the action most likely to produce the desired goal. It involves deliberation, judgment, and choice. Decision making is important in the problem-solving process, but not all decisions involve problem solving. Problem-solving and diagnostic reasoning are discussed in Chapter 4.

Creative thinking involves the ability to establish new relationships and concepts and find new solutions to problems. It is more associative than systematic. Unlike problem solving and decision making, creative thinking may not establish logical explanations for actions and may not consider possible outcomes.

Critical thinking is goal-oriented, purposeful thinking that involves a number of mental skills, such as determining what data is relevant, evaluating the credibility of sources, and making inferences. It is essential to making good clinical judgments. Critical thinking is further explained in Chapter 2.

Qualities Needed for Successful Use of Nursing Process

Interpersonal Skills

Interpersonal skills are the verbal and nonverbal activities used in person-to-person communication. Your success in developing a trusting relationship with patients depends on your ability to communicate—to listen and to convey compassion, interest, and information.

Example: Elsa Banayos is the primary nurse for a team of patients. When she notices that the nursing assistant is not using correct body mechanics to help Mr. Davis out of bed, she draws on her interpersonal skills. She must intervene for the safety of both Mr. Davis and the assistant without embarrassing the assistant or undermining Mr. Davis's confidence in her.

Technical Skills

Nurses use psychomotor skills to carry out various procedures and to work with high-technology equipment, such as heart monitors and respirators. They must master technical and psychomotor skills in order to bring about the desired results for clients and gain their trust.

Example: Turning a patient smoothly to minimize pain will help establish trust and rapport. If you are clumsy with this operation, the patient may not think you are competent and will be less likely to trust you in other situations. He may hesitate to ask you for information or help, and you may not be able to get important data from him.

Creativity and Curiosity

Vision and insight are needed to find new and better ways of doing things. Always ask yourself, "*Why* are we doing this? Why are we doing it *this* way?" The excellent nurse understands the rationale for every nursing activity. If she cannot find a reason for the activity or cannot show that it is having the desired effect, she works to have it discontinued.

Example: Mauricio Rossini works on a unit where most of the patients are ambulatory. One day as he was changing bed linens for a patient, he wondered, "Why am I using this draw sheet? These patients are ambulatory, and we use fitted bottom sheets." When the unit manager realized this piece of linen served no useful purpose, it was discontinued, saving both money and nursing time.

Adaptability

Always enter a situation with a tentative plan, but be flexible enough to adapt to the demands of the situation. Realize that nursing care must be adjusted as the client's needs change.

Example: According to the care plan, Mr. Akers was to be up in a chair for 15 minutes. However, as soon as he was out of bed he became pale and dizzy, so his nurse helped him back to bed instead of continuing toward the chair.

BENEFITS OF NURSING PROCESS

Using nursing process as the framework for planning and giving care provides benefits for the client, the nurse, and the nursing profession.

Benefits to the Client

Because the client is the focus of nursing, the most important reasons for using the nursing process are the ways in which it benefits clients.

Continuity of Care
A written care plan provides continuity and coordination of care. Hospitals are staffed 24 hours a day, so patients are usually cared for by at least two or three RNs during a 24-hour day, depending on the staffing schedule. Each of these nurses might be competent, but if the staff does not function in a coordinated manner, patients may not perceive them as competent and begin to lose confidence that their needs will be met.

Example: Janelle Washington has just had her first baby and is having difficulty breastfeeding. The evening nurse has told her she should wake the baby up and try to feed him every two hours. The day nurse tells Ms. Washington to feed the baby on demand, because he will wake up when he gets hungry. Ms. Washington is becoming confused and discouraged. She tells her husband, "Maybe we should bottle feed the baby; this is really hard to do."

Prevention of Omission and Duplication
A systematic approach improves the quality of care by preventing omissions and duplications. Duplication of care wastes time that could be spent productively. Furthermore, it can be tiring and irritating for clients.

Example: Melissa Carpenter has just had a baby and is on a postpartum unit where the nurses use written care plans with a checklist for teaching needs. When the evening nurse arrives, she sees that the day nurse has already marked off the section on episiotomy care, so she does not reteach that information. Instead, she spends her time helping Ms. Carpenter learn to bathe her baby.

Individualized Care
The nursing process promotes individualized care. Each person is unique, and human responses to a disease (or any stressor) are infinitely variable. Some people are reassured by receiving a lot of detailed information; others are made anxious by it. Some people react to pain by crying and moving about; others withdraw and become very still. With a care plan to point out the client's specific, unique needs, the tendency to categorize and care for clients solely on the basis of their medical diagnosis can be avoided.

Example: On a women's care unit, the usual care of a client with a hysterectomy includes monitoring for complications and providing client teaching. Because Carol Wu's care plan stated that she had a hearing problem, the nurses were careful to position themselves so that Ms. Wu could read their lips and understand the discharge teaching.

Notice that the interventions for Ms. Wu's hearing deficit were unrelated to her most obvious stressor (hysterectomy). Because the nurses focused on the individual (Ms. Wu) instead of the diagnosis (hysterectomy), the client's needs were successfully met.

Increased Client Participation

In the present health care environment, cost-cutting is a priority. Therefore, most patients are admitted to the hospital for a short time only. They must quickly regain their independence and ability to provide self-care because dismissal from the hospital does not necessarily mean that they are in good health. Treatments frequently continue even after patients return home—in fact, home care commonly includes complex care such as intravenous therapy and mechanical ventilation. The nursing process encourages clients to participate more actively in their care. Clients are involved at each step of the nursing process; for instance, they provide assessment data, validate the nursing diagnoses, and give input for goal setting. Clients realize that their contributions are important and as they learn more about their bodies, they are more able to make wise health decisions.

Taking all of the above into account, you can see that the basic benefit to clients is that the nursing process improves the quality of care they receive. When the nursing process is implemented, continuous evaluation of care occurs, assuring that the client's changing needs are met.

Benefits to the Nurse

The nursing process benefits not only the client, but the nurse as well.

Job Satisfaction

Using the nursing process can increase your job satisfaction. Many of the rewards in nursing come from realizing that you have helped someone. As you begin to see how the nursing process increases your ability to help, you will benefit from the satisfaction of a job well done. Additionally, good care plans will save you time, energy, and frustration, thereby increasing your ability to find creative solutions to client care. Creativity helps prevent the burnout that can result from a repetitive, "cookbook" approach to your daily work.

Continual Learning

Effective use of the nursing process fosters inquiry and continued learning by increasing your awareness of accountability to the client. As this awareness stimulates you to further develop your knowledge and skills, you will grow in your nursing role and gain pride in your professional achievements.

Increased Self-Confidence

Using care plans will increase your confidence and comfort in the nursing role. Good care plans define client problems specifically, state goals that are important to the client, and give directions for accomplishing them. This kind of specific guidance helps you to feel secure with the interventions you make.

Staffing Assignments

Nurses use written care plans when making staffing assignments. They allow quick reference to the amount and type of nursing care needed without lengthy perusal of the client's chart. This enables the nurse to assign the staff member best suited for each client. Some clients need an experienced professional nurse; for other clients an aide might provide most of the care with supervision from the professional nurse.

Standards of Practice

Successful use of the nursing process will help assure you of meeting the standards of practice for your profession. As mentioned before, the ANA and CNA have developed standards for nursing practice. These are the standards to which you will be held accountable. Other organizations have developed additional standards for specialty areas of nursing. For instance AWHONN (the Association of Women's Health, Obstetric, and Neonatal Nurses) sets standards that apply especially to nursing care of women and infants. The ability to use the nursing process is a part of the standards of practice of all these organizations.

Benefits to the Profession

Proper use of the nursing process *promotes collaboration* among members of the nursing team as they work together to implement the care plan. Communication improves when all team members value a systematic, organized approach. As teamwork progresses, and everyone begins to feel the satisfaction of delivering effective, individualized care, the work atmosphere becomes more positive.

By improving communication, the nursing process *prevents errors and expedites diagnosis and treatment* of health problems. This in turn means fewer and shorter hospital stays and lower costs for health care institutions. In order for their services to be valued by employers, nurses must demonstrate that they contribute to better patient outcomes and decreased cost.

The nursing process *helps people to understand what nurses do*. Because of the complex nature of nursing, nurses sometimes find it difficult to define their role specifically to someone outside the profession. It is important to clearly demonstrate to the public and to other professions the contributions that nurses make to the health of individuals and to the general public. Nurses do much more than help the doctor, give medicine, and fetch the bedpan—which is how some people think of them. You can use the nursing process to show how careful assessment and problem intervention benefits clients, prevents complications, and hastens recovery.

Critical Thinking Questions

✓ Are all registered nurses professional nurses?
✓ Are all professional nurses registered nurses?
✓ The term "professional nurse" is used often. Who are the "nonprofessional" nurses, and what are they doing?

NURSING PROCESS AND WELLNESS

The nursing process is applicable in health as well as illness. Under pressure for cost-containment, health care is shifting from hospitals to outpatient clinics, surgicenters, schools, the workplace, and the home. The nature of hospitals is changing dramatically, and nurses are increasingly working in nontraditional settings. Nurses in such settings frequently work with well clients and focus on health promotion, health protection, and disease prevention. **Health-promotion** activities (e.g., daily exercise) are directed toward achieving a higher level of wellness; they are not aimed at avoiding any particular disease. **Health protection** focuses on activities that decrease environmental threats to health (e.g., air pollution). **Disease prevention** involves actions that help to prevent specific health problems or diseases (e.g., immunizations, prenatal care).

While most of the national health budget is still spent on care and treatment of illnesses, health-promotion initiatives are receiving attention from government agencies. The U.S. Public Health Service, in *Healthy People 2000* (1990), outlines a national strategy for improving the health of the nation during this decade. In this report, they acknowledge that health promotion and disease prevention provide the best opportunities for preserving our health care resources. The broad goals outlined in this report follow:

1. Increase the span of healthy life for Americans.
2. Reduce health disparities among population groups.
3. Achieve access to preventive services for all Americans.

Consider how the nursing process might work in the following case study. Phases of the nursing process are underlined.

Case Study: Judy Witkowski is a 40-year-old corporate executive. Her company requires her to have an annual physical exam, so she has come to the company nurse. The nurse takes a complete health history (<u>assessment</u>), which reveals no past medical problems, except that Ms. Witkowski's father died of a heart attack when he was 62 years old. The nurse performs a complete physical examination (<u>assessment</u>) and discovers no physical problems: Ms. Witkowski's blood pressure is 120/74 and her pulse is 84; she is 10 lb. overweight. The nurse also asks her about her health habits and lifestyle. He discovers that Judy works long hours and often takes work home; her only exercise is an occasional golf game; she eats a balanced diet and gets about 7 hours of sleep a day; and she smokes a pack of cigarettes per day. Ms. Witkowski's lab results and chest X ray provide no indication of an existing health problem.

If nursing were concerned only with ill persons, Ms. Witkowski's nurse would analyze this data, diagnose that no problem exists, and conclude that no interventions are needed (<u>diagnosis</u>). However, he takes a holistic perspective rather than a disease-oriented one, and understands the importance of nursing in disease prevention and health promotion. The nurse diagnoses that Ms. Witkowski has unmet health-promotion needs (<u>diagnosis</u>). Using input from Ms. Witkowski, he sets broad goals (<u>planning</u>) that she will (1) become aware of ways in which her lifestyle can either increase or decrease her risk of disease and (2) experience improved health status, as evidenced by quitting smoking,

Overview of Nursing Process

instituting an exercise program, and maintaining her present weight. The nurse does not include a goal that she will reduce her work hours, since Judy insists that she needs to work long hours, that she enjoys it, and that she has no interest in changing that behavior.

The nurse writes the goals on Ms. Witkowski's care plan and chooses nursing orders (<u>planning</u>) aimed at meeting the goals. To reach Goal 1, the nurse will talk with Judy about the effect of smoking on coronary and peripheral circulation, and about the relationship of exercise and diet to weight control. To meet Goal 2, he will give her printed information about basic food groups, a "Stop Smoking" pamphlet, and a booklet of suggested aerobic exercises. He also encourages her to attend the company-sponsored Stop Smoking Clinic (<u>implementation</u>). He does not refer her to a dietitian, since she seems adequately informed and motivated to avoid gaining weight when she stops smoking. Judy and the nurse include in the plan that she will return in a month to be weighed. At that time, they will also evaluate her efforts to stop smoking and institute an exercise program (<u>evaluation</u>). If goals are being met, the nurse plans to assess Judy's stress level and coping mechanisms to see what effect, if any, her strenuous work schedule may be having on her. At that point, modifications may be made in her care plan (<u>evaluation</u>).

ETHICAL CONSIDERATIONS

Professional standards of practice require you to apply the nursing process in an ethical manner. For example, you are ethically responsible for evaluating the quality of the care you give and maintaining the knowledge you need to give good care. Standard V of the ANA *Standards of Professional Performance* (ANA, 1991) specifically requires that nurses' decisions and actions be made in an ethical manner (Box 1–3). The other standards indirectly imply the ethical nature of nursing practice (Box 1–4). The JCAHO (Joint Commission on Accreditation

---

Box 1–3. Standard V. Ethics

The nurse's decisions and actions on behalf of clients are determined in an ethical manner.
Measurement Criteria
1. The nurse's practice is guided by the *Code for Nurses*.[1]
2. The nurse maintains client confidentiality.
3. The nurse acts as a client advocate.
4. The nurse delivers care in a nonjudgmental and nondiscriminatory manner that is sensitive to client diversity.
5. The nurse delivers care in a manner that preserves/protects client autonomy, dignity, and rights.
6. The nurse seeks available resources to help formulate ethical decisions.

[1]American Nurses Association (1985). *Code for Nurses with Interpretive Statements.* Kansas City, MO: ANA.

Source: American Nurses Association, *Standards of Clinical Nursing Practice: Standards of Professional Performance* (1991). Kansas City, MO.: ANA, p. 15. Used with permission.

Box 1–4. American Nurses Association Standards of Professional Performance

Standard I.   **Quality of Care.**   The nurse systematically evaluates the quality and effectiveness of nursing practice.

Standard II.   **Performance Appraisal.**   The nurse evaluates his/her own nursing practice in relation to professional practice standards and relevant statutes and regulations.

Standard III.   **Education.**   The nurse acquires and maintains current knowledge in nursing practice.

Standard IV.   **Collegiality.**   The nurse contributes to the professional development of peers, colleagues, and others.

Standard V.   **Ethics.**   The nurse's decisions and actions on behalf of clients are determined in an ethical manner.

Standard VI.   **Collaboration.**   The nurse collaborates with the client, significant others, and health care providers in providing client care.

Standard VII.   **Research.**   The nurse uses research findings in practice.

Standard VIII.   **Resource Utilization.**   The nurse considers factors related to safety, effectiveness, and cost in planning and delivering client care.

Source: American Nurses Association, *Standards of Clinical Nursing Practice* (1991). Kansas City, MO.: ANA. Used with permission.

---

of Healthcare Organizations) *Standards Related to Ethics* also requires nurse participation in ethical matters: "3.2. Nursing staff members have a defined mechanism for addressing ethical issues in patient care" and "3.2.1. When the hospital has an ethics committee or other defined structures for addressing ethical issues in patient care, nursing staff members participate" (1992, p. 3.7).

SUMMARY

Nursing process
- ✓ is a systematic problem-solving approach to delivering holistic care to well and ill clients.
- ✓ benefits clients, nurses, and the nursing profession.
- ✓ consists of five interrelated steps—assessment, diagnosis, planning, implementation, and evaluation.
- ✓ is client centered, goal directed, systematic, and universally applicable.
- ✓ requires special nursing knowledge and skills in order to be used successfully.
- ✓ must be used in an ethical manner in order to meet standards of professional practice.

Applying
Nursing Process

1. Brian Callaway <u>has smoked two packs of cigarettes a day for the past 30 years</u>. He has just been told that his chest X ray shows some suspicious <u>lesions on his lung</u> and that he will need a <u>biopsy</u> to see if he has lung cancer. Mr. Callaway says <u>he coughs a lot</u> and that <u>he becomes short of breath when climbing stairs</u>. Which of the underlined data items are appropriate phenomena of concern to the nurse, and which ones are medical concerns?

   Nursing Concerns   *Medical Concerns*

2. Match each stage of the nursing process with the examples of activities that occur in that stage.

   a. Assessment   **1.** _C_ Writing short-term objectives

   b. Diagnosis   **2.** _A_ Conducting a nursing interview

   c. Planning   **3.** _C_ Writing nursing orders on the care plan

   d. Implementation   **4.** _D_ Carrying out the nursing orders

   e. Evaluation   **5.** _D_ Charting the care given to the client

                            6. _A_ Performing a physical examination

                            7. _D_ Giving the client a bedbath

                            8. _E_ Using client data to decide whether goals have been met

                            9. _B_ Stating the client's problem and its cause

3. What qualities of the nurse are being demonstrated in the following examples? Choose the correct quality from the list below:

Adaptability   Interpersonal skills
Creativity and curiosity   Technical skills
Intellectual skills

a. _interpersonal skills_ The nurse sits quietly while an elderly client reminisces about old friends.

b. _technical skills_ The student nurse practices catheterization in the school lab.

c. _intellectual skills_ The student nurse performs the critical thinking activities in this text.

d. _Creativity + curiosity_ The head nurse works on a unit with ambulatory patients. All the beds have draw sheets on them. When he discovers no one can give a reason for using the draw sheets, the nurse has the staff stop using them, saving time and money for the hospital.

e. _adaptability_ The care plan says the patient's dressing should be changed at 0900 and 2100. At 0900, Mr. Sanchez has the first visitor he has had in his three-week hospital stay. His nurse decides to postpone his dressing change until his visitor leaves.

4. Read the following case study.

   Alma Boiko had been in an intermediate care facility since having a stroke that left her unable to care for herself. When she developed pneumonia, she was transferred to a hospital. Juan Apodaca, RN, settled her comfortably in bed and briefly interviewed her about her symptoms. He obtained a temperature of 101° F, pulse 120, respirations 32, and B/P of 100/68. Juan examined Ms. Boiko's chart to obtain a history of her illness and a record of her nursing care. He applied oxygen by nasal cannula, as ordered by the physician. When performing the physical examination, Juan noticed a reddened area over Ms. Boiko's coccyx.

   Because she was unable to move about in bed, he wrote a diagnosis of "Risk for Impaired Skin Integrity over coccyx related to constant pressure to bony prominences caused by inability to move about in bed." He set a goal that the skin on Ms. Boiko's coccyx would remain intact, and that the redness would be gone within 2 days. <u>He wrote nursing orders for skin care</u>, a schedule for turning Ms. Boiko every 2 hours, and orders for frequent, continued observation of her skin.

Two days later, while <u>bathing Ms. Boiko</u>, Juan <u>observed that her coccygeal area was still red</u>, a small area of skin was peeling off, and there was some serous drainage. Juan <u>concluded that the goal had not been met</u>. He was sure his data was adequate, and he changed his nursing diagnosis to "Impaired Skin Integrity over coccyx. . . ." The other staff members assured Juan that the 2-hour turning schedule had been carried out, except for 6 hours at night when Ms. Boiko was left to sleep undisturbed. Even though turning every 2 hours while awake was a standard of care on that unit and had been adequate for other clients, Juan concluded that this was not often enough for Ms. Boiko. <u>He decided to change the order on the care plan</u> to read "Turn every 2 hours around the clock."

a. Label the underlined activities *A, D, P, I,* or *E,* according to the step of the nursing process represented by the activity.

b. List below all the client data (human responses) Juan obtained.

c. Circle the activities that show the cyclic nature of the nursing process.

d. List all the nursing orders described in the case. (Note that some are summarized in the case study instead of being fully written out in nursing-order format.)

e. Where in the case study do you see the most obvious example of overlapping in the nursing process steps?

f. How did Juan demonstrate the nursing qualities of creativity and adaptability in Ms. Boiko's care?

g. Ordering a turning schedule that was more frequent than usual for Ms. Boiko benefited her by providing which of the following?

(1) Continuity of care
(2) Freedom from omission and duplication
(3) Individualized care
(4) Maximum client participation in care

REFERENCES

American Nurses Association. (1973). *Standards of Nursing Practice.* Kansas City, MO: ANA.

American Nurses Association. (1980). *Nursing: A Social Policy Statement.* Kansas City, MO: ANA.

American Nurses Association. (1985). *Code for Nurses with Interpretive Statements.* Kansas City, MO: ANA.

American Nurses Association. (1991). *Standards of Clinical Nursing Practice.* Kansas City, MO: ANA.

Benner, P., and Wrubel, J. (1989). *The Primacy of Caring: Stress and Coping in Health and Illness.* Menlo Park, CA: Addison-Wesley Publishing Co.

Canadian Nurses Association. (1987). *A Definition of Nursing Practice: Standards for Nursing Practice.* Publication No. ISBNB 0-919 108-51-2. Ottawa: CNA.

Hall, L. (1955). Quality of nursing care. *Public Health News* (June). New Jersey State Department of Health.

Johnson, D. (1959). A philosophy for nursing diagnosis. *Nursing Outlook, 7:* 198–200.

Johnson, D. (1961). The significance of nursing care. *American Journal of Nursing, 61*(11): 63–66.

Johnson, D. (1980). The behavioral system model for nursing. In Riehl, J., and Roy, C., eds., *Conceptual Models for Nursing Practice.* 2nd ed. New York: Appleton-Century-Crofts, 207–16.

Joint Commission on Accreditation of Healthcare Organizations. (1992). *Accreditation Manual for Hospitals.* Oakbrook Terrace, IL: JCAHO.

Leininger, M. M. (1978). *Transcultural Nursing: Concepts, Theories, and Practice.* New York: Wiley.

Neuman, B. (1972). The Betty Neuman model: A total person approach to viewing patient problems. *Nursing Research, 21*(3): 264–69.

Neuman, B. (1980). The Betty Neuman health-care systems model: A total person approach to patient problems. In Riehl, J., and Roy, C., eds., *Conceptual Models for Nursing Practice.* New York: Appleton-Century-Crofts.

Nightingale, F. (1969). *Notes on Nursing. What It Is, What It Is Not.* New York: Dover Publications. Originally published in 1859.

Orem, D. (1971). *Nursing: Concepts of Practice.* New York: McGraw-Hill.

Orlando, I. (1961). *The Dynamic Nurse-Patient Relationship.* New York: G. P. Putnam's Sons.

Parse, R. (1974). *Nursing Fundamentals.* Flushing, New York: Medical Examination Publishing.

Parse, R. (1981). *Man-Living-Health: A Theory of Nursing.* New York: John Wiley & Sons.

Parse, R. (1987). *Nursing Science: Major Paradigms, Theories, and Critiques.* Philadelphia: W. B. Saunders.

Peplau, H. (1952). *Interpersonal Relations in Nursing.* New York: G. P. Putnam's Sons.

Rogers, M. (1970). *The Theoretical Basis of Nursing.* Philadelphia: F. A. Davis.

Rogers, M. (1980). Nursing: A science of unitary man. In Riehl, J., and Roy, C., eds., *Conceptual Models for Nursing Practice.* 2nd ed. New York: Appleton-Century-Crofts.

Roy, C. (1970). A conceptual framework for nursing. *Nursing Outlook, 18*(3): 42–45.

Roy, C. (1976). *Introduction to Nursing: An Adaptation Model.* Englewood Cliffs, NJ: Prentice Hall.

Roy, C. (1980). The Roy adaptation model. In Riehl, J., and Roy, C., eds., *Conceptual Models for Nursing Practice.* 2nd ed. New York: Appleton-Century-Crofts.

U.S. Department of Health and Human Services, Public Health Service. (1990). *Healthy People 2000.* DHHS Publication No. (PHS) 91-50212. Washington, DC: Superintendent of Documents, U.S. Government Printing Office.

Watson, J. (1988). *Nursing: Human Science and Human Care. A Theory of Nursing.* National League for Nursing Publication No. 15-2236. New York: National League for Nursing.

Wiedenbach, E. (1963). The helping art of nursing. *American Journal of Nursing, 63*(11): 54–57.

Wright, K. (1992). An overview of nursing process. *Gastroenterology Nursing, 15*(1):14–17.

CHAPTER 2

CRITICAL THINKING
AND NURSING PROCESS

OBJECTIVES

On completing this chapter, you should be able to do the following:
• Define critical thinking.
• Explain the importance of critical thinking for nurses.
• Discuss the relationship between critical thinking and nursing process.
• Describe some important critical thinking skills and attitudes.
• Critically examine the merits of nursing process and its use in nursing practice.

WHY NURSES NEED TO THINK CRITICALLY

Learning how to do nursing requires more than just storing up facts. In day-to-day practice nurses use information to make decisions, generate new ideas, and solve problems. The ability to translate nursing knowledge to nursing practice is closely associated with critical thinking, or the purposeful mental activity in which ideas are produced and evaluated and judgments are made. In this chapter we will examine how nurses acquire knowledge and how they can effectively apply what they learn to specific patient situations.

Consider the following real-life exemplar presented by an expert nurse:

". . . How do you choose between a butterfly or an IV intracath? [You] have to consider why you want that line in. And just learning the insertion alone is difficult. You take into consideration the length of time you will be leaving the line in and the kinds of medications that will be given, or whether it's a short-term, keep-open IV with limited medications, then the butterfly IV is more comfortable and presents less of a threat of phlebitis. Doctors vary in their preferences as well, and you have to take that into consideration. And of course, the condition of the patient and his veins makes a great deal of difference. For example, with older patients special skill is required. They look as if they are going to be so easy to get in because the veins look large, but they are so fragile. If you do not use a very, very slight tourniquet, the thin membrane of the older patient's vein will just pop open" (Benner, 1984, pp. 124–125).

Critical Thinking and Nursing Process

Types of Nursing Knowledge

Critical thinking is not exercised in a vacuum. It is used to apply a basic core of knowledge to each client situation. The nurse's fund of knowledge affects her ability to use cognitive, interpersonal, or technical skills effectively. Four "patterns of knowing" make up the basic core of nursing knowledge: nursing science, nursing art, nursing ethics, and personal knowledge (Carper, 1978; Chinn and Kramer, 1991).

Nursing Science

In the field of nursing, scientific knowledge consists of research findings and conceptual models of nursing (e.g., Roy's Adaptation model, 1980; Neuman's Systems model, 1972), as well as theoretical explanations and research findings from other fields and disciplines (e.g., physiology, psychology). It is used to describe, explain, and predict.

Scientific knowledge includes an understanding of the nature of helping relationships and verbal and nonverbal communication. Nurses use interpersonal knowledge to interact with patients, families, and other health team members (for instance, to communicate caring and support to a client during a technical procedure).

Another example of scientific knowledge is understanding the effect of sociocultural and developmental factors on client behavior (for example, understanding how a client's religious or cultural beliefs may influence willingness to cooperate with treatment plans). When working directly with clients or when supervising other team members who are performing delegated tasks, knowledge of change theory and motivational theory are also useful scientific knowledge.

Scientific knowledge also includes the facts and information necessary for performing technical skills (i.e., principles of the skill, steps of the procedure, knowledge of the equipment). Technical skills (also called psychomotor skills) are hands-on skills. They are often task-oriented and involve direct contact with the client. For well clients, the nurse might use technical skills to operate a slide projector when teaching a high school class about sexually transmitted diseases, for example. When procedures are done skillfully, nursing actions are more likely to be successful (e.g., if bed linens are not taut and wrinkle-free, the plan to protect the client's skin integrity may fail).

Nursing Art

The art of a profession is the *way* in which its practitioners express their knowledge. Scientific knowledge is acquired by scientific investigation; art involves feelings gained by subjective experience. Scientific knowledge can be verified and explained to others; but nursing art is more difficult to describe. It is through the art of nursing that nurses express caring; therefore it must include affective considerations, such as attitudes, beliefs, and values.

Sensitivity and **empathy** (the ability to imagine what another person is feeling) are important facets of this mode of knowing. They enable the nurse to be aware of the client's perspective and attentive to verbal and nonverbal cues to his psychological state. A nurse who is highly skilled in empathizing with patients has a wider range of interventions available for providing effective, satisfying nursing care (Carper, 1978).

Examples of Interpersonal Knowledge
- ✓ Active listening
- ✓ Conveying interest
- ✓ Giving clear explanations
- ✓ Comforting
- ✓ Making referrals
- ✓ Sharing attitudes, feelings, and knowledge
- ✓ Managing
- ✓ Delegating
- ✓ Supervising

Examples of Technical Skills
- ✓ Changing dressings
- ✓ Teaching CPR
- ✓ Giving injections
- ✓ Turning and positioning patients
- ✓ Attaching a heart monitor
- ✓ Suctioning a tracheostomy

Nursing Ethics

Ethical knowledge refers to knowledge of accepted professional standards of conduct. It is concerned with matters of obligation, or what ought to be done, and it consists of information about basic moral principles and processes for determining right and wrong actions. Nurses are accountable to clients and to each other for the ethical performance of their work. Whether developed formally or informally, the ethics of a profession represent the traditions and values of the group.

A **professional code of ethics** is a formal set of written statements reflecting the goals and values of the profession. Formal codes define professional expectations and provide a framework for making ethical decisions. Appendix A, the American Nurses Association "Code for Nurses" (1985), is an example of one formal code of ethics for nurses.

The informal ethics of a profession are based on **conventional moral principles**—those that are widely held in a profession, expressed in practice, and enforced by rewards and sanctions (e.g., approval or disapproval of fellow professionals). The conventional moral principles of nursing are those unwritten values that are rooted in nurses' more general moral views, their experiences, and the history of the profession. The following are four important conventional principles of the nursing profession:

✓ Nurses have an obligation to be competent.
✓ The good of patients should be the nurse's primary concern.
✓ Nurses should not use their positions to exploit patients.
✓ Nurses should be loyal to each other. (Jameton, 1984, p. 73)

Personal Knowledge

Personal knowing is concerned with encountering, knowing, and actualizing one's *self*. It involves knowing self in relation to another human being and interacting on a person-to-person rather than a role-to-role basis. This pattern of knowing enables nurses to approach patients as people rather than objects and to establish therapeutic relationships. The more highly developed the nurse's self-awareness and self-knowledge, and the better her self-concept, the more attuned to the patient she is likely to be (Carper, 1978).

Practice Wisdom

Practice wisdom is acquired from intuition, tradition, authority, trial and error, and experience (Ziegler et al., 1986). It provides the basis for much of the nursing care that is given during the implementation step. As a broader, research-based body of knowledge is developed, nurses will come to depend less on practice wisdom. Meanwhile, you should refine and use your critical thinking skills to evaluate strategies based on practice wisdom, and continue to seek new scientific and ethical knowledge as it becomes available.

Nursing Draws on Knowledge from Other Fields

Some professionals, like chemists or mathematicians, are concerned almost exclusively with the single body of knowledge that makes up their field. This is not the case for nurses. Because nursing deals holistically with human responses, nurses must draw meaningful information from other subject areas (such as physiology, nutrition, psychology) in order to understand the meaning of client

Critical Thinking and Nursing Process

data and plan effective interventions. Using insight from one subject to shed light on another, as nurses do, requires critical thinking skills.

Nurses Deal with Change in Stressful Environments

The rapidly changing situations in which nurses work make it especially important for them to think critically. Treatments, medications, and technology change constantly, and a patient's condition may change from minute to minute. Therefore, routine behaviors, or "the usual procedure," may not be adequate for the situation at hand. Knowing the routine for giving nine o'clock medications may not help you to deal with a patient who is frightened of injections, or one who does not wish to take a medication. The clinical environment is fast-paced and sometimes hectic; nurses must base their decisions on knowledge and rational thinking in order to respond appropriately under stress.

Nurses Make Frequent, Varied, and Important Decisions

During the course of a workday, a nurse makes decisions of many kinds. These are not trivial decisions; they often involve a client's well-being, even her survival, so it is important that the decisions be good ones. Nurses use critical thinking skills to collect and interpret information and make sound judgments that contribute to good decisions. They must use good judgment to decide which of their many observations to report to physicians and which to handle on their own. While the level of decision-making may vary, all health care personnel need to use critical thinking.

Example: Part of Edna Chin's assignment as a nursing assistant is to answer patients' call lights. She has been told in report which patients are on bed rest and which ones need help to ambulate. She has helped Ms. Porter to the bathroom three times in the past 3 hours. Realizing that Ms. Porter usually does not void this often, Edna decides to give this information to the RN immediately instead of waiting until the end-of-shift report.

THE NATURE OF CRITICAL THINKING

By now you may be wondering, What is critical thinking? Do I do it? How can I tell when I and others are doing it? Box 2–1 contains standards that can help you evaluate and develop your thinking.

Definition

Critical thinking is both an attitude and a reasoning process involving a number of intellectual skills. According to Paul (1988b), critical thinking is disciplined, self-directed, rational thinking that "certifies what we know and makes clear wherein we are ignorant. . . ." It is "the art of thinking about your thinking while you're thinking so as to make your thinking more clear, precise, accurate, relevant, consistent, and fair" (pp. 2–3).

Critical thinking is both an attitude and a skill. As you might expect of such a complex behavior, there is no single, simple definition for it. However, it has some characteristics that will help you to know when it is taking place.

Characteristics

Critical thinking involves conceptualization. Conceptualization is the intellectual process of forming a concept. A **concept** is a mental image of reality. In conceptualization, an abstract idea is generalized from particular instances and exists as a symbol in the mind. Concepts are ideas about events, objects, and properties, as well as the relationships between them.

Nursing uses concepts about two kinds of reality: (1) **properties**, or the way things are; and (2) **processes**, or the way things happen. A property concept, for example, might be about the patient's level of anxiety, or whether the patient's incision is infected. A process concept might be about how morphine works in the central nervous system, or what patients experience when they are in pain (Kim, 1983, pp. 8–10).

Critical thinking is rational and reasonable. This is the most obvious feature of critical thinking. Reason and **rationality** refer to the fact that the thinking is based on reasons rather than prejudice, preferences, self-interest, or fears. Suppose you decide to vote for the Democratic candidate in an election because your family has always voted for Democrats. That decision is based on preference, prejudice, and, possibly, self-interest. On the other hand, suppose you had taken time to reflect on what the candidate said about the issues in the election and had based your choice on that. In that case, even though you might still have voted for the Democrat, you would have been thinking rationally, using facts and observations to draw your conclusions.

Box 2–1. Are You a Critical Thinker?

Do you:
- ✓ Explore the thinking and assumptions that underly your emotions and feelings?
- ✓ Base your judgments on facts and reasoning, not personal feelings or self-interest?
- ✓ Suspend judgment until you have all the necessary data?
- ✓ Support your views with evidence?
- ✓ Evaluate the credibility of sources you use to justify your beliefs?
- ✓ Differentiate among facts, opinions, and inferences?
- ✓ Distinguish relevant from irrelevant data and important from trivial data?
- ✓ Ask for clarification when you don't understand?
- ✓ Use knowledge from one subject, discipline, or experience to shed light on other situations?
- ✓ Turn mistakes into learning opportunities by determining what went wrong and thinking of ways to avoid that mistake in the future?
- ✓ Fight the tendency to believe that you should have all the answers?

**Critical Thinking
and Nursing Process**

Critical thinking is reflective. This means that the person who thinks critically does not jump to conclusions or make a hurried decision, but takes the time to collect data and then think the matter through in a disciplined manner, weighing facts and evidence.

Critical thinking is, in part, an attitude. It is an attitude of inquiry. A critical thinker examines existing claims and statements to see if they are true or valid rather than blindly accepting them. In response to a claim like, "Fords are better than Chevrolets," a critical thinker might ask: (1) What do you mean by "better than"; better in what ways? and (2) What information do you have that this is so? Critical thinkers are skeptical, but constructively so. They ask, "Why?" and "How?"

Critical thinking is autonomous thinking. Critical thinkers think for themselves. They do not passively accept the beliefs of others, but analyze the issues and decide which authorities are credible. For example, they use critical thinking to examine beliefs they acquired as children, accepting them for rational reasons or rejecting those they have been holding for the wrong reasons. Because they will not accept or reject a belief they do not understand, critical thinkers are not easily manipulated.

Critical thinking includes creative thinking. Traditionally, nursing practice and education have not encouraged creativity. Nurses were taught the "one right way" to perform procedures, and test questions asked for the "one right answer." This is changing. You will be expected to question the status quo often and appropriately—to find new and better ways of doing things. **Creative thinking** is a productive intellectual skill that creates original ideas by establishing relationships among thoughts and concepts. It involves the ability to break up and transfer a concept to new settings or uses. For example, the concept of *brick* could be thought of along the lines of its molecular structure, its dimensions, its color, its effect on the economy, its hardness, its ability to transfer heat, and so on. Whatever the idea is, the creative thinker is able to transfer it—to find it again in other settings (e.g., a remembered smell, a relationship, a psychomotor procedure). Creative thinkers do not simply memorize and evaluate existing knowledge; they create alternative courses of action, make reasonable hypotheses, and finds new solutions to problems.

Creative thinking involves more or less random thought and occurs at different levels of consciousness. It may not establish logical explanations for actions, especially when the problem is unusual; nor does it necessarily consider possible outcomes in forming the new idea. Creative thinking, however, is directed, even though it is more random than systematic. **Directed thinking** is purposeful and goal-directed, unlike **associative thinking**, which involves random, unstructured thoughts (for example, daydreaming).

Critical thinking is fair thinking. Critical thinkers attempt to remove bias and one-sidedness from their own thinking and to recognize it in others. This requires critical thinkers to examine the reasons for their choices and decisions. It also requires an awareness of their own values and feelings and a willingness to examine the basis for them.

Critical thinking focuses on deciding what to believe or do. Critical thinking is used to evaluate arguments and conclusions, create new ideas or alternative courses of action, decide on a course of action, produce reliable observations, draw sound conclusions, and solve problems.

CRITICAL THINKING: SKILLS AND ATTITUDES

Critical thinking involves both cognition (thinking) and attitude (feeling). To think critically, you must have both the cognitive skills and the motivation or desire to use them. Examples of critical thinking skills are listed in Box 2–2.

Critical Thinking Attitudes

Several interdependent traits of mind (attitudes) are essential to critical thinking (Paul, 1988b), and they are best developed simultaneously. It may take *courage*, for instance, to become aware of the limits of your knowledge and develop *intellectual humility*.

Thinking Independently

Critical thinking requires that you think for yourself. People acquire many beliefs as children because they are rewarded for believing or because they do not question, not because they have rational reasons for believing. As they mature and acquire knowledge, critical thinkers examine and analyze their beliefs holding those they can rationally support and rejecting those they cannot. Being an independent thinker does not mean ignoring what others think and doing whatever you please. Rather, following the ideas of others makes you dependent only if you accept the ideas without question. Therefore, critical thinkers consider a wide range of ideas, learn from them, and then make their own judgments about them. Nurses must be willing to challenge orders, activities, and rituals that have no rational support.

Example: Nurses traditionally wore white, starched caps. Originally, the caps were designed to prevent hair or hair-borne contaminants from getting on patients and equipment. However, these head coverings evolved into small caps perched on the top of the head. Eventually, most nurses and institutions gave up the cap when they realized it no longer served the original purpose.

Box 2–2. Examples of Critical-Thinking Cognitive Skills

Defining a problem	Making valid inferences
Formulating relevant hypotheses	Critical analysis
Recognizing assumptions	Generating problem solutions
Making decisions	Categorizing information
Developing criteria for evaluation	Reasoning inductively
Making criterion-based judgments	Reasoning deductively

**Critical Thinking
and Nursing Process**

Intellectual Humility

Intellectual humility involves being aware of the limits of your knowledge and being sensitive to the fact that the mind can function self-deceptively. Critical thinkers are willing to seek new information and to rethink their conclusions in light of new knowledge; they are not afraid to admit they don't know. Admitting lack of knowledge or skill can enable the nurse to grow professionally.

> *Example:*   A nurse working on a new unit feels insecure and unsure about how to proceed. As a critical thinker, he requests a meeting with the nurse-manager to discuss professional strengths and areas of inexperience and to develop strategies for gaining the needed knowledge and skills. Admitting insecurity and requesting help enabled the nurse to obtain support and learn unit policies and procedures more rapidly.

Intellectual Courage

Intellectual courage involves the willingness to listen to, and examine fairly, ideas or views to which you may have a strong, negative reaction. This type of courage comes from recognizing that beliefs are sometimes false or misleading. Rational beliefs are those that have been examined and found to be supported by good reasons and evidence. Inevitably, after such examination, you will come to see some truth in ideas previously considered false or dangerous and some questionable elements in ideas previously held to be true. You need courage to be true to your thinking in such cases, especially if social penalties for non-conformity are severe.

> *Example:*   Evelyn White is a nurse in a community where there is a negative attitude toward homosexuality and acquired immune deficiency syndrome (AIDS). Her friends believe that the homosexual lifestyle is unacceptable and that AIDS is a punishment. In caring for clients with AIDS, Evelyn learns to view them as individuals rather than labels. Because some of her friends have difficulty accepting her view, Evelyn risks losing them. It requires courage for her to stand up for what she knows to be right.

Intellectual Empathy

Intellectual empathy is the ability to imagine oneself in the place of others in order to understand them and their actions and beliefs. People frequently make the mistake of believing that the way they see things is the way they really are. It is easy to misinterpret the words or actions of a person who is from a different cultural, religious, or socioeconomic background. It is difficult to understand the actions and feelings of a person experiencing a situation that you have not experienced yourself. For instance it is difficult for a nurse to understand the feelings of a hospitalized client if the nurse has never been ill or hospitalized.

> *Example:*   Marta Chavez has cancer. Her husband does not want her to be told of the diagnosis. Dave Glen, Marta's nurse, believes that Marta has a right to know, and his initial reaction is irritation with Mr. Chavez. However, as he begins to consider what his own actions should be, Dave thinks, "I wonder why Mr. Chavez has made this decision. What is their relationship like? What is Mr. Chavez's view about caring, the right to know, the marital relationship? What was his reasoning?"

Intellectual empathy will enable you to reason and understand from the perspective of others.

Intellectual Integrity

Intellectual Integrity requires you to apply the same rigorous standards of proof to your own evidence that you apply to others' evidence. Critical thinkers are consistent in the standards they apply. They honestly admit inconsistencies and error in their own thought and actions. By nature, people tend to be inconsistent. For example, we tend to overrate someone who likes us, and judge more harshly those who dislike us.

Intellectual Perseverance

Nurses who are critical thinkers show perseverance in finding effective solutions to client and nursing problems. Determination and perseverance enable them to clarify concepts and sort out related issues, in spite of difficulties and frustrations, even when others are opposed to their search. Confusion and frustration are uncomfortable, but critical thinkers resist the temptation to find a quick and easy answer. Important questions tend to be complex and confusing and therefore require a great deal of thought and research, perhaps over a long period of time.

Faith in Reason

Critical thinkers recognize the power of reason. They are confident that it is in everyone's best interest to develop, and to encourage others to develop, the ability to think rationally. Faith in reason implies the belief that people can, and should, learn to think for themselves and become reasonable, despite tendencies of the mind to do otherwise. Reason does not negate the value of intuition; rather reason allows us to distinguish intuition from prejudice.

Fairmindedness

Fairness requires that we assess all viewpoints with the same standards and not base judgments on personal or group bias or prejudice. Critical thinkers also realize it is unfair to judge new ideas before fully understanding them. They consider opposing points of view and listen with an open mind to new ideas. (Note that this also requires intellectual courage and empathy.) In the following example, a student reasons from the viewpoint of his instructor:

Example: Todd Mubarik's nursing instructor had assigned him to care for a client who required very little physical care. Todd was eager to use some of his newly acquired psychomotor skills, so he was at first annoyed. "This is a complete waste of my clinical time," he thought. But then his sense of fairness surfaced. "I wonder what reasons my instructor had for assigning this client," he thought. As he considered the instructor's viewpoint, it occurred to him that he had been focusing intensely on technical skills, perhaps to the point of overlooking the client's psychosocial needs. "Maybe," he thought, "this is an opportunity for me to concentrate more on communicating with my client. With this client, I can focus on identifying and meeting *his* needs, rather than my own need to practice skills."

Exploring Thoughts and Feelings

Although we distinguish between thought and feeling in an effort to understand them, in reality they are inseparable. All feelings are based on some kind of

**Critical Thinking
and Nursing Process**

thinking, and all thought creates some level of feeling. The feelings you have in response to a situation would be different if you had a different understanding of the situation.

   Example: In the preceding example, Todd at first felt disappointed and angry with his instructor. But, as his understanding (thoughts) of the situation changed, so did his feelings. He was still disappointed that he would not have a chance to give an injection, but he was no longer angry.

When confronted with someone else's feelings critical thinkers consider what thoughts the person might have that contribute to those feelings. They think, "Why is he angry? How is he interpreting this situation? Would I feel the same if I were in his place? Are his feelings rational?" Critical thinkers ask similar questions about their own feelings.

Cognitive Skills

Cognitive skills are the complex, active intellectual processes used in activities such as critical analysis, problem solving, and decision making. For example, when solving problems, nurses make inferences, differentiate facts from opinions, evaluate the credibility of information sources, and use many other cognitive skills (see Box 2–2 on page 29). Although the terms *problem solving* and *decision making* are sometimes used interchangeably, they are separate processes that are related in some situations.

Decision Making

Decision making is a critical thinking process for choosing the best actions to meet a desired goal. Strader has defined it as "the process of establishing criteria by which alternative courses of action are developed and selected" (1992, p. 233). A decision must be made whenever there are two or more mutually exclusive choices. For example, in the United States a person who wishes to become a nurse can attend a diploma, associate degree, or baccalaureate program. The person must make a decision.

   At least one author defines the nursing process as "a series of decisions made by the nurse in interaction with the client" (Young-Meyer, 1993, p. 230). Nurses

---

Critical Thinking Questions

Critical thinkers reject force and manipulation as ways of changing another's mind. However, manipulation is not always done selfishly. We may realize that if someone does not do as we wish, serious harm may come to him. For example, if a friend was drinking but still insisted on driving, you might trick her into giving you her car keys.

✓ Recall an experience when you were forced or tricked into changing your mind about something. How did you feel when you discovered you had been manipulated?

✓ What are some ways in which nurses might manipulate patients into doing something "for their own good"?

✓ What do you think about the statement, "If you don't do your breathing exercises, you may get pneumonia"?

do make decisions in each step of the nursing process. However, as a nurse you will also make decisions in situations that do not involve problem solving. You will make value decisions (e.g., to keep client information confidential); time management decisions (e.g., taking clean linens to the patient's room at the same time as the medication in order to save steps); scheduling decisions (e.g., to bathe the client before visiting hours); and priority decisions (e.g., which interventions are most urgent or which can be delegated).

Problem-Solving Methods

Problem solving is the process of identifying a problem and then planning and taking steps to resolve it. In addition to the nursing process, three of the most commonly used methods are trial and error, intuition, and scientific method (research process).

In the **trial-and-error** method you would try a number of solutions until you found one that worked. However, without considering alternatives systematically, you cannot know why that solution worked and another did not. This method is not recommended for nurses because it is inefficient and because the patient might suffer harm if the approach is inappropriate.

Intuition is the "direct apprehension of a situation based upon a background of similar and dissimilar situations and embodied intelligence or skill" (Benner, 1984, p. 295). It is the "immediate knowing of something without the conscious use of reason" (Schraeder and Fisher, 1987, p. 46). Using intuition, you would rely on an inner sense to provide the solution to the problem. Experienced nurses describe instances in which they sensed something was wrong, even though they could not say what prompted the feeling.

Intuition is neither systematic nor data-based. It has not been considered an appropriate basis for nursing decisions because it has been viewed as a form of guessing. However, it is gaining credibility as an essential and legitimate aspect of expert clinical judgment that is acquired through knowledge and experience with similar types of situations (Benner and Tanner, 1987). For example, nurses develop expertise in a specialty area, such a cardiovascular nursing, through continuous and meaningful experience with clients experiencing cardiovascular problems. The experienced nurse's knowledge base enables her to recognize the cues and patterns encountered in clinical practice and begin to intuitively make correct decisions. Intuition is not a valid problem-solving method for novices or students, because they usually lack the knowledge base and clinical experience on which to base a sound judgment. As a beginning practitioner, you should be cautious about flashes of intuition and discuss them with colleagues before acting on them.

The **scientific method** is a systematic, logical approach to problem solving, based on data and hypothesis testing. You may recall from Chapter 1 that the nursing process is similar to the scientific method. Formal, deliberative problem solving is used primarily in the diagnosis and planning steps. The implementation step parallels hypothesis testing in the scientific method: in this step the nursing orders (hypotheses) are actually put into action (tested) to see if they achieve the client goals (if the hypothesis is valid).

The **nursing process** is also a problem-solving method. It is discussed in the following section and in the remainder of the text.

*Critical Thinking
and Nursing Process*

RELATIONSHIP TO NURSING PROCESS

Recall from Chapter 1 that the nursing process is a problem-solving method that involves decision making. Critical thinking is an essential part of problem solving and decision making. Therefore, it is essential to the nursing process. However, even though critical thinking and the nursing process are closely related, they are not identical. People use critical thinking in many situations outside the nursing process and in many situations in which there is no problem to solve. For example, you think critically about what television commercials ask you to believe, and about the claims made by politicians. Figure 2–1 illustrates the relationship between critical thinking and the nursing process. Consider some examples of ways in which nurses use critical thinking in the different steps of the nusing process.

Assessment

In the assessment phase of the nursing process, nurses gather data about the patient and *validate* what the patient says with what they observe. They must *make reliable observations* and *distinguish relevant from irrelevant and important from unimportant data*. These are basic critical thinking skills. **Relevant** data is that which pertains to the topic; **Irrelevant** data is that which does not. Data can be accurate and relevant, yet unimportant, as the following example illustrates.

> *Example:* In assessing Mr. Wiley's skin, Martin Fry, RN, notes that it is dry, thin, and inelastic. This is *relevant information* that Martin will use in diagnosing Risk for Impaired Skin Integrity. Martin also notices that Mr. Wiley has a 4-inch, white, contracted scar on his lower abdomen. It is obviously an old scar and is now *irrelevant* to Martin's nursing diagnosis. In the same assessment, Martin noticed that Mr. Wiley, age 50, is balding. This data is *relevant* because it pertains to the topic, skin. However, it is a normal finding, and *not important* in making this nursing diagnosis.

Critical
Thinking

Nursing
Process

Figure 2.1. Relationship of critical thinking to the nursing process

During the assessment phase, nurses *organize and categorize* the relevant, important data in some useful manner, usually according to a theory-based nursing framework.

Diagnosis

People make inferences when they tentatively assign meaning to data they see, hear, or otherwise sense. They may not know what the data means but may think they do, perhaps on the basis of past experience. For example, if you hear a siren, you may infer that it is an ambulance even though you do not see the vehicle. When making nursing diagnoses, nurses examine the data they have organized to *look for patterns and relationships among the various cues* and *make sound inferences* about them.

> *Example:* The nurse observes that a patient is grimacing and moving about restlessly in bed. The nurse's knowledge and previous experience suggest that these symptoms mean the client is in pain. This is only an *inference* and, until verified, neither a fact nor a nursing diagnosis.

Critical thinkers are careful to *suspend judgment when they do not have enough data*. This is what nurses do when they write a "possible" rather than an "actual" nursing diagnosis. They weigh the data and decide whether their conclusions are warranted, based on the data they have. In the preceding example, the nurse needs more data to be certain the inference is correct. She should question the patient to *validate her observations.*

Conceptualization is important in diagnosing because each of the diagnostic labels in the North American Nursing Diagnosis Associations (NANDA) tax-onomy (e.g., inside the covers of this text) is actually a concept. People use concepts to distinguish one kind of thing from another, relate one kind of thing to another, and describe things to people who have the same understanding of the concept. When a nurse reports that a client has Altered Oral Mucous Membrane, for example, other nurses immediately have an idea of the cluster of symptoms associated with that NANDA diagnosis.

When looking for patterns and relationships among the various pieces of patient data, nurses *use both inductive and deductive reasoning.* **Inductive reasoning** begins with specific details and facts and uses them to arrive at conclusions and generalizations. You form concepts by generalizing from personal experience, impressions, theories, and other knowledge. When you see patterns in a set of particular examples, such as dog, cat, bear, and elephant, you generalize to form the concept *animal.* A **generalization** is the relationship between two or more concepts, such as the qualities dogs, cats, bears, and elephants have in common that makes them fit the concept *animal.* When reasoning inductively, you assume that what is true of a sufficient number of individual cases is true of all cases or that certain pieces of data, when they occur together, suggest a particular interpretation.

Example: If you observe in a large number of cases that ice melts when warmed to 32° F, you will reason that all ice melts at 32° F.

Example: A nurse who observes that a client has oral pain, a coated tongue, dry mouth, decreased salivation, and halitosis (bad breath), will conclude that the client has Altered Oral Mucous Membrane (a nursing diagnosis).

The validity of an inductive conclusion depends on the number of observations made, and on the quality of those observations. Think about the difference in the certainty of the conclusions drawn in the two examples above. When scientific induction leads to conclusions that are almost invariably true (e.g., ice melts at 32° F), those conclusions can be used as the major premises for deductive reasoning.

Deductive reasoning begins with a major theory, generalization, fact, or *major premise* that generates the specific details and predictions. You reason from the universal to the particular—what is true of a class of things is true of each member of that class.

Example:

Fact (major premise)	All ice melts at 32° F.
Fact (premise)	It is warmer than 32° F in this room.
Conclusion	The ice in the patient's water pitcher will melt.

**Critical Thinking
and Nursing Process**

Example:

Premise   In a nursing diagnosis, *fear* is defined as a feeling of dread related to an identifiable source that the person validates. The defining characteristic is the ability to identify the object of fear.

Fact   Billy Adams' mother tells the nurse he is afraid of "shots".

Conclusion   The nurse makes a diagnosis of Fear; so when she goes to Billy's room to draw blood, she is careful not to frighten him further. When Billy screams and tries to run away, the nurse recognizes this as a sign of Fear, and she observes for other signs such as an increased pulse and dilated pupils.

In deductive reasoning, if the facts in the premises are true, then the conclusion must be true. However, we sometimes assume that generalizations are true when they may not be. The following is an example of wrongly assuming (generalizing) that a major premise (the first statement) is always true.

Premise   All infections cause fever.
Fact   Mr. Annas's temperature is 102° F.
Incorrect conclusion Mr. Annas has an infection.

First of all, not all infections produce fever, although most do. Secondly, something other than an infection can produce fever (e.g., heat prostration). An error in reasoning may also be made if the *minor premise* (the second statement, or the patient data) is incorrect. For example, if Mr. Annas had a hot drink before his temperature was taken, the 102° reading would be incorrect. You might again conclude incorrectly that he has an infection.

In the preceding example, you would incorrectly conclude that Mr. Annas has an infection if you incorrectly assumed that all infections cause fever. An **assumption** is an idea or concept that you take for granted (e.g., people used to assume the world was flat). Assumptions can be true or false, as seen in the sample of Mr. Annas's fever. In the diagnosis step, nurses must try to *recognize and examine their assumptions* about patient situations and about the meaning of the data.

Planning

When planning care with clients, nurses use knowledge and reasoning skills to *develop evaluative criteria.* They use the goals or outcomes developed in this stage as criteria for evaluating the client's progress and the success of the nursing actions. They use the skill of *forming valid generalizations, explanations, and predictions* in developing goals and choosing nursing interventions. Nurses *make interdisciplinary connections* when they use their knowledge of subjects such as physiology, psychology, and sociology to choose appropriate nursing orders and provide rationales for them. And finally, nurses *hypothesize* that certain nursing interventions will relieve the patient's problem and/or help achieve the stated health goals. Generating nursing interventions is similar to generating hypotheses in the scientific method.

Implementation

Relationship to Nursing Process

In this phase nurses *apply their knowledge* and principles from nursing and related courses to each specific patient-care situation. As mentioned before, the ability to apply, not simply memorize, principles is a mark of critical thinking.

> **Example:** A nursing student has learned the principles *Heat is lost through evaporation* and *The normal newborn is at risk for cold stress.* Although she has never bathed a newborn and has not memorized the procedure for doing so, she prevents cold stress by uncovering only the parts she is bathing, and drying the infant well.

Carrying out the nursing orders in the implementation phase can be compared to *hypothesis testing* in the scientific method. The nursing orders must be translated into action (or tested) in order to decide whether they were successful.

Evaluation

In the evaluation phase, the nurse uses new observations to determine whether patient goals have been met, that is, whether the nursing orders (hypotheses) were successful (correct). *Using criterion-based evaluation* (see implementation above) is a critical thinking skill.

> **Example:** When bathing the newborn, the student realizes she must evaluate the results of her actions; that is, she must determine whether she has kept the infant warm enough. The most obvious criterion to use is that the infant's body temperature should be at least 98° F. Although no rule states that she should take the baby's temperature after a bath, she does so in order to evaluate whether she has achieved the goal of avoiding cold stress.

Table 2–1 provides a summary and questions for checking your thinking in each step of the nursing process.

Table 2–1. Examples of Critical Thinking in the Nursing Process

Nursing Process Step	Critical Thinking Skills	Questions to Check Your Thinking
Assessment	Making reliable observations Distinguishing relevant from irrelevant data Distinguishing important from unimportant data Validating data Organizing data Categorizing data according to a framework Recognizing assumptions	What assumptions am I making about the patient? Is my data correct and accurate? How reliable are my sources? What data is important? Relevant? What biases do I have that might cause me to miss important information? Am I listening carefully to get the patient's and family's perspective? Do I have all the facts? What other data might I need?

Table 2–1. Examples of Critical Thinking in the Nursing Process (continued)

Nursing Process Step	Critical Thinking Skills	Questions to Check Your Thinking
Diagnosis	Finding patterns and relationships among cues Identifying gaps in the data Making inferences Suspending judgment when lacking data Making interdisciplinary connections Stating the problem Examining assumptions Comparing patterns with norms Identifying factors contributing to the problem	Do I know what is within normal limits for this data? Do I have enough data to make a valid inference? What biases might I have that could affect how I see the patient's problems? Do I have enough data to make a nursing diagnosis or should I make a "possible" diagnosis? What other problems might this data suggest other than the one that seems most obvious to me?
Planning	Forming valid generalizations Transferring knowledge from one situation to another Developing evaluative criteria Hypothesizing Making interdisciplinary connections Prioritizing client problems Generalizing principles from other sciences	Do I need help to plan interventions, or am I qualified to do it? Did I remember to give high priority to the problems the patient and family identified as important? What are the most important problems we need to solve? What interventions worked in similar situations? Is this situation similar enough to merit using them with this patient? Are there other plans that might be more agreeable to the patient, and therefore more likely to work? Why do I expect these interventions to be effective? Based on what knowledge?
Implementation	Applying knowledge to perform interventions Using interventions to test hypotheses	Has the patient's condition changed since the plan was made? Have I overlooked any new developments? What is the patient's initial response to the intervention? Are there any safety issues I have overlooked?

Table 2–1. Examples of Critical Thinking in the Nursing Process (concluded)

Nursing Process Step	Critical Thinking Skills	Questions to Check Your Thinking
Evaluation	Deciding whether hypotheses are correct Making criterion-based evaluations	What are the patient responses after the interventions? Have I overlooked anything? Does the data indicate that goals were met? Does the patient feel the goals were met? Does the patient trust me enough to give honest answers? Am I sure the problem is really resolved? What might we have done that would have been more effective? What nursing care is still needed, if any?

HOW CAN CRITICAL THINKING BE DEVELOPED?

Critical thinking is not an "either-or" phenomenon; it exists on a continuum, along which people develop and use it more or less effectively. Some people make better evaluations than others; some people believe information from nearly any source; and still others seldom believe anything without carefully evaluating the credibility of the source. Critical thinking is not easy, but with practice you can develop a critical attitude and good thinking skills. Most of the exercises in this book require you to practice critical thinking skills, even though they don't always state which ones you are using. In addition, a special "Critical Thinking" exercise appears at the end of every chapter. Each of these explains a different critical thinking skill and asks you to apply it. The exercise at the end of this chapter applies to the material in Chapter 1, which had no critical thinking exercise because the subject had not yet been presented.

Nurses need to use critical thinking in applying the nursing process and achieving the purpose of nursing. You are taking the first steps along the path to critical thinking when you believe in the importance of understanding rather than memorizing, and when you trust your own ability to make sense of evidence and principles. As you increase your critical thinking abilities, you will find that your thinking is no longer limited by the influences of your unexamined beliefs, feelings, and values. This will enhance your efforts to bring about good outcomes for your clients.

**Critical Thinking
and Nursing Process**

SUMMARY

Nurses

✓ must be critical thinkers because of the nature of their work.

✓ use critical thinking skills in each step of the nursing process.

Critical thinking

✓ involves both attitudes and reasoning processes.

✓ includes decision-making and problem-solving processes.

✓ can be improved with practice.

Critical thinkers

✓ use logic.

✓ recognize the difference between fact and inference.

✓ consider issues before forming an opinion.

✓ believe in their ability to think things through and make decisions.

✓ are able to apply knowledge and principles to specific situations.

Five types of nursing knowledge are: nursing science, nursing art, nursing ethics, personal knowledge, and practice wisdom.

Critical Thinking Practice

Discuss this exercise with your classmates. Compare your thinking with theirs. You will not be able to find "the one right answer" in the text because this is a *thinking* exercise.

Recall that an assumption is an idea or concept we take for granted, and that assumptions can be true or false. You can better evaluate someone's reasoning if that person tells you the assumptions on which it is based. In each step of the nursing process nurses must recognize and examine their assumptions about clients, about the data, and about the meanings they attach to the data. In order to evaluate assumptions—yours or someone else's—you must first be able to recognize them. Make it a habit to look for hidden, unstated assumptions. Start with this text! To help you begin, an assumption in Chapter 1 is that nurses ought to use the nursing process.

> **Recognizing Assumptions**

1. Why is that statement an assumption? Could you say it is a fact instead? Why or why not?

2. What evidence does the chapter give that the assumption is true?

3. How could you prove to yourself that this assumption is (or is not) true? What further evidence is needed?

4. What other assumptions can you find in Chapter 1? Write them here.

Applying
Nursing Process

---

1. This chapter gave reasons to justify the assertion that nurses need to be critical thinkers; these are listed below. Write the letters that match them to the correct examples.

____ C ____ Nursing is an applied discipline.

____ B ____ Nursing draws on knowledge from other subjects and fields.

____ A ____ Nurses deal with change in stressful environments.

____ D ____ Nurses make frequent, varied, and important decisions in their work.

a. Sally Sims works in an intensive-care unit. Today she performed neurological checks on her patient every hour. When her client stopped breathing she helped resuscitate him and put him on a ventilator. He has three different intravenous solutions running. She also had to attend an in-service meeting to learn how to use the new IV pump. When she returned to the unit, she learned that her client was to receive a new, experimental medication and now needed neuro checks every 15 minutes.

b. Patrick Patel is taking a psychology course because he wants to understand his patients better. Today at work, he looked up a new medication in a pharmacology book. He also reviewed the inflammatory process in a physiology text.

c. Recalling that local lack of nutrients and oxygen results in tissue damage, Roberto Saldona turns his immobile patient at least every 2 hours to prevent pressure sores.

d. Today Samantha Wiles chose to use a smaller-than-usual needle to inject a client with frail tissues and little muscle mass. She decided to let a patient's family stay past visiting hours because the patient needed their support. When another patient had symptoms of low blood sugar, she decided to give him some juice and wait to see how he responded before calling the physician.

2. Look at each of the responses to the case below. Which nurse(s) demonstrated critical thinking? Circle the correct nurse(s) (A, B, C, or D).

Case. The night nurse has just reported as follows: "Mr. Stewart doesn't look very good to me. He said he felt 'sick' when I took his vital signs at 0600. Probably he just needs some orange juice." The day nurse is floating to a new unit and does not know any of her patients today. She knows from the night report that Mr. Stewart is 80 years old, he is diabetic, and his vital signs were within normal limits at 0600.

Nurse A, realizing that the regular staff probably knew the patients better than she did, followed the night nurse's advice and immediately gave Mr. Stewart some orange juice before making rounds on her other patients. After making rounds she returned to see if he was feeling better.

Nurse B, realizing that she was not an expert on diabetes, immediately called Mr. Stewart's physician and relayed the night report so that she could get orders about how to proceed.

Nurse C went to Mr. Stewart's room immediately after report, took his vital signs, listened to his heart and lungs, and asked him to describe how he was feeling. Unable to recall the symptoms of low blood sugar, he looked them up in a nursing text before giving Mr. Stewart the orange juice. His plan was to call the physician if Mr. Stewart's condition did not improve within the hour.

Nurse D gave Mr. Stewart the orange juice immediately. She then charted that Mr. Stewart had a hypoglycemic reaction (low blood sugar) and initiated a care plan for that problem, including nursing orders to give orange juice as needed and to reassess the patient within 30 minutes.

3. In the situations above, for each nurse who did not use critical thinking, explain what the nurse did wrong. In your explanations, use the information from "The Nature of Critical Thinking" in Chapter 2.

4. Which thinking does the situation demonstrate: critical, creative, associative, or directed?

   a. _____ Mr. Adams is having difficulty understanding the calorie content of different foods, so his nurse thinks of an entirely new way to present the information to him.

   b. _____ The nurse determines that a client is too weak to sit at the lavatory and assigns an aide to bathe him.

   c. _____ Prior to surgery, Ms. Morris's nurse notices that her facial expression is tense and her hands are trembling. The nurse analyzes the relationship between these cues and recognizes that the client is anxious.

   d. _____ The nurse notices that Ms. Ginsburg is left alone in the corridor to wait for surgery. She imagines how lonely the client must feel, and she is reminded of the time her mother was in the hospital. She wonders if her mother is still following her low-salt diet. She pats Ms. Ginsburg's hand as she walks by to another client's room.

5. Enter the letter for the kind of knowledge demonstrated by the following examples:

   (S) Scientific, (E) Ethical, (P) Practice wisdom, (A) Nursing art, (SK) Self-knowledge

   a. __ The nurse is having lunch with colleagues who are discussing her client's personal life. One of them says, "I heard she made all that money in real estate. Is that true?" The nurse replies, "I can't discuss personal data about her, especially where it could be overheard."

   b. __ Mr. Castaneda is reading his wife's chart, which was accidentally left at her bedside. The nurse says, "I'm sorry, Mr. Castaneda, but I must have Ms. Castaneda's permission in order to give you information that is in the chart."

   c. __ After reading several research reports, the head of the newborn nursery discontinued the requirement that parents must wear special gowns when holding the infants.

   d. __ The nurses on a surgical floor urge patients to ambulate to help promote the return of peristalsis after surgery. No one can say exactly how it helps, but they all remember patients who passed flatus after ambulating (and some who didn't).

REFERENCES

American Nurses Association. (1985). *Code for Nurses with Interpretive Statements*. Kansas City, MO: ANA.

Bandman, E., and Bandman, B. (1995). *Critical Thinking in Nursing*. 2nd ed. Norwalk, CT: Appleton and Lange.

Benner, P. (1984). *From Novice to Expert: Excellence and Power in Clinical Nursing Practice*. Menlo Park, CA: Addison-Wesley.

Benner, P., and Tanner, C. (1987). How expert nurses use intuition. *American Journal of Nursing, 87*:23–31.

Brookfield, S. (1987). *Developing Critical Thinkers*. San Francisco: Jossey-Bass, Inc.

Carper, B. (1978). Fundamental patterns of knowing in nursing. *Advances in Nursing Science, 1*:(October)13–23.

Case, B. (1994). Walking around the elephant: A critical-thinking strategy for decision making. *Journal of Continuing Education in Nursing, 25*(3):101–109.

Chaffee, J. (1990). *Thinking Critically*. 3rd ed. Boston: Houghton Miffin.

Chinn, P., and Kramer, M. (1991). *Theory and Nursing*, 3rd ed. St. Louis, MO: Mosby Year Book.

Doona, M. (1992). Judgment: The nurse's key to knowledge. *Journal of Professional Nursing, 8*(4):231–238.

Eggen, P., and Kauchak, D. (1988). *Strategies for Teachers: Teaching Content and Thinking Skills*. 2nd ed. Englewood Cliffs, NJ: Prentice Hall.

Gordon, M., Murphy, C., Candee, D., and Hiltunen, E. (1994). Clinical judgment: An integrated model. *Advances in Nursing Science, 16*(4):55–70.

Halpern, D. (1984). *Thought and Knowledge: An Introduction to Critical Thinking*. Hilldale, NJ: Lawrence Erlbaum Associates.

Hamers, J., Abu-Saad, H., and Halfens, R. (1994). Diagnostic process and decision making in nursing: A literature review. *Journal of Professional Nursing, 10*(3):154–163.

Jameton, A. (1984). *Nursing Practice: The Ethical Issues*. Englewood Cliffs, NJ: Prentice Hall, pp. 71–79.

Jenks, J. M. (1993). The pattern of personal knowing in nurse clinical decision making. *Journal of Nursing Education, 32*:399–405.

Jones, J. (1988). Clinical reasoning: Ethic, science, art. *Journal of Advanced Nursing, 13*(2):185–192.

Jones, S., and Brown, L. (1993). Alternative views on defining critical thinking through the nursing process. *Holistic Nursing Practice, 7*(3):71–76.

Kim, H. (1983). *The Nature of Theoretical Thinking in Nursing*. Norwalk, CT: Appleton-Century-Crofts.

Kramer, M.K. (1993). Concept clarification and critical thinking: Integrated processes. *Journal of Nursing Education, 32*:406–414.

Neuman, B. (1972). The Betty Neuman model: A total person approach to viewing patient problems. *Nursing Research, 21*(3):264–69.

Norris, S. (1985). Synthesis of research on critical thinking. *Educational Leadership*, (May):40–45.

Paul, R. (1988a). *The Critical Student and Person*. From The Eighth Annual and Sixth International Conference on Critical Thinking and Educational Reform. The Center for Critical Thinking and Moral Critique, Sonoma State University, Rohnert Park, CA 94928.

Paul, R. (1988b). *What, Then, Is Critical Thinking?* From The Eighth Annual and Sixth International Conference on Critical Thinking and Educational Reform. The Center for Critical Thinking and Moral Critique, Sonoma State University, Rohnert Park, CA 94928.

Roy, C. (1980). The Roy adaptation model. In Riehl, J. and Roy, C., eds., *Conceptual Models for Nursing Practice*. 2nd ed. New York: Appleton-Century-Crofts.

Ruggiero, V. (1991). *The Art of Thinking: A Guide to Critical and Creative Thought*. 3rd ed. New York: HarperCollins.

Schmieding, N. J. (1993). *Ida Jean Orlando: A Nursing Process Theory*. Newbury Park, CA: Sage Publications.

Schraeder, B., and Fischer, D. (1987). Using intuitive knowledge in the neonatal intensive care nursery. *Holistic Nursing Practice, 1*(3):45–51.

Snyder, M. (1993). Critical thinking. A foundation for consumer-focused care. *Journal of Continuing Education in Nursing*, *24*(5):206–210.

Strader, M. (1992). Critical thinking. In Sullivan, E. J., and Decker, P. J. *Effective Management in Nursing*, 3rd ed. Redwood City, CA: Addison-Wesley Nursing, pp. 225–248.

Tschikota, S. (1993). The clinical decision-making processes of student nurses. *Journal of Nursing Education, 32*:389–398.

Wurzbach, M. (1991). Judgment under conditions of uncertainty. *Nursing Forum, 26*(3):27–34. Young-Meyer, V. (1993). A Two-level approach to nursing process. *Journal of Nursing Staff Development, 9*(5):230–235.

Ziegler, S., Vaughan-Wrobel, B., and Erlen, J. (1986) *Nursing Process, Nursing Diagnosis, Nursing Knowledge: Avenues to Autonomy*. Norwalk, CT. Appleton-Century-Crofts.

CHAPTER 3

ASSESSMENT

OBJECTIVES

On completing this chapter, you should be able to do the following:
- Relate the assessment step to the other steps of the nursing process.
- Differentiate between subjective and objective data.
- Compare initial and ongoing assessment.
- Describe effective interview techniques.
- State the contents of the initial comprehensive nursing assessment of a client.
- Use a nursing framework to structure data collection.
- Give examples of a "special purpose" assessment.
- Describe nursing assessments that are pertinent to well clients.
- Explain why and how data should be validated.
- Explain the need for honesty and confidentiality when collecting data.
- Explain why critical thinking is important in the assessment step.

ASSESSMENT: THE FIRST STEP OF THE NURSING PROCESS

Assessment, the first step in the nursing process, is the systematic gathering of relevant and important patient data. Nurses use data to: (1) identify health problems, (2) plan nursing care, and (3) evaluate patient outcomes. **Data** is the set of information or facts about the patient. During the assessment step, the nurse collects, validates, records, and organizes data into predetermined categories (see Box 3–1 on page 48 and Figure 3–1).

    Standards of Practice Standard I of the American Nurses Association *Standards of Nursing Practice* (1991b, p. 9) outlines nurses' accountability for assessment. Adhering to the criteria in Box 3–2 on page 49 will help assure you that you are collecting data in a professional manner. Keep the criteria in mind as you work through this chapter.

The Purpose of Nursing Assessment

The purpose of nursing assessment is to provide data about patient, family, and community patterns of health and illness, deviations from normal, strengths, coping abilities, and risk factors for health problems. The nursing assessment

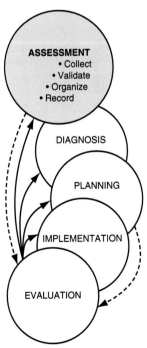

Figure 3–1. The Assessment Step

Assessment

Examples of patient data:
✓ Blood-pressure reading
✓ Urine color, clarity
✓ Patient's verbal statements
✓ Results of lab tests

Examples of family data:
✓ Genogram
✓ Interactions among members
✓ Family income
✓ Type of housing

Examples of community data:
✓ Physical environment: air, water
✓ Culture and subcultures
✓ Morbidity and mortality rates
✓ Employment patterns

focuses on patient responses to health problems—unlike the medical assessment, which focuses on disease processes and pathology. A nursing assessment may produce information about a medical diagnosis, but this is not the focus of the assessment. For example, when admitting a patient to the hospital for surgery, the nurse is interested in his disease symptoms and the nature of the surgery, but her primary interest is in how the symptoms affect his ability to care for himself, what he expects to result from the surgery, how his recovery period will affect his life, and what his main concerns are at this time.

Relationship to Other Steps of the Nursing Process

Recall from Chapter 1 that even though the steps of the nursing process are discussed separately for ease in understanding them, they are actually interrelated and overlapping. This is especially true of the assessment step. Assessment data must be accurate and complete because it forms the basis for the decisions made in the remaining steps of the nursing process. The usefulness and validity of the nursing diagnoses depend greatly on the quality of the data collected in the assessment phase. When planning goals and nursing orders, the nurse uses patient data to decide which goals are realistic and which nursing orders will be most effective.

In effect, assessment is a continuous process carried out during all phases of the nursing process. The nurse may begin to formulate a tentative problem in her mind while she is still collecting data. Assessment overlaps with the implementation and evaluation steps in that the nurse continues to collect patient data as she is carrying out these steps.

Example: As the nurse is bathing a patient (implementation), she is observing his skin condition and joint mobility. After the nursing orders have been carried out, during the evaluation phase, the nurse collects data to determine patient progress toward goal achievement (e.g., she observes the skin to see if turning and positioning the patient have prevented pressure sores).

Using Nursing Frameworks in Assessment

A **nursing model** or **theoretical framework** is a set of interrelated concepts that represents a particular way of thinking about nursing, clients, health, and the environment. In the literature, such sets of concepts may be called theories, models, frameworks, or conceptual frameworks. These terms differ in meaning, depending on the extent to which the set of concepts has been used and tested in practice and on its level of detail and organization. For the purposes of this chapter, you do not need to determine whether a theorist's ideas are a framework, a model, or a theory. Any level of organized concepts can be used to guide data collection.

A theoretical framework indicates which data is significant and guides the nurse in selecting which client characteristics to observe. It tells you what to assess and why. The major concepts of the framework provide the categories for collecting and organizing data, and they help to ensure that data collection is complete. A nursing model will produce data useful in planning nursing care; a medical model will result in data useful for medical diagnoses and treatments. Gordon's framework, for example, directs nurses to collect data about common patterns of behavior that contribute to health, quality of life, and achievement of human potential (Gordon 1994, p. 69). Particular nursing models are discussed in more detail under "Organizing the Data" later in this chapter.

Assessment is the systematic gathering of relevant and important patient information for use in identifying health problems and planning and evaluating nursing care.

Critical Thinking in Assessment

Assessment is more than just writing information on an assessment form. You will need critical thinking skills and a good knowledge base to decide which assessments to make, how much information you need, where and how to get that information, and which data is meaningful. When performing assessments, you will use your experience and knowledge from nursing and other courses to apply principles and theories about basic human needs, anatomy and physiology, disease processes, human growth and development, human behavior,

---

BOX 3–2. ANA Standard I: Assessment

The nurse collects client health data.

Measurement Criteria

1. The priority of data collection is determined by the client's immediate condition or needs.

2. Pertinent data are collected using appropriate assessment techniques.

3. Data collection involves the client, significant others, and health care providers when appropriate.

4. The data collection process is systematic and ongoing.

5. Relevant data are documented in a retrievable form.

Abstracted from American Nurses Association, *Standards of Clinical Nursing Practice* (Kansas City, MO: ANA, 1991, p. 9). Used with permission.

Assessment

socioeconomic patterns and trends, and various cultures and religions. Recall from Table 2–1 on p. 37 that the following critical thinking skills are used in the assessment phase:

> Making reliable observations
> Distinguishing relevant from irrelevant data
> Distinguishing important from unimportant data
> Validating data
> Organizing data
> Categorizing data

These skills can be developed through knowledge and practice. The exercises at the end of each chapter provide some of the practice you need to develop critical thinking skills.

COLLECTING THE DATA

Data collection is the process of gathering information about a client's health status. Nurses collect data of various types, from a number of sources, and at different times during the patient's illness. This section will help you develop your data-collection skills.

Types of Data

Data is classified as subjective and objective. Subjective data is sometimes called **covert data** or **symptoms;** objective data is sometimes called **overt data** or **signs.** Both types of data are needed for a thorough assessment.

Subjective data can be verified only by personal experience. Such data is not measurable or observable; it can be obtained only from what the client tells you. Subjective data includes the client's thoughts, beliefs, feelings, sensations, and perceptions of self and health (e.g., pain, dizziness, nausea, sadness, and happiness).

You may not always be able to obtain subjective data. Some clients, such as infants, unconscious people, or the cognitively impaired, may not be able to provide subjective data, or their data may be unreliable. Although you will usually obtain subjective data from the client, data from significant others and other health professionals may also be subjective if it consists of opinion and perception rather than fact. See Table 3–1 for factors that may make it difficult to obtain subjective data.

Objective data can be detected by someone other than the client. You will usually obtain it by observing and examining the client. Examples of objective data include the following:

Pulse rate
Urine output
Results of diagnostic tests or X rays

Skin color
Skin turgor
Posture

When used in the nursing process, the terms *subjective* and *objective* have the special meanings described above. *Subjective* does not suggest biased information or personal interpretation of meaning, as it does in common use, and *objective* does not necessarily carry the common meaning of *impartial*.

Table 3–1. Factors That May Interfere with the Ability to Obtain Subjective Data

Patient Factor	Effect	Nursing Action
Language difficulty (e.g., not fluent in English)	Unable to clearly communicate vital information	Use simple, clear language; obtain an interpreter.
High anxiety	Rapid, incoherent speech; distortion of information	Try to reduce anxiety by speaking slowly and quietly. Emphasize that accurate information is needed to give appropriate help.
Fear that illness is incapacitating	May deny certain symptoms or deliberately give misleading facts	Explore discrepancies between client statements and physical findings or data from other sources.
Acute illness and/or pain	Short responses; primary concern is intervention to alleviate problem.	Provide required intervention (e.g., give pain medication) before obtaining data. Ask closed questions; obtain only essential data.
Limited mental capacity	Possibility of inaccurate, unreliable information	Encourage client to provide as much information as able; then use secondary sources.
Previous negative experience with health care professionals	Resists providing data. Believes, "It won't help me anyway. It didn't do any good before."	Acknowledge previous experience and the imperfection of health professionals. Request another chance to help. Convey competence. Respect client's thoughts and feelings.

From Kozier et al., *Fundamentals of Nursing,* 5th ed. (Redwood City, CA: Addison-Wesley Nursing, 1995).

Assessment

Sources of Data

The nurse may gather data from a variety of sources, which fall into two broad categories: *primary* and *secondary*. You should use the most reliable source of data, whether it is the client or a significant other, and you should indicate the source on the client's record.

The client is the **primary** data source; all other data sources are **secondary.** Primary source data can be subjective or objective; that is, it can be obtained from what the client tells you or by observation and examination.

Secondary data is obtained from sources other than the client (e.g., other people, client records). It can be subjective or objective. *Significant others*, such as family or friends, can supplement and validate data obtained from the client. They are especially valuable sources when the client is a child or has difficulty communicating. When possible, you should get the client's consent before collecting data from significant others.

Other health care providers, such as the physician, social worker, and respiratory therapist, can provide information about the areas of client functioning with which they are involved. Sharing information among disciplines is especially important when the client is being transferred from one institution to another (e.g., from a nursing home to a hospital) or discharged from the institution for follow-up care at home.

The client's written record from present and past hospitalizations can be used to help plan the initial nursing assessment and to confirm the other data. Reading the records, or chart, before you see the client can help you to formulate goals for the interview and prevent you from covering topics already assessed by someone else. Be aware, however, that it can also give you predetermined ideas about the client. Failure to approach the client with an open mind can cause you to miss some data. Whatever your choice, the client's record should be reviewed early in the data-collection process.

Information from nursing and other literature may be important to the assessment process, especially for students and beginning practitioners. For example, if you have never cared for a client with trigeminal neuralgia, it would be important to read the textbook picture of the disease in order to know what signs and symptoms to look for when assessing the client. The literature also provides helpful information about developmental norms, cultural differences, and spiritual practices to use as a guide during data collection. Table 3–2 summarizes types and sources of data.

Initial Versus Ongoing Assessment

Assessment begins with the nurse's first contact with the client and continues throughout all subsequent nurse-client encounters. Although initial and ongoing assessment both involve data collection, they differ in purpose and, usually, in scope.

Initial Assessment

The **initial assessment** is made during the first nurse-client encounter. Except in emergency situations, the initial assessment is comprehensive, consisting of all subjective and objective data pertinent to the client's present health status.

When the assessment is performed on admission of the client to a health care agency, it is called the **admission assessment.** The JCAHO (1994) recommends that each client have an initial assessment to determine the need for and type of care and the need for further assessment.

The Nursing Data Base The end product of the initial comprehensive assessment is the **nursing data base**; in fact the initial assessment is also called **data base assessment.** Figure 3–2 illustrates the place of the data base in the overall scheme of the assessment step. The complete data base consists of the nursing history and physical examination, as well as data from the patient's records, consultations, and a review of the literature. Figure 3–3 on page 56 is an example of a nursing data base, as are Appendices B and C.

The **nursing history** is obtained by interviewing the patient. It contains subjective data about the effects of the illness on the patient's daily functioning and ability to cope. It considers the whole person, including data about all the patient's basic needs, not just the biological ones. The specific content of a nursing history varies in different settings (e.g., a long-term care facility would require different information than a walk-in clinic) and with different nursing models. Regardless of setting or model, a nursing history usually includes the general content areas shown in Box 3–3, on page 55.

The **nursing physical examination** is a systematic assessment of all body systems, using observation and examination skills. It is concerned with identifying strengths and deficits in the client's functional abilities rather than with identifying pathology. The physical examination produces objective data.

*Collecting
the Data*

Table 3–2. Types and Sources of Data		
Types of Data		
	Subjective	**Objective**
Description	*Covert data, symptoms.* Can be perceived and verified only by the patient. What the patient says.	*Overt data, signs.* Can be observed by others or tested against a standard.
Examples	Itching, pain, feelings of worry. "I'm afraid." "It hurts here."	Pulse rate, skin color, urine output, X-ray results, skin turgor, posture.
Sources of Data		
	Primary	**Secondary**
Description	Subjective or objective information obtained directly from the patient.	Information about the patient obtained from the family, verbal reports from other health care professionals.
Examples	Itching, pulse rate, skin color, statements of pain or anxiety.	X-ray results in the chart, statements from records or other people that the client is not eating.

Assessment

Ongoing Assessment

Ongoing assessment consists of data gathered after the data base is completed—ideally, during every nurse-patient interaction. The data is used to identify new problems and to evaluate the status of problems that have already been identified. See Table 3–3 on page 58 for a summary comparison of initial and ongoing assessment.

Comprehensive Versus Focus Assessment

A **comprehensive assessment** provides an overall picture of the client's health status. The nurse obtains data about all the client's body systems and functional abilities, without necessarily having a particular health problem in mind. The initial assessment of a client is usually comprehensive and follows the agency's printed assessment form (e.g., Figure 3–3 on page 56).

In a **focus assessment**, the nurse gathers data about an actual, potential, or possible problem that has been identified (Alfaro-Le Fevre, 1994; Carpenito, 1993). The assessment focuses on a specific topic or particular area of the body instead of the client's overall health status. Data from focus assessments is used to evaluate the status of existing problems and to identify new problems.

Figure 3–2. Overview of Assessment

Example: *Evaluation of an existing problem.* The care plan for Hassim Asad included the problem of Fluid Volume Deficit. When performing ongoing assessment during Mr. Asad's bath, the nurse noted that his oral mucous membranes were moist and that he had good skin turgor—signs that his fluid-volume problem was resolving.

Example: *Identification of a new problem.* After his bath, Mr. Asad mentioned that his head was beginning to hurt. He had not mentioned headaches before. The nurse took his blood pressure and questioned him about the nature and onset of the pain. Mr. Asad's blood pressure was elevated, and he was having blurred vision. The nurse elevated the head of the bed, relieving his pain somewhat, and notified the physician of this new development.

A focus assessment is not limited to ongoing data collection; it can also be used in the initial assessment when the client reports a symptom or other unusual findings. Any symptom or difficulty the client reports should be expanded on by

---

Box 3–3. Components of a Nursing Health History

Component	Example or Explanation
Biographical information	Age, sex, marital status
Chief complaint or reason for visit	Specifically, what initiated the patient to seek help (e.g., chest pain, weight loss, check-up)
History of present illness	Includes usual health status, chronology of the illness, and effect of the illness on the client's daily life
Past health status	Previous hospitalizations or surgeries, childhood diseases
Review of systems and their effect on client's functioning	Subjective data regarding body systems such as respiratory system (cough, shortness of breath, etc.). Difficulties with activities such as dressing, grooming, eating, and elimination
Social and family history	Family relationships, friendships; ethnic affiliation; occupational history; economic status; home and neighborhood conditions; exposure to toxic materials
Lifestyle, including usual habits and patterns of daily living	Personal habits, such as alcohol and tobacco use; usual diet; sleep/rest patterns; exercise
Spirtual well-being	Client's source of strength or hope
Psychological data	Major stressors; usual coping pattern; available supports; communication style; self-concept
Client's perception of health status and illness	Does the client realize the implications of the illness (e.g., does he think his arthritis can be cured)?
Client's expectations of caregivers	What the client thinks will be done for him. What he wants the nurses to do to help

<table>
<tr><td colspan="2">

ADMISSION DATA

Date 4-16-95 Time 3:15p.m Primary Language English
Arrived Via: ☐ Wheelchair ☐ Stretcher ☑ Ambulatory
From: ☐ Admitting ☐ ER ☑ Home ☐ Nursing Home ☐ Other
Admitting M.D. R. Katz   Time Notified 5 p.m.

ORIENTATION TO UNIT

	YES	NO		YES	NO
Arm Band Correct	☒	☐	Visiting Hours	☒	☐
Allergy Band	☒	☐	Smoking Policy	☒	☐
Telephone	☒	☐	TV, Lights, Bed Controls,		
Electrical Policy	☒	☐	Call Lights, Side Rails	☒	☐
Educational Mat'l	☒	☐	Nurses Station	☒	☐
(TV Brochure)	☒	☐			

Family M.D. R. Katz
Weight 125 lb. Height 5ft. 2in.   BP:R — L 122/80
Temp. 103 F Pulse 92. weak Resp.28. shallow
Source Providing Information ☑ Patient ☐ Other
Unable to Obtain History ☐
Reason for Admission (Onset, Duration, Pt.'s Perception) "Chest cold" X2 weeks S.O.B on exertion. "Lung pain, fever," "Dr. says I have pneumonia."

</td></tr>
</table>

PSYCHOSOCIAL HISTORY

Recent Stress None
Coping Mechanism Not assessed because of fatigue
Support System Husband. co-workers, friends
Calm: ☑ Yes ☐ No
Anxious: ☐ Yes ☐ No Facial muscles tense; trembling
Religion Catholic, Would want Last Rites
Tobacco Use: ☐ Yes ☑ No
Alcohol Use: ☐ Yes ☑ No
Drug Use: ☐ Yes ☑ No

NUEROLOGICAL

Oriented: ☑ Person ☑ Place ☑ Time ☐ Confused ☐ Sedated
☐ Alert ☐ Restless ☑ Lethargic ☐ Comatose
Pupils: ☑ Equal ☐ Unequal ☑ Reactive ☐ Sluggish
☐ Other 3mm.
Extremity Strength: ☑ Equal ☐ Unequal
Speech: ☑ Clear ☐ Slurred ☐ Other

MUSCULO-SKELETAL

Normal ROM of Extremities ☑ Yes ☐ No
☑ Weakness ☐ Paralysis ☐ Contractures ☐ Joint Swelling ☑ Pain
☐ Other ↘ related to fatigue   when coughing

ALLERGIES & REACTIONS

Drugs Penicillin
Food/Other
Signs & Symptoms rash, nausea
Blood Reaction ☐ Yes ☑ No Dyes/Shellfish ☐ Yes ☑ No

RESPIRATORY

Pattern: ☐ Even ☐ Uneven ☑ Shallow ☑ Dyspnea
☑ Other diminished breath sounds
Breathing Sounds: ☐ Clear ☑ Other inspiratory crackles
Secretions: ☐ None ☑ Other pink. thick sputum
Cough: ☐ None ☑ Productive ☐ Nonproductive

MEDICATIONS

Current Meds	Dose/Freq.	Last Dose
Synthroid	0.1 mg. daily	4-16. 8 a.m.

Disposition of Meds: ☒ Home ☐ Pharmacy ☐ Safe *At Bedside

CARDIOVASCULAR

Pulses: Apical Rate 92-W ☑ Reg. ☐ Irregular ☐ Pacemaker
S = Strong W = Weak A = Absent D = Doppler
Radial R 92 L ___ Pedal R ___ L ___
Edema: ☑ Absent ☐ Present Site
Perfusion: ☐ Warm ☐ Dry ☑ Diaphoretic ☐ Cool (Hot)

MEDICAL HISTORY

☑ No Major Problems   ☐ Gastro
☐ Cardiac   ☐ Arthritis
☐ Hyper/Hypotension   ☐ Stroke
☐ Diabetes   ☐ Seizures
☐ Cancer   ☐ Glaucoma
☐ Respiratory   ☑ Other Childbirth-1992

Surgery/Procedures	Date
Appendectomy	1978
Partial thyroidectomy	1991

GASTROINTESTINAL

Oral Mucosa ☐ Normal ☑ Other pale and dry
Bowel Sounds: ☑ Normal ☐ Other Abd. soft
Wt. Change: ☐ ☑ N/V Stool Frequency/Character 1/day:soft
Last B/M 4-15-95 ☐ Ostomy (type)
Equip.

GENITOURINARY

Urine: Last Voided This morning
☐ Normal ☐ Anuria ☐ Hematuria ☐ Dysuri ☐ Incontinent
☒ Other amount & frequency since ill
☐ Catheter (type)   Other
LMP 4-1-95   ☐ Vaginal/Penile Discharge
Other

SPECIAL ASSISTIVE DEVICES

☐ Wheelchair ☐ Contacts ☐ Venous ☐ Dentures
☐ Braces ☐ Hearing Aid Access ☐ Partial
☐ Cane/Crutches ☐ Prosthesis Device ☐ Upper
☐ Walker ☐ Glasses ☐ Epidural Catheter ☐ Lower
☐ Other None

SELF CARE

Need Assist with: ☐ Ambulating ☐ Elimination
☐ Meals ☒ Hygiene ☐ Dressing
While fatigued

ADDRESSOGRAPH PLATE

Luisa Sanchez. [F. age 28]
#4637651

VALUABLES

Patient informed Hospital not responsible for personal belongings.
Valuables Disposition: ☐ Patient ☐ Safe ☐ Given to
Patient/SO Signature None

✿ **NORTH BROWARD HOSPITAL DISTRICT**
NURSING ADMINISTRATION ASSESSMENT

Figure 3–3. Assessment for Luisa Sanchez
(Nursing assessment tool courtesy of North Broward Hospital District, Broward County, Florida. Reprinted with permission.)

NUTRITION	General Appearance: ☑ Well Nourished ☐ Emaciated ☐ Other _____ Appetite: ☐ Good ☐ Fair ☑ Poor -x2 days Diet _Liquid_ Meal Pattern _3/day_ ☐ Feeds Self ☐ Assist ☐ Total Feed	1. What do you know about your present illness? _"Dr. says I have pneumonia." "I will have an I.V."_ 2. What information do you want or need about your illness? _____ 3. Would you like family/SO involved in your care? _Husband, Michael_ 4. How long do you expect to be in the hospital? _"1-2 days"_ 5. What concerns do you have about leaving the hospital? _____

SKIN ASSESSMENT

Color: ☐ Normal ☐ Flushed ☑ Pale ☐ Dusky ☐ Cyanotic ☐ Jaundiced ☑ Other _Cheeks flushed, hot_

General Description _Surgical scars: RLQ abdomen; anterior neck_

_____
_____
_____

Note Cultures Obtained _____
_____
_____
_____

PRESSURE SORE "AT RISK" SCREENING CRITERIA

OVERALL SKIN CONDITION
Grade
☐ 0	Turgor (elasticity adequate, skin warm and moist)
☑ 1	Poor turgor, skin cold & dry
☐ 2	Areas mottled, red or denuded
☐ 3	Existing skin ulcer/lesions

BOWEL AND BLADDER CONTROL
Grade
☑ 0	Always able to ask for bedpan
☐ 1	Incontinence of urine
☐ 2	Incontinence of feces
☐ 3	Totally incontinent Confined to bed

REHABILITATIVE STATE
Grade
☐ 0	Fully ambulatory
☑ 1	Ambulated with assistance
☐ 2	Chair to bed ambulation only
☐ 3	Confined to bed
☐ 4	Immobile in bed

NUTRITIONAL STATE
Grade
☐ 0	Eats all
☑ 1	Eats very little
☐ 2	Refuses food often
☐ 3	Tube feeding
☐ 4	Intravenous feeding

MENTAL STATE
Grade
☑ 0	Alert and clear
☐ 1	Confused
☐ 2	Disoriented/senile
☐ 3	Stuporous
☐ 4	Unconcious

CHRONIC DISEASE STATUS (i.e. COPD, ASCVD, Peripheral Vascular Disease, Diabetes, or Renal Disease, Cancer, Motor or Sensory Deficits, Elderly, Other)
Grade
☑ 0	Absent
☐ 1	One Present
☐ 2	Two Present
☐ 3	Three or more Present

TOTAL _____ Refer to Skin Care Protocol

FALLS SCREENING

If one or more of the following are checked institute fall precautions/plan of care
☐ History of Falls ☐ Unsteady Gait ☐ Confusion/Disorientation ☐ Dizziness

If two or more of the following are checked institute fall precautions/plan of care
☐ Age over 80 ☐ Utilizes cane, walker, w/c ☐ Sleeplessness
☐ Impaired vision ☐ Impaired hearing ☐ Urgency/frequency in elimination
☐ Multiple Diagnoses ☐ Medication/Sedative /Diuretic etc.
☐ Inability to understand or follow directions

EDUCATION/DISCHARGE PLANNING

CHECK APPROPRIATE BOX
Will patient need post discharge assistance with ADLs/physical functioning? ☐ Yes ☑ No ☐ Unknown
Does patient have family capable of and willing to provide assistance post discharge?
☑ Yes ☐ No ☐ Unknown ☐ No family
Is assistance needed beyond that which family can provide?
☐ Yes ☑ No ☐ Unknown
Previous admission in the last six months?
☐ Yes ☑ No ☐ Unknown
Patient lives with _Husband and 1 child_
Planned discharge to _Home_
Comments: _Fatigue and anxiety may have interfered with learning. Re-teach anything covered at admission, later._

Social Services Notified ☐ Yes ☑ No

NARRATIVE NOTES

S--c/o sharp chest pain when coughing and dyspnea on exertion. States unable to carry out regular daily exercise for past week. Coughing relieved "if I sit up and sit still." Nausea associated with coughing. Having ocasional "chills." Occasionally becomes frightened, stating, "I can't breathe." Well groomed but "too tired to put on make-up."

O--Chest expansion < 3cm, no nasal flaring or use of accessory muscles. Breath sounds and insp. crackles in Ⓡ upper and lower chest.
    Assesses own supports as "good" (eg, relationship ī husband). Is "worried" about daughter. States husband will be out of town until tomorrow. Left 3-year-old daughter with neighbor. Concerned too about her work (is attorney). "I'll never get caught up." Had water at noon—no food today. Informed of need to save urine for 24 hr. specimen. IV D₅W LR 1000 mL started in Ⓡarm, 100 mL/hr. Slow capillary refill. Keeping head of bed↑ to facilitate breathing.

NURSE SIGNATURE/TITLE	DATE	TIME
Mary Medina, RN	4-16-95	3:30pm
NURSE SIGNATURE/TITLE	DATE	TIME

✹ **NORTH BROWARD HOSPITAL DISTRICT**
NURSING ADMINISTRATION ASSESSMENT

Figure 3–3. Concluded

Assessment

asking further questions about it (e.g., When did it begin? What makes it worse? What relieves it?). When a client needs repeated in-depth assessment of a particular problem area, most agencies have special assessment forms for recording the ongoing focus assessment (e.g., a flow sheet for hourly neurological assessments).

Use of Computers in Assessment

Many health care agencies use computerized information systems to facilitate data collection. In some automated assessment systems, patients actually respond directly to interview questions on the computer screen. In other systems, the nurse interviews the patient and enters the data into a bedside terminal. Nurses may also use bedside terminals to prompt them through a systematic and complete physical examination of a patient. And finally, nurses use computers to record the interview and examination data.

Data-Collection Methods

Three methods of collecting data are used in both comprehensive and focus nursing assessments: observation, physical examination, and interview.

Observation

Observation is the conscious, deliberate use of the physical senses to gather data from the patient and his environment. Train yourself to begin observing as you first enter the patient's room. What is he doing? Does he show signs of distress, such as restlessness or pallor? What is in the environment? Are the side rails up? Are there any safety hazards? Is all the equipment working? Is the intravenous solution running? Who are the people in the room and how do they interact with the patient? Closer observations will disclose data such as skin temperature, breath sounds, and drainage odors.

Physical Examination

A complete data base requires both subjective and objective data. **Physical examination** provides objective data that can be used to validate the subjective data obtained in the interview or clarify the effect of the patient's disease on her ability to function. The data from the initial physical examination serves as a baseline for comparing the client's later responses to nursing and medical interventions.

Observation Examples

✓ Seeing pink, serous drainage on a cast.

✓ Hearing quiet breathing.

✓ Smelling fruity odor on a patient's breath.

✓ Feeling that the skin is warm and dry.

Table 3–3. Initial Versus Ongoing Assessment	
Initial Assessment	**Ongoing Assessment**
Admission assessment	Focus assessment
Data base assessment	Focuses on specific problems, activities, or behaviors
Comprehensive assessment	
Can include focus assessment	Focuses on identified problems (can also be used to identify new problems)
Data is used to make initial problem list	Data is used to evaluate goal achievement and problem resolution

In a complete physical examination, the nurse assesses all body parts in an orderly, systematic manner. One approach is to proceed from *head to toe*. In this case, the head and neck would be examined first, and then the shoulders, chest (including heart and lungs), and back. Another approach is to examine each of the *body systems* in a predetermined order, for example, respiratory, neurological, cardiovascular, musculoskeletal, and so on. Whatever approach you choose, the examination should follow the same order each time to prevent omission of data.

In an admission assessment, the nurse usually conducts a complete physical examination, but this can vary depending on the severity of the illness and the kind of information needed. During ongoing assessment, the nurse examines specific body areas, systems, or functions, instead of the entire body. These examinations are made to obtain data related to the patient's complaints, previously identified problems, and responses to nursing and medical interventions.

> *Example:* A client who is taking an antibiotic complains, "I itch all over." The nurse examines his skin for rash or discoloration.

You will use the techniques of inspection, auscultation, palpation, and percussion when performing a physical examination. Like the nursing process, these require practice. Refer to a text on the fundamentals of nursing or physical assessment for in-depth discussion of these techniques and other aspects of the physical exam.

Inspection is done visually, either with the naked eye or with instruments such as an otoscope, which is used in examining the ears. Abdominal distention and skin pallor are examples of data found on inspection. Inspection is an active process in that the nurse must know what to look for. It is also a systematic process, more thorough and detailed than observation.

Auscultation uses the nurse's hearing. Using *direct* auscultation with the unaided ear the nurse can hear sounds such as the client's coughing. A stethoscope is used for *indirect* auscultation to amplify the sounds made within the client's body, such as crackles and wheezes in the lungs.

Percussion is the striking of a body surface, usually with the tip of the finger, to elicit sound or vibration. Different sounds are produced, depending on whether the finger strikes over a solid, fluid-filled, or air-filled area. It is useful, for instance, in determining whether a patient's abdomen is distended with air or fluid.

Palpation uses the sense of touch. The finger pads are usually used because they are the most sensitive to tactile stimulation. The nurse uses palpation, for example, to check for bladder distention and to obtain the patient's pulse rate and strength.

Interview

A **nursing interview** is a planned, structured communication in which the nurse questions a patient to obtain subjective data. An admission interview is formal and planned. During ongoing assessment, interviews may be informal, brief, narrowly focused interactions between nurse and patient, but they are still purposeful, structured communication.

Purpose During the initial assessment, the main purpose of the interview is to obtain subjective data for the nursing history. At the same time, the nurse usually orients the patient to her surroundings and gives her some information

Collecting the Data

Examination Examples
- ✓ Taking a patient's pulse
- ✓ Weighing a patient
- ✓ Listening to heart sounds
- ✓ Palpating the abdomen
- ✓ Auscultating bowel sounds

Assessment

about her stay (e.g., how to call for help, where to put her belongings). In addition to asking questions, the nurse should provide enough teaching and counseling to relieve some of the patient's anxieties. For both nurse and patient, impressions gained in the initial interview form the basis for the beginning of the nurse-patient relationship.

Preparing for the Interview As a rule, you should begin by reviewing the chart, so you will know who the patient is and what you want to accomplish; but be careful not to form preconceived ideas. After forming some goals for the interview, think of some initial leading questions. Schedule a time when you will be free from interruptions—not too close to mealtime, treatment time, or visiting hours. Provide privacy, wait until visitors are gone, or ask them to leave the room. Be sure the patient is comfortable: ask if he is thirsty or needs to use the bathroom. Consider the patient's emotional state, as well. If he is very anxious or frightened, you may need to relieve his anxiety before proceeding with the interview.

Types There are two basic types of interview: directive and nondirective. A **directive interview** is highly structured. The nurse controls the subject matter and asks questions in order to obtain specific information. This is an efficient way to obtain factual, easily categorized information, such as age, sex, and analysis of symptoms. A directive interview uses mainly **closed questions**, which call for brief, specific responses. Closed questions are especially effective in emergency situations or when the patient is very anxious. Remember, however, that a directive interview and closed questions are not very effective in helping a patient to express emotion, nor in getting information about personal or emotionally charged matters.

A **nondirective interview** allows the patient to talk about whatever she wishes, in the order and at the pace she chooses. The nurse clarifies, summarizes, and uses open-ended questions and comments to encourage communication. An **open-ended question** may specify the topic of discussion, but it is broad and requires elaboration from the patient. Such questions are good for eliciting feelings, attitudes, and beliefs. Nondirective interviewing is time-consuming and can result in a great deal of irrelevant data; however, it is useful in helping a patient to express feelings and in promoting communication.

The nursing interview requires a combination of directive and nondirective techniques. Use directive questioning to obtain the more specific information on the nursing history (e.g., biographical information, previous surgeries, childhood diseases). Then use broad statements to guide the patient to talk about other topics, such as sleep patterns, pain, and usual routines; finally, follow up or clarify those responses with specific, directive questions.

Example:

(Closed question)	*Nurse:*	How many times have you been pregnant?
	Patient:	Four.
(Closed question)	*Nurse:*	Were there any problems with your other deliveries?
	Patient:	Yes, with my last one.

(Open-ended question, directing topic)	*Nurse:*	What happened?
	Patient:	I was in labor a long time, and then something happened to the baby's heart rate. They did an emergency cesarean section.
(Open-ended question)	*Nurse:*	What plans have you made for this delivery?

The last, broad question elicits information about a topic of the nurse's choice. A more directive, closed question along the same lines would be, "Do you plan to have a C-section again this time?" If the nurse wanted to explore the patient's feelings, she might have said, "What are your concerns for *this* delivery?"

Table 3–4 lists some common interviewing problems, along with some suggestions for handling them. Along with Box 3–4 on page 64, these suggestions should help you improve the quality of your interviews.

VALIDATING THE DATA

Validation is the act of "double-checking" or verifying data to confirm that it is accurate and factual. Critical thinkers validate data in order to:

✓ Ensure that assessment information is complete, accurate, and factual
✓ Eliminate their own errors, biases, and misperceptions of the data
✓ Avoid jumping to faulty conclusions about the data

To collect data accurately, you must be aware of your own biases, values, and beliefs, and be able to separate fact from interpretation and assumption. For example, a nurse seeing a man holding his arm to his chest might assume that he is experiencing chest pain, when in fact he has a painful hand. The acceptance of assumptions is called **premature closure**. To avoid premature closure and build an accurate data base, the nurse should ask the client why he is holding his arm to his chest. The client's response may validate the nurse's assumption (of chest pain) or prompt further questioning. Not all data require validation. For example, data such as height, weight, birth date, and most laboratory studies can be accepted as factual. As a rule, you should validate data when:

1. *Subjective and objective data (or interview and physical examination data) do not agree.*

   Example: Ms. Dolan states she has never had high blood pressure. However, the nurse obtains a reading of 190/100.

2. *The client's statements differ at different times in the assessment.*

   Example: At first a labor patient stated that this was her first pregnancy. Later, when the nurse asked about prior hospitalizations, she said, "Once, in 1990, to have my appendix removed; and in 1992 when I had a miscarriage." The nurse realized that a miscarriage is counted as a pregnancy, making this the patient's second pregnancy.

Table 3–4. Common Interviewing Problems

Source of Problem	Explanation	Suggested Nursing Actions
Interviewer's own discomfort	1. You may feel you are imposing on the patient, perhaps because you do not clearly know how the information will be used. (Especially true for students.)	1. Do your "homework." Be sure you understand the purpose of the interview; explain it to the patient during the introduction phase.
	2. You may feel uncomfortable asking personal questions of a stranger.	2. Remember that nurses are concerned with the whole person and that the data is needed in order to give comprehensive care. Early in the interview, tell the patient to respond only as he feels comfortable. Remember that patients can choose what they wish to tell you, so they have some power to preserve their own privacy. Remind yourself that patients are usually at ease if you are at ease. Also, it may be that the patient has felt the need to talk about the subject, did not know how to bring it up, and is relieved that you have done so.
	3. Knowing that patients may respond to some questions with tears or anger, you may be afraid to ask such questions.	3. It may be hard to accept another's expressions of feelings, but it is important that you learn to do so. Avoiding potentially upsetting topics can leave large gaps in the data base. Remember that the patient usually feels better after expressing emotions—even though you may be uncomfortable.
Interviewer's curiosity	There is a fine line between interest and curiosity. Patients appreciate interest, but resent curiosity. This may cause them to be less inclined to talk to you.	Don't become too emeshed in the details of the patient's story. Focus on getting the information you need for planning care.
Patients' family and visitors inhibit responses	1. The client may be embarrassed to discuss personal information in front of others, or it may be information clients do not wish others to know (e.g., a wife may not want her husband to know that she was treated for a sexually transmitted disease before they were married).	1. Unless the visitor is an important source of information (e.g., when the patient is a small child), ask the visitor to step out for a few minutes, or postpone the interview until the visitor leaves.

Table 3–4. Common Interviewing Problems (concluded)		
Source of Problem	**Explanation**	**Suggested Nursing Actions**
	2. Spouses often answer the questions you address to the patient.	2. Thank the spouse for the information, but remind them that it is important for you to get the information from the patient's perspective.
Nurse is not culturally sensitive	There are cultural variations in communication (e.g., in some cultures social courtesies must be established before personal topics are discussed).	Be aware of differences in the meaning of phenomena such as touch, facial expressiveness, use of silence, and need for physical space. For example: ✓ In some cultures, strangers do not make direct eye contact. ✓ Men of all cultures require more space than women, as a rule.

3. *The data seems extremely abnormal.*

   Example: The client has a resting pulse of 50 beats/minute and a blood pressure of 190/100.

4. *Factors are present that interfere with accurate measurement.*

   Example: A crying infant will have a higher than normal respiratory rate and should be quieted in order for assessment data to be correct.

The following are some ways in which you can validate data:

✓ Clarify vague or ambiguous statements by asking the patient more questions (e.g., "What, exactly, did your son *do* when he started 'acting strange'?").
✓ Recheck your measurement to be sure it is accurate (e.g., take the blood pressure a second time in the opposite arm).
✓ Check to be sure your measuring device is working correctly, or use a different piece of equipment (e.g., take the client's temperature with two different thermometers).
✓ Ask someone else to collect the same data to confirm your findings (e.g., ask a more experienced nurse).
✓ Always compare subjective and objective data to verify the client's statements with your observations (e.g., compare pain behaviors to patient's statements about the pain).

Assessment

ORGANIZING THE DATA

ANA Standard I requires that data collection be systematic (see Box 3–2). This means that in addition to collecting and validating the data, the nurse organizes related cues into predetermined categories. Grouping related data helps the nurse to find the patterns necessary for identifying client strengths, health problems, and risk factors. Most health care agencies and schools of nursing have printed forms for the nursing data base. These forms organize the nursing history and the physical examination according to the framework or nursing theory the

---

Box 3–4. Guide for Interviewing

1. Prepare for the interview.
- ✓ Read the chart. Think of some initial leading questions.
- ✓ Provide privacy: Ask visitors to leave; pull the bed curtain.
- ✓ Schedule a block of time for the interview.
- ✓ Reduce distractions (e.g., turn off the television).
- ✓ Be sure the client is comfortable.

2. Set the stage.
- ✓ Use the patient's name. Ask what name she prefers you to use.
- ✓ Introduce yourself. Sit down. Make eye contact. Listen.
- ✓ Set a time limit at the beginning of the interview.

3. Obtain the data.
- ✓ Start the client's main complaint ("Why are you here?").
- ✓ Next, ask about nonthreatening subjects and symptoms. Introduce personal or threatening material later in the interview, when you and the patient are more at ease.
- ✓ Don't mechanically "fill out the form." Follow client leads for expanding on or introducing a topic.

4. Use good communication techniques.
- ✓ Say *I*, not *we* (as in "*We* need some information from you"). *We* indicates lack of personal involvement and creates psychological distance between you and the client.
- ✓ Don't use endearing names, such as "grandma, dear, sweetie." Most people feel belittled by this.
- ✓ Use language the patient can understand. Many patients do not know the meaning of *void* or *vital signs*. Check the patient's understanding of a word by saying, for example, "Explain what happens when you have diarrhea."
- ✓ Don't "talk down" to the patient (e.g., "I need to feel your tummy").
- ✓ Don't ask too many questions; you may seem curious instead of concerned. Use neutral statements and reflection to get information (e.g., instead of, "Where do you work?" say, "Tell me about your job").
- ✓ Avoid closed questions that require only a one-word or yes/no answer.
- ✓ Avoid "why" questions (e.g., "Why have you been unable to stop smoking?"). For many people, *why* connotes disapproval and may provoke a defensive response.
- ✓ Encourage the patient to continue by nodding or saying, "Um-hmm," or "Yes . . . ." or "Go on."
- ✓ If the patient is rambling, allow him to finish a sentence before interrupting. Then try to redirect the conversation by saying something like, "You hadn't finished telling me about . . ."
- ✓ Use and accept silence. Give the client time to search for and organize thoughts.

agency prefers. Using these forms (e.g., Figure 3–3) enables you to organize the data at the same time you collect and record it, making the assessment more efficient. For ongoing assessments, you will not always have a data-collection form, so you will need to organize the data after you collect it. Frameworks are used to organize both initial and ongoing assessment data. This section describes some different frameworks for organizing data.

A *framework* is, very simply, a way of looking at something. Suppose a patient is trembling. A nurse using only a psychological framework might conclude the patient is frightened; a nurse using only a biological framework might conclude that the patient is cold. A variety of frameworks are useful in collecting and organizing patient data: some focus on human needs, some on adaptive responses, others on self-care abilities, and so on. No matter which model you use, it is important to use it consistently in order to become familiar with it. Even if you do not use a form to collect data, you will still classify related cues according to your chosen framework when you are finished. Using a framework gives you a special way to view the patient, helps you to make thorough, systematic assessments, and makes the data more meaningful.

Nursing Models

In order to maintain a holistic approach, it is best to use a nursing model. Using a *body systems* model, for instance, leads you to focus on problems of system and organ function, which are usually medical rather than nursing problems. A *nursing* model enables you to identify problems *nurses* can address.

Gordon established a framework of 11 *Functional Health Patterns* "that contribute to . . . health, quality of life, and achievement of human potential" (1994, p. 69). Using this framework to organize assessment data, the nurse notes emerging patterns and determines whether the client's functioning in each of the patterns is functional or dysfunctional. See Table 3–5 and Appendix C.

Orem's (1991) *Self-Care Model* focuses on the client's abilities to perform self-care activities to maintain life, health, and well-being. Using this framework, the nurse identifies self-care deficits that require nursing intervention. See Table 3–6 on page 67.

Roy's (1984) *Adaptation Model* describes patients as biopsychosocial beings, constantly adapting to external and internal demands. Using this framework, the nurse would note patterns indicating the client's inability to adapt in one of four modes: physiological, self-concept, social role, and interdependence. See Table 3–7 on page 68 and Appendix B.

The North American Nursing Diagnosis Association (NANDA) characterizes each person by a unique organization of nine *Human Response Patterns*, which reflect the whole person in interaction with the environment. Note that this is not, strictly speaking, a nursing theory, but a framework for assessing and diagnosing. See Table 3–8 on page 69.

Nonnursing Models

Frameworks from other disciplines may also be helpful for clustering data. Maslow's *Hierarchy of Needs* clusters data according to basic human needs that are common to all people. This model theorizes that basic needs

Assessment

Body Systems Model
Integumentary system
Respiratory system
Nervous system
Musculoskeletal system
Gastrointestinal system
Genitourinary system
Reproductive system

(e.g., physiological) must be met before a person can meet higher needs (e.g., self-esteem). See Table 3–9 on page 70 for an example of data organized according to Maslow's model.

Nonnursing models are more narrowly focused than nursing models; therefore, you will usually need to combine them with other approaches. For example, you might combine Maslow's hierarchy of needs with a **body systems (medical) model,** which focuses on abnormalities of body systems.

RECORDING THE DATA

ANA Standard I (See Box 3–1) requires that assessment data be accessible, communicated, and *recorded.* An additional consideration is that the nursing data base becomes a part of the client's permanent record. Therefore, you

Table 3–5. Organizing Data According to Gordon's 11 Functional Health Patterns		
Functional Health Pattern	**Pattern Describes**	**Examples**
Health Perception/ Health Management	Client's perceived pattern of health and well-being and how health is managed.	Compliance with medication regimen, use of health-promotion activities such as regular exercise, annual check-ups.
Nutritional-Metabolic	Pattern of food and fluid consumption relative to metabolic need and pattern; indicators of local nutrient supply.	Condition of skin, teeth, hair, nails, mucous membranes; height and weight.
Elimination	Patterns of excretory function (bowel, bladder, and skin). Includes client's perception of "normal" function.	Frequency of bowel movements, voiding pattern, pain on urination, appearance of urine and stool.
Activity-Exercise	Patterns of exercise, activity, leisure, and recreation.	Exercise, hobbies. May include cardio-vascular and respiratory status, mobility, and activities of daily living.
Cognitive-Perceptual	Sensory-perceptual and cognitive patterns.	Vision, hearing, taste, touch, smell, pain perception and management; cognitive functions such as language, memory, and decision making.
Sleep-Rest	Patterns of sleep, rest, and relaxation.	Client's perception of quality and quantity of sleep and energy, sleep aids, routines client uses.

Table 3–5. Organizing Data According to Gordon's 11 Functional Health Patterns (continued)

Functional Health Pattern	Pattern Describes	Examples
Self-Perception/ Self-Concept	Client's self-concept pattern and perceptions of self.	Body comfort, body image, feeling state, attitudes about self, perception of abilities, objective data such as body posture, eye contact, voice tone.
Role-Relationship	Client's pattern of role engagements and relationships.	Perception of current major roles and responsibilities (e.g., father, husband, salesman); satisfaction with family, work, or social relationships.
Sexuality-Reproductive	Patterns of satisfaction and dissatisfaction with sexuality pattern; reproductive pattern.	Number and histories of pregnancy and childbirth; difficulties with sexual functioning; satisfaction with sexual relationship.
Coping/Stress Tolerance	General coping pattern and effective of the pattern in terms of stress tolerance.	Client's usual manner of handling stress, available support systems, perceived ability to control or manage situations.
Value-Belief	Patterns of values, beliefs (including spiritual), and goals that guide client's choices or decisions.	Religious affiliation, what client perceives as important in life, value-belief conflicts related to health, special religious practices.

Adapted with permission from Gordon, *Nursing Diagnosis: Process and Application,* 3rd ed. (St. Louis: C.V. Mosby, 1994, p. 70).

Table 3–6. Organizing Data According to Orem's Self-Care Model

Group data into the following categories of "universal self-care requisites."

1. The maintenance of a sufficient intake of air
2. The maintenance of a sufficient intake of water
3. The maintenance of a sufficient intake of food
4. The provision of care associated with elimination processes and excrements
5. The maintenance of a balance between activity and rest
6. The maintenance of a balance between solitude and social interaction
7. The prevention of hazards to human life, human functioning, and human well-being
8. The promotion of human functioning and development within social groups in accord with human potential, known human limitations, and human desire to be normal. (Normalcy is used in the sense of that which is essentially human and that which is in accord with the genetic and constitutional characteristics and the talents of individuals.)

Source: Orem, *Nursing: Concepts of Practice,* 4th ed. (St. Louis: Mosby-Year Book, 1991, p. 126).

Assessment

should record the assessment in ink on the form provided by the agency, on the same day the client is admitted. Write neatly and legibly, using only the abbreviations approved by the agency. Do not try to write everything the client says word for word, as this is likely to interfere with the communication between you and the client.

For both comprehensive and focus assessment record subjective data in the client's own words when possible, using quotation marks. You may paraphrase or summarize what the client says, but do not use quotation marks in that case. Be sure to record the data, not what you think it means. Do not record judgments, opinions, or conclusions. Record **cues** (what the client tells you and what you see, hear, feel, smell, and measure); not **inferences** (your judgment or interpretation of what the cues mean). Table 3–10 on page 70 compares subjective and objective cues with conclusions (inferences).

Critical thinkers use concrete, specific terms to describe data. Avoid vague generalities such as *good, normal, adequate,* or *tolerated well.* These words mean different things to different people. Suppose a nurse writes, "Vision adequate." Does this mean the client can read newsprint without eyeglasses? Or when she is wearing glasses? Or that she can see well enough to ambulate without assistance? It would be better to record "Able to read newsprint at 24 inches while wearing glasses."

Table 3–7. Organizing Data According to Roy's Adaptation Model

Categories (Adaptive Modes)	Explanation
1. Physiological needs Activity and rest Nutrition Elimination Fluid and electrolytes Oxygenation Protection Regulation: temperature Regulation: the senses Regulation: endocrine system	Balance must be maintained in each of the subcategories.
2. Self-concept Physical Self Personal Self	Adaptation means developing a positive self-concept, including the physical self, moral-ethical self, and self-ideal. Includes self-esteem and psychological integrity.
3. Role Function	Ability to function in various roles, such as parent, spouse, worker, and so on.
4. Interdependence	Achieving balance between dependence and independence.

Source: Roy and Andrews, *The Roy Adaptation Model: The Definitive Statement* (Norwalk, CT: Appleton & Lange, 1991, pp. 15–17).

SPECIAL PURPOSE ASSESSMENTS

Special Purpose Assessments

In some situations you will wish to perform an in-depth assessment of certain areas of a client's functioning. Most agencies have forms developed for special assessments. For example, you may be asked to gather in-depth data about a client's nutritional status, using a form provided by your school. Or you may use a special form to monitor the level of consciousness, pupil reaction, and limb movement of a comatose patient. This section discusses self-care, cultural, spiritual, and wellness assessments.

Self-Care Assessment

The JCAHO and other reimbursement agencies mandate patient education and discharge planning. Thorough data about the patient's knowledge and self-care abilities enables the nurse to develop an individualized teaching plan. However,

Table 3–8.   NANDA Human Response Patterns

Pattern and Description	Examples of Assessments
1. *Exchanging*—Involves mutual giving and receiving	Nutritional status, temperature, elimination, oxygenation, circulation, fluid balance, condition of skin and mucous membranes, risk factors for injury/accidents, body systems.
2. *Communicating*—Involves sending messages	Ability to express thoughts verbally; orientation, physical impairments to speech; language barrier.
3. *Relating*—Involves establishing bonds	Type of social interactions; relationships with significant others; support system; ability to perform roles, including parenting; sexual functioning; family functioning; financial support.
4. *Valuing*—Involves the assigning of relative worth	Religious preference; relationship with deity; perception of suffering; acceptance of illness; religious practices; cultural orientation and practices.
5. *Choosing*—Involves the selection of alternatives	Ability to accept help; adjustment to health status; desire for dependence/independence; denial of problem; adherence to therapies; ability to make decisions.
6. *Moving*—Involves activity	Tolerance to activity; ability to care for self; sleep patterns; diversional activities; history of disability; home environment; safety needs; breastfeeding.
7. *Perceiving*—Involves the reception of information	Body image; self-esteem; ability to see, hear, feel, smell, taste; amount of hopefulness; perceived ability to control current situation.
8. *Knowing*—Involves the meaning associated with information	Amount of knowledge about current illness or therapies; previous illnesses; risk factors; expectations of therapy; cognitive abilities; readiness to learn; orientation; memory.
9. *Feeling*—Involves the subjective awareness of information	Pain; grieving; capacity or risk for violence; level of anxiety; emotional integrity.

Adapted by permission from the North American Nursing Diagnosis Association, *Classification of Nursing Diagnoses,* Proceedings of the Fifth Conference, Kim, McFarland, and McLane, eds. (St. Louis: C. V. Mosby, 1986, p. 29).

Assessment

the nurse has less time than ever before to focus on the patient as an individual. One way to overcome this obstacle is to have the patient do a self-assessment, using a checklist. One such tool assesses patients' self-care abilities with regard to the items at the top of page 71 (Johannsen, 1992).

Table 3–9. Organizing Data According to Maslow's Basic Human Needs

Data Categories (Needs)	Examples of Data
Physiological (Basic survival needs)	Oxygen, nutrition, fluids, body temperature regulation, warmth, elimination, shelter, sex
Safety and Security (Need to be safe and comfortable)	Physical safety (infection, falls, drug side effects); psychological security (knowledge of procedures, bedtime rituals, usual routines, fear of isolation dependence needs); pain
Love and Belonging (Need for love and affection)	Information about significant others, social supports
Esteem and Self-Esteem (Need to feel good about self)	Changes in body image (e.g., puberty, surgery); changes in self-concept (e.g., ability to perform usual role in family); pride in capabilities
Self-Actualization (Need to achieve one's maximum potential; need for growth and change)	Extent to which potential is being achieved, autonomy, motivation, problem-solving abilities, ability to give and accept help, feelings about accomplishments, roles

Source: Maslow, *Motivation and Personality,* 2nd ed (New York: Harper & Row, 1970).

Table 3–10. Comparison of Data and Conclusions (Cues and Inferences)

Cues (Data)		Inferences (Conclusions)
Subjective	**Objective**	
"My back really hurts." (Paraphrase: Patient states his back hurts.)	Lying rigidly in bed. Facial grimacing observed.	Patient is in pain.
"My armband is too tight and my arm is really sore." (Paraphrase: Patient says his armband is too tight and his arm is sore.)	Left arm is hot, red, and swollen in a 4' × 4' area around the IV insertion site.	Left arm is infected at IV site.
"I'm not sure I should have this surgery. It might not even help, and it is very dangerous. I guess I'm scared."	Tearful. Facial muscles tense. Pulse rate 100. Hands trembling.	Patient is afraid of having surgery.

Remember: You should record cues, not inferences.

- ✓ Seeking and securing medical assistance
- ✓ Understanding and attending to the effects of illness
- ✓ Effectively carrying out the therapeutic regimen
- ✓ Regulating discomfort/harmful effects of the regimen
- ✓ Living with the illness in a style conducive to health
- ✓ Modifying self-concept

Special Purpose Assessments

For each of those abilities, clients check responses to indicate what information they have, their perceptions and feelings about it, and what they actually do.

Cultural Assessment

Because nurses are expected to provide individualized care, you must understand how the client's cultural beliefs and practices can affect his or her health and illness (ANA, 1991a, p. 1). Box 3–5 provides an overview of six phenomena that must be assessed in order to provide culturally competent nursing care (Giger and Davidhizar, 1995). **Cultural competence** requires knowledge of the values, beliefs, and practices of various cultures, along with attitudes of awareness, openness, and sensitivity. Figure 3–4 is a heritage assessment that analyzes the degree to which a person identifies with the dominant culture and with a traditional culture (Spector, 1994). You may wish to use this tool with clients or as a self-assessment to discuss with your peers.

Spiritual Assessment

A holistic assessment includes information about the client's spiritual well-being. For well clients, the spiritual dimension is important to overall well-being. When a client is ill, spirituality can be either a source of support or a source of difficulty. Nurses usually elicit spiritual data as a part of the general history. It is best to do

---

Box 3–5. Six Phenomena of Cultural Assessment

- ✓ **Communication.** A continuous process by which one person may affect another through written or oral language, gestures, facial expressions, body language, space, or other symbols.
- ✓ **Space.** The area around a person's body that includes the individual, body, surrounding environment, and objects within that environment.
- ✓ **Social organization.** Includes the family and other groups within a society that dictate culturally accepted role behaviors of different members of the society and rules for behavior. Behaviors are prescribed for significant life events, such as birth, death, childbearing, childrearing, and illness.
- ✓ **Time.** Refers to the meaning and influence of time from a cultural perspective. Time orientation refers to an individual's focus on the past, the present, or the future. Most cultures combine all three time orientations, but one orientation is more likely to dominate.
- ✓ **Environmental control.** Refers to the ability or perceived ability of an individual or persons from a particular cultural group to plan activities that control nature, such as illness, causation, and treatment.
- ✓ **Biologic variations.** Refers to the biologic differences among racial and ethnic groups; can include physical characteristics, such as skin color; physiologic variations, such as lactose intolerance; or susceptibility to specific disease processes, such as sickle cell anemia.

Source: As seen in *Fundamentals of Nursing,* Fifth Edition, by Kozier et al. Copyright 1995 by Addison-Wesley Publishing Company. Summarized from Giger and Davidhizar, *Transcultural Nursing: Assessment and Intervention* (St. Louis: Mosby-Year Book, 1991).

Heritage Assessment

I. Demographic Data

1. Location_____

2. (a) Age_____
   (b) Date of Birth_____
   (c) Place of Birth_____

3. Sex
   (1) Female   (2) Male

4. What is the highest grade completed in school?_____

5. Are you
   (1) Married   (2) Widowed
   (3) Divorced   (4) Separated
   (5) Never married

II. Heritage Assessment: Your Ethnic, Cultural, and Religious Background

1. Where was your mother born?
   _____

2. Where was your father born?
   _____

3. Where were your grandparents born?:
   a. Your mother's mother?
   _____
   b. Your mother's father?
   _____
   c. Your father's mother?
   _____
   d. Your father's father?
   _____

4. How many brothers do you have?_____ sisters_____

5. In what setting did you grow up?
   Urban   Rural   Suburban

6. In what country did your parents grow up?
   Father_____
   Mother_____

7. How old were you when you came to the United States?
   _____

8. How old were your parents when they came to the U. S.?
   Mother_____
   Father_____

9. When you were growing up, who lived with you?_____
   _____

10. Have you maintained contact with:
    a. Aunts, uncles, cousins   Yes No
    b. Brothers and sisters?   Yes No
    c. Parents   Yes No
    d. Your own children?   Yes No

11. Did most of your aunts, uncles, cousins live near to your home?
    Yes No

12. Approximately how often did you visit your family members who lived outside of your home?
    (1) Daily   (2) Weekly (3) Monthly
    (4) Once a year or less (5) Never

13. Was your original family name changed?   Yes No

14. What is your religious preference?
    (1) Catholic   (2) Jewish
    (3) Protestant   (4) Denomination
    (5) Other   (6) None

15. Is your spouse the same religion as you?   Yes No

16. Is your spouse the same ethnic background as you?
    Yes No

17. What kind of school did you go to?
    (1) Public   (2) Private
    (3) Religious

18. As an adult, do you live in a neighborhood where the neighbors are the same religion and ethnic back ground as yourself? Yes No

19. Do you belong to a religious institution?   Yes No

20. Would you describe yourself as an active member?   Yes No

21. How often do you attend your religious institution?
    (1) More than once a week
    (2) Weekly   (3) Monthly
    (4) Special holidays only (5) Never

22. Do you practice your religion in your home?   Yes No
    (if yes, please specify)
    (1) Praying   (2) Bible reading
    (3) Diet
    (4) Celebrating religious holidays

23. Do you prepare foods of your ethnic background? Yes No

24. Do you participate in ethnic activities?   Yes No
    (if yes, please specify)
    (1) Singing
    (2) Holiday celebrations
    (3) Dancing   (4) Festivals
    (5) Costumes   (6) Other

25. Are your friends from the same religious background as you?
    Yes No

26. Are your friends from the same ethnic background as you?
    Yes No

27. What is your native language?
    _____

28. Do you speak this language?
    (1) Prefer (2) Occasionally
    (3) Rarely

29. Do you read your native language?
    Yes No

III. Beliefs and Practices Regarding Personal Health and Illness
(Note: Use a separate sheet of paper for long answer questions.)

1. How do you describe "health"?

2. How do you rate your health?
   (1) Excellent (2) Good
   (3) Fair   (4) Poor

3. How do you describe "illness"?

4. What do you believe causes illness?
   (1) Poor eating habits?   Yes No
   (2) Incorrect food combinations? Yes No
   (3) Viruses, bacteria, "germs?" Yes No
   (4) God's punishment for sin? Yes No
   (5) The "Evil Eye?"   Yes No
   (6) Other people's hexes or spells?   Yes No
   (7) Witchcraft?   Yes No
   (8) Changes in environment, i.e.. cold/hot weather? Yes No
   (9) Exposure to drafts   Yes No
   (10) Overwork?   Yes No
   (11) Underwork?   Yes No
   (12) Grief and loss?   Yes No
   (13) Other

5. What did your mother do to keep you from getting sick?

6. How do you keep yourself from getting sick?

7. What home remedies did your mother use to treat illness?

8. What home remedies do you use?

9. Describe in 200-300 words an incident in your nursing practice when cultural differences (religious, ethnic, or lay/nursing) caused a problem for you.

Figure 3–4. Heritage assessment (Courtesy of Rachel E. Spector, PhD, RN, CTN. Reprinted with permission.)

the spiritual assessment at the end of the interview, once you have developed a relationship with the client. The following questions may be helpful when working with clients who indicate a religious affiliation:

✓ Please tell me about any particular religious practices that are important to you.
✓ Will being here (or being ill) interfere with your religious practices?
✓ Do you feel your faith is helpful to you? In what ways is it important to you right now?
✓ How can I help you carry out your faith? For example, would you like me to read your prayer book to you?
✓ Would you like a visit from your spiritual counselor, minister, or the hospital chaplain?

Nurses sometimes hesitate to ask questions about spirituality because they are afraid they may impose their own ideas of spirituality on the patient; or perhaps they fear that using "religious language" would alienate a client who does not express his spirituality in such language (e.g., "Do you pray regularly?" or "Are you saved?"). It may help to think of spirituality in a broad sense, not as limited to religion. The following are some questions and observations that may help you to assess the client's spiritual status without asking direct, spiritual questions (Cathell, 1991; Stoll, 1979):

1. *The patient's concept of "God."* All people are religious in the sense that they need something to give meaning to their life. For some, "God" is the religious meaning of God; for some it is their work; for others it is their lifestyle, their children, and so on. Listen to what the patient says about how he spends his time and energy. Observe the books at his bedside and the programs he watches on television. Does the patient's life have meaning, value, and purpose? Does he seem to be at peace with himself?

2. *The patient's source of hope and strength.* This might be God in the traditional sense; it may be a family member; or the client may describe an "inner source" of strength. Notice who the client talks about most often; or ask, "Who is important to you?" or "Where do you go to feel loved and understood?"

3. *The significance of religious practice and rituals.* In addition to asking specific questions, notice whether the client seems to be praying when you enter the room, before meals, or during procedures. Observe whether he is visited by a clergy member. Look for such items as religious literature, pictures, rosaries, church bulletins, and religious get-well cards at the bedside. These provide clues to the kind of spiritual support that are meaningful to the client.

4. *The patient's thoughts about the relationship between spiritual beliefs and his state of health.* Is the client questioning the meaning of his illness: "Why did God let this happen to me?" Some people believe illness is a punishment for some wrong they have done. Others may see illness as a test of their faith. Still others may see their faith as therapy for their illness: "If I have faith, I will get well."

5. *The patient's fear of alienation, loneliness, or solitude.* This can take many forms. Instead of appearing lonely, patients may use distancing behaviors such as joking. Some patients are overly sophisticated about their illness. They talk about it in terms of lab values, pathophysiology, and medications, but

Assessment

Health Promotion Behaviors

Sleeping 7–8 hours per night, regularly

Eating breakfast regularly

Eating regular meals

Little or no snacking

Maintaining optimal weight

Frequent exercise

Moderate alcohol consumption

Avoiding smoking

Practicing safer sex

Stress management

do not say how they feel about it or what it means in their life. Other clients may pace the halls, have sleep disturbances, or seem angry, apathetic, or preoccupied.

Wellness Assessment

A thorough assessment of the client's health status is basic to health promotion. **Health promotion** is more than avoidance or prevention of disease. It includes activities undertaken for the purpose of improving well-being and achieving a higher level of health (e.g., stress management and physical fitness). See Table 3–11 for a summary of the components of a wellness assessment (Pender, 1987, p. 103).

ETHICAL CONSIDERATIONS

As in all aspects of care, nurses must be aware of their ethical responsibilities when assessing clients. According to the ANA "Code for Nurses" (1985),

> the nurse provides services with respect for human dignity and the uniqueness of the client. . . . The nurse safeguards the client's right to privacy by judiciously protecting information of a confidential nature.

Honesty and confidentiality are the issues most frequently encountered during this step of the nursing process. These issues involve the moral principles of veracity and autonomy.

Honesty

The moral principle of **veracity** holds that we should tell the truth and not lie. In assessing patients, this means that you should be honest about how you will use the data: to plan the patient's care, for research, for a student paper, and so forth. Remember when you introduce yourself to the patient to tell him what to expect from the interview and how the information will be used.

Truthfulness also affects the patient's autonomy. The moral principle of **autonomy** holds that a person has the right to be independent and to determine for himself what is to happen to him. If the patient does not know how the data will be used, he cannot make a truly informed choice about whether to participate in the interview and thereby loses some of his autonomy.

Confidentiality

Treat assessment data as confidential. Failure to do so robs the patient of his autonomy, since it removes his control over how data is used and shared. Among other things, confidentiality means that assessment notes should be kept in the patient's chart, not lying about where anyone else can read them. It also means that you should not talk about patient data at the desk, in the halls, or in the lunchroom, where casual observers might overhear.

A client may tell you something in confidence that you feel you must tell in order to protect her; for example, a client might tell you of her plans for suicide. If you believe you cannot keep the information confidential, then you are

Table 3–11. Using a Wellness Framework to Organize Data

Assessment Categories	Explanation and Examples
Physical-Fitness Assessment	Exercise tolerance (e.g., step test), general apparance, muscle strength, joint flexibility, body proportions, percent of body fat
Nutritional Assessment	Comparison of weight to body build and height, muscle mass, 24-hour recall of food intake, knowledge of nutrition, effect of socio-cultural beliefs on diet, use of the Food Guide Pyramid and Recommended Daily Allowances of essential nutrients.
Health Risk Appraisal	Assessment of a client's risk of disease or injury over the next 10 years by comparing his characteristics with the characteristics and mortality risk of the corresponding age, sex, and racial group. Several tools have been developed for this purpose. Pender's (1987, pp. 119, 123–129) tool assesses five categories of risk: (1) cardiovascular disease, (2) malignant disease, (3) automobile accidents, (4) suicide, and (5) diabetes.
Lifestyle Assessment	Categories usually assessed are physical activity; nutritional practices; stress management; personal habits such as smoking, alcohol consumption, drug use; safety and health-care practices (e.g., last Pap smear, last chest X ray). Figure 3–5 is an example of a lifestyle assessment.
Health Beliefs	The client's perception of his ability to control his own health status. Clients who believe they have a major influence on their own health status are more likely to take the initiative in health promotion and disease prevention (e.g., breast self-examination). Motivation to engage in health behaviors is based on a person's beliefs that (a) one is vulnerable to the health problem, (b) the illness is a threat, (c) the recommended health action will reduce the threat without substantial inconvenience, and (d) people should be generally concerned about health matters (Becker et al. 1972, p. 852).
Life Stress Review	Stress can be defined as a stimulus, life event, or set of circumstances causing a disrupted response (Lyon & Werner, 1987). People who have a high level of stress are often more prone to illness and have a lowered ability to cope with illness. Several scales have been developed to document a person's relatively recent experiences, such as divorce, pregnancy, and retirement, which can be considered stressful. This includes both positive and negative events.

Sources: Becker et al., (1972), Motivation as predictors of health behavior, *Health Services Reports, 87*:852–62; Edelman and Mandle, *Health Promotion throughout the Lifespan*, 3rd ed. (St. Louis: Mosby, 1994); Kozier et al., *Concepts and Issues in Nursing Practice*, 2nd ed. (Redwood City, CA: Addison-Wesley Nursing, 1992, pp. 278–286); Lyon and Werner, Stress, In Fitzpatrick and Taunton, eds., *Annual Review of Nursing Research* (New York: Springer Publishing Co., 1987, 5: 3–22); Pender, N., *Health Promotion in Nursing Practice*, 2nd ed. (Norwalk, CT: Appleton & Lange, 1987); and Pinnell and de Meneses, *The Nursing Process: Theory, Application, and Related Processes* (Norwalk, CT: Appleton-Lange, 1986, pp. 89-90).

healthstyle: *a self-test*

All of us want good health. But many of us do not know how to be as healthy as possible. Health experts now describe lifestyle as one of the most important factors affecting health. In fact, it is estimated that as many as seven of the ten leading causes of death could be reduced through common-sense changes in lifestyle. That's what this brief test, developed by the Public Health Service, is all about. Its purpose is simply to tell you how well you are doing to stay healthy. The behavior is covered in the test are recommended for most Americans. Some of them may not apply to persons with certain chronic diseases or handicaps, or to pregnant women. Such persons may require special instructions from their physicians.

	Almost Always	Sometimes	Almost Never
Cigarette Smoking			
If you <u>never smoke,</u> enter a score of 10 for this section and go to the next section on *Alcohol and Drugs.*			
1. I avoid smoking cigarettes.	2	1	0
2. I smoke only low tar and nicotine cigarettes *or* I smoke a pipe or cigars.	2	1	0
Smoking Score:_____			
Alcohol and Drugs			
1. I avoid drinking alcoholic beverages or I drink no more than 1 or 2 drinks a day.	4	1	0
2. I avoid using alcohol or other drugs (especially illegal drugs) as a way of handling stressful situations or the problems in my life.	2	1	0
3. I am careful not to drink alcohol when taking certain medicines (for example, medicine for sleeping, pain, colds, and allergies), or when pregnant.	2	1	0
4. I read and follow the label directions when using prescribed and over-the-counter drugs.	2	1	0
Alcohol and Drugs Score:_____			
Eating Habits			
1. I eat a variety of foods each day, such as fruits and vegetables, whole grain breads and cereals, lean meats, dairy products, dry peas and beans, and nuts and seeds.	4	1	0
2. I limit the amount of fat, saturated fat, and cholesterol I eat (including fat on meats, eggs, butter, cream, shortenings, and organ meats such as liver).	2	1	0
3. I limit the amount of salt I eat by cooking with only small amounts, not adding salt at the table, and avoiding salty snacks.	2	1	0
4. I avoid eating too much sugar (especially frequent snacks of sticky candy or soft drinks).	2	1	0
Eating Habits Score:_____			

	Almost Always	Sometimes	Almost Never
Exercise/Fitness			
1. I maintain a desired weight, avoiding overweight and underweight.	3	1	0
2. I do vigorous exercises for 15–30 minutes at least 3 times a week (examples include running, swimming, brisk walking).	3	1	0
3. I do exercises that enhance my muscle tone for 15–30 minutes at least 3 times a week (examples include yoga and calisthenics).	2	1	0
4. I use part of leisure time participating in individual, family, or team activities that increase my level of fitness (such as gardening, bowling, golf, and baseball).	2	1	0
Exercise/Fitness Score:_____			
Stress Control			
1. I have a job or do other work that I enjoy.	2	1	0
2. I find it easy to relax and express my feelings freely.	2	1	0
3. I recognize early, and prepare for, events or situations likely to be stressful for me.	2	1	0
4. I have close friends, relatives, or others whom I can talk to about personal matters and call on for help when needed.	2	1	0
5. I participate in group activities (such as church and community organizations or hobbies that I enjoy.	2	1	0
Stress Control Score:_____			
Safety			
1. I wear a seat belt while riding in a car.	2	1	0
2. I avoid driving while under the influence of alcohol and other drugs.	2	1	0
3. I obey traffic rules and the speed limit when driving.	2	1	0
4. I am careful when using potentially harmful products or substances (such as household cleaners, poisons, and electrical devices).	2	1	0
5. I avoid smoking in bed.	2	1	0
Safety Score:_____			

Figure 3–5. Healthstyle: A Self Test (Courtesy of National Health Information Clearinghouse, Washington, D.C.)

What Your Scores Mean to YOU

Scores of 9 and 10

Excellent! Your answers show that you are aware of the importance of this area to your health. More important, you are putting your knowledge to work for you by practicing good health habits. As long as you continue to do so, this area should not pose a serious health risk. It's likely that you are setting an example for your family and friends to follow. Since you got a very high test score on this part of the test, you may want to consider other areas where your scores indicate room for improvement.

Scores of 6 to 8

Your health practices in this area are good, but there is room for improvement. Look again at the items you answered with "Sometimes" or "Almost Never." What changes can you make to improve your score? Even a small change can often help you achieve better health.

Scores of 3 to 5

Your health risks are showing! Would you like more information about the risks you are facing and about why it is important for you to change these behaviors. Perhaps you need help in deciding how to successfully make the changes you desire. In either case, help is available.

Scores of 0 to 2

Obviously, you were concerned enough about your health to take the test, but your answers show that you may be taking serious and unnecessary risks with your health. Perhaps you are not aware of the risks and what to do about them You can easily get the information and help you need to improve, if you wish. The next step is up to you.

Figure 3–5. (concluded)

obligated (by the principle of veracity) to tell the client that, in her best interest, you must share the information with other caregivers. A similar situation arises when a client tells you something that you feel you must reveal in order to protect someone else. There is no rule about when to tell and when not to tell. You will, each time, have to balance the need to preserve autonomy against the need to protect the client or others.

In both instances, it is better from an ethical standpoint to stop the client from telling you something you cannot keep confidential. Of course this is not always possible, but often you can pick up clues from the client that she is about to disclose this kind of information. If you do, you might say something like, "This sounds like something I may not be able to keep confidential. Are you *sure* you want to go on with it?"

SUMMARY

Assessment
- ✓ is the collection, validation, organization, and recording of data using interview, observation, and examination.
- ✓ requires critical thinking skills, a good knowledge base, and an awareness of ethical issues.
- ✓ uses directive and nondirective interviewing techniques, adapting to the special needs of the client.
- ✓ may be comprehensive or focused.
- ✓ may involve various conceptual frameworks to collect and organize data.
- ✓ may include in-depth assessment for special purposes (e.g., wellness assessment).
- ✓ should consider the moral principles of honesty and confidentiality.

When a state studies its transportation problems, the planners classify the various means of transportation in a few categories such as cars, trucks, buses, planes, and trains. This is done so that the large bulk of information about how each kind of vehicle fits into the state's transportation picture can be summarized. Generalities about each class of vehicle are more valuable in planning than the mass of unorganized data about each kind of vehicle. Also, such classification can produce new information by identifying common features of the vehicles in each category.

Similarly, when collecting patient data, nurses classify it according to their chosen theoretical framework (e.g., Maslow, Gordon, NANDA). Unclassified data about a patient might look something like this:

Harold Sims is a 35-year-old carpenter. He is married and has three children. There is a 2-inch scar on his forearm. He states he has been "short of breath" on exertion and is coughing frequently. Scattered wheezes are auscultated throughout his lungs. He is able to read newsprint without glasses. Active bowel sounds are auscultated in all four quadrants of his abdomen.

Practice in Critical Thinking: Classifying

Now look at the data again, listed with the related cues in bold print:

Age 35
Works as a carpenter
2-inch scar on forearm
States he has been "**short of breath**" on exertion.
States having frequent **cough**
Scattered wheezes auscultated throughout lungs
Able to read newsprint without glasses
Married; has 3 children
Active bowel sounds auscultated in all 4 quadrants

This is only a small part of the total data collected on a patient. Notice how difficult it is to find the related items, even when they are in bold print. With a framework for data collection, related items are classified together naturally, making the data more meaningful and the patterns more obvious. A framework also helps prevent omission of data, since categories with scant or no data will be obvious when you have finished your assessment.

Learning the Skill of Classification

Start with a simple example. Classify the various jobs in your community into the following categories. List some local jobs that fit each classification.

Agricultural

Technical

Health care

Clerical

Other

Compare your answers with those of your classmates and discuss any differences you may have in your classifications. Explain why each job fits in its category.

Applying the Skill

Classify the following patient data using two different frameworks: Gordon's and NANDA's. Review the discussion in Chapter 3 about these frameworks and refer to Tables 3–4 and 3–5 as needed.

Discuss your answers with your classmates individually or in class. There is no answer key for this exercise because the emphasis is not on whether your answers are *correct*, but on the thinking process you used to arrive at the answers—that is, the skill of *classifying*. The only way to evaluate your thinking process is to discuss it with others and get feedback from them.

Patient Data

Age 37

States having continual vaginal bleeding for the past 6 months

States has never been pregnant

Skin warm and dry

Hears normal speech at 10 feet

Takes iron pills

Weighs 130 lb.

States "light social drinker"

States she is not concerned about effect of hysterectomy on her sexuality

Works as a hairdresser

"I sleep a lot" when under stress

Blood sugar—124

Chest X ray normal

Manages all activities of daily living independently

Takes a bulk-forming laxative daily

Blood pressure 120/80

Oriented to time, place, and person

Wants to see hospital chaplain before surgery

States vision is 20/20 with glasses

Good skin turgor

Full range of motion of neck

Hemoglobin 9.5

5 feet, 5 inches tall

Has smoked 1/2 pack per day for 16 years

Lungs clear to auscultation

Allergic to penicillin

States eats 3 meals a day, but snacks often

States mother had cervical cancer

Has frequent headaches, takes aspirin to relieve

Unmarried

Urinates 5–6 times per day, "No difficulty"

Temperature 100°

Drinks "lots of water"

Hospitalized in 1980 for appendectomy

One formed stool per day; occasional constipation

1. **Classify the data, using Gordon's framework.** Refer to Table 3–5 on pages 66-67 as needed. (A few items have been classified for you. Notice that some of the data appears in more than one pattern.)

Patterns	Data
Health Perception/ Health Management	Takes iron pills
Nutritional-Metabolic	Takes iron pills
Elimination	
Activity-Exercise	States she has asthma
Cognitive-Perceptual	
Sleep-Rest	
Self-Perception/ Self-Concept	
Role-Relationship	
Sexuality-Reproductive	
Coping/ Stress-Tolerance	
Value-Belief	
Other	Age 37

Notice that in some categories (or patterns) you may have entered no data. If you have classified the data correctly, this would indicate to you, as a practicing nurse, that your data collection is incomplete.

2. **Classify the same data using one of the following frameworks.** Make your own table using the categories of the model you choose.

   ✓ Orem's Self-Care Model, Table 3–6 on page 67
   ✓ Roy's Adaptation Model, Table 3–7 on page 68
   ✓ NANDA Human Response Patterns, Table 3–8 on page 69
   ✓ Maslow's Basic Needs, Table 3–9 on page 70
   ✓ The body systems model, on page 66

Adapted from *Critical Thinking Worksheets,* a Supplement of *Addison-Wesley Chemistry,* by Wilbraham et al. (Menlo Park, CA: Addison-Wesley Publishing Company, 1990).

Applying Nursing Process

1. Listed below are data-collection practices observed on various nursing units. You are the quality-control nurse. Place a check mark beside the practices that meet ANA Standard I.

   a. ___ Admission data is recorded on a printed form in predetermined categories.

   b. ___ There is an admission assessment in the chart. The nursing progress notes on two different days list care given to the patient, but no assessment data about the patient.

   c. ___ The nurses record the comprehensive assessment in paragraph form on the nursing progress notes; they do not all record the data in the same order.

   d. ___ Each patient's chart contains a nursing history and physical examination. A divider with a tab makes these easy to locate.

2. Place a *C* beside the cues. Place an *I* beside the inferences.

 a. ___ The client's blood pressure is 140/80.

 b. ___ The client states he is in pain.

 c. ___ The client is afraid.

 d. ___ The client is depressed.

 e. ___ The client's wife says he forgets to take his pills.

 f. ___ The incision is draining pink fluid.

 g. ___ The incision is infected.

3. Classify the data below by placing the letters in the appropriate columns. Note that most letters will be placed in *two* columns (subjective/objective and primary/secondary). The first one is done for you.

Subjective Data	Objective Data	Primary Source	Secondary Source
	a		a

a. You read in the chart that the client's blood pressure is 140/80.

b. Client's wife says he doesn't sleep well.

c. You observe that the client is pale.

d. The aide tells you the client is pale.

e. You palpate the client's pulse. It is 84 bpm.

f. Mrs. Jones says, "I can't sleep."

g. The nursing progress notes say, "Client is breathing rapidly."

h. The night nurse reports the client's temperature is 98.6°

i. The client is coughing.

j. Client states he is cold.

k. The client is walking with a limp.

l. Urine output measured at 100 mL.

m. You feel the dressing. It is dry.

n. Client says she cannot void.

o. You auscultate wheezes in the patient's lungs.

p. Anesthetist tells you the pulse is weak and thready.

q. You palpate a weak, thready pulse.

r. Patient tells you his leg hurts.

4. Suppose your instructor gives you the following patient assignment for the next day.

You are to perform the admission assessment, including interview and physical examination, on Melissa Bourque, who is being admitted for cosmetic surgery. Patient is a 45-year-old female. Her preoperative lab work has been done and will be on the chart, along with her medical records from the physician's office.

Will you read Ms. Bourque's chart before doing the nursing interview? Why or why not?

5. Indicate whether the *nurse* (you) obtained the data by interview (*I*), observation (*O*), or physical examination (*E*).

a. ___ You read in the chart that the client's blood pressure is 140/80.

b. ___ Client's wife says he doesn't sleep well.

c. ___ You see that the client is pale.

d. ___ You feel the dressing. It is dry.

e. ___ You count the client's pulse at 84 bpm.

f. ___ You hear the client cough.

g. ___ Client states he is cold.

h. ___ Urine output is measured at 100 mL.

i. ___ Client says she cannot void.

j. ___ You auscultate wheezes in the client's lungs.

k. ___ Anesthetist tells you the pulse is weak and thready.

6. Identify the type of question: *C* = Closed, *O* = Open-ended.

a. ___ Would you like a backrub?

b. ___ Where would you like me to begin?

c. ___ Did you sleep well?

d. ___ How did you sleep?

e. ___ What do you think kept you from sleeping well?

f. ___ Are you hearing voices?

g. ___ Tell me about the voices.

h. ___ Are you worried about the operation?

i. ___ How do you feel now?

j. ___ Tell me about the delivery.

7. The client says, "I have this pain in my stomach." Write examples of questions the nurse could ask to find out more about it.

   a. A closed question:

   b. An open-ended question:

8. You need to perform the data base assessment for Stella Contini. You have read her chart and know that she is 50 years old, unmarried, and has no children. She has severe arthritis in several joints and is being admitted for a total knee replacement. Her mother and sister are at the bedside. Ms. Contini has a roommate in the adjoining bed.

   a. To *prepare* for the interview, what do you need to do?

   b. There is a section on the assessment form labeled "Reason for Hospitalization." What would you say to Ms. Contini to elicit this information?

   c. There is a section on the form labeled "Usual sexual functioning" and another labeled "Changes in sexual functioning since illness." Would you ask these questions? Why or why not?

9. Place a check mark beside the data that should be validated.

    a. ___ The patient tells you he is not anxious about the barium enema. He is lying quietly in bed with no obvious muscle tension. His hands are still. His skin is warm and dry.

    b. ___ The patient says, "On a scale of 1 to 10, the pain is a 10. Worst I can imagine." Less than five minutes ago, you observed the patient talking on the telephone in a normal tone of voice.

    c. ___ The patient says he smokes two packs of cigarettes a day. You observe that his teeth and fingers are brown-stained.

    d. ___ The client tells you on admission that she lives alone. In a later conversation, she refers to her roommate.

    e. ___ The data was obtained early in the interview, and then the client became confused and began to ramble incoherently.

    f. ___ The mother says her little boy "eats like a horse." You observe that the child is thin and small for his age.

10. Some of the following nursing progress notes consist of data. Others are judgments about the data or conclusions drawn by the nurse. Draw a line through each of the judgments/conclusions.

    a. Patient stated, "I feel sick."

    b. Vomited 100 mL green-tinged fluid.

    c. Patient is nauseated.

    d. Patient was tearful during the interview.

    e. Client is disoriented.

    f. Tolerated clear liquids well.

    g. Ambulated to bathroom with no dizziness.

    h. Ms. Benitez is extremely fearful of this surgery.

    i. Abdomen is distended.

    j. Client states he is confused about the medication schedule.

    k. Respirations normal.

    l. Vision is poor.

    m. Drinking adequate amount of fluids.

11. Write the correct word in the blank: Is the situation a question of *honesty, confidentiality,* or *neither?*

a. _____ The nurse asks the patient whether he prefers a bedbath or a whirlpool bath.

b. _____ Before beginning the interview, the nurse tells the patient she needs the information to help plan his care.

c. _____ Nora Morenz is collecting data about pain relief measures for a research project. Because it does not change the patients' care and because they are not mentioned by name, she decides not to tell them she is collecting data for research.

d. _____ A patient's wife overhears the staff discussing information about her husband in the lunchroom.

e. _____ The client tells the nurse she has a knife hidden in the room and that "Someone is going to be sorry." The nurse looks for the knife, but cannot find it. She tells the client, "I am afraid for you and for the other patients. I'm sorry, but I will have to share what you've told me with the rest of the staff."

REFERENCES

Alfaro-LeFevre, R. (1994). *Applying Nursing Process.* 3rd ed. Philadelphia: J. B. Lippincott Company.

American Nurses Association. (1991a). *Position Statement on Cultural Diversity in Nursing Practice.* Kansas City, MO: ANA.

American Nurses Association. (1991b). *Standards of Clinical Nursing Practice.* Kansas City, MO: ANA.

American Nurses Association. (1985). *Code for Nurses with Interpretive Statements.* Kansas City, MO: ANA.

Andrews, H., and Roy, C. (1986). *Essentials of the Roy Adaptation Model.* Norwalk, CT: Appleton-Century-Crofts.

Becker, M., Drachman, R., and Kirscht, J. (1972). Motivation as predictors of health behavior. *Health Services Reports, 87*:852–62.

Bestard, S., and Courtenay, M. (1990). Focusing on wellness. *Canadian Nurse, 86*(11):24–25.

Carpenito, L. (1993). *Nursing Diagnosis: Application to Clinical Practice.* 5th ed. Philadelphia: J. B. Lippincott Company.

Cathell, D. (1991). A spiritual assessment without asking spiritual questions. Lecture. Shawnee Mission Medical Center, Merriam, KS.

Edelman, C., and Mandle, C. (1994). *Health Promotion Throughout the Life Span.* 3rd ed. St. Louis: Mosby.

Ellis, A., and Cavanagh, S. (1992). Aspects of neurosurgical assessment using the Glasgow Coma Scale. *Intensive and Critical Care Nursing, 8*:94–99.

Giger, J., and Davidhizar, R. (1995). *Transcultural Nursing: Assessment and Intervention.* St. Louis: Mosby.

Gordon, M. (1994). *Nursing Diagnosis: Process and Application.* 3rd ed. St. Louis: Mosby.

Gordon, M., Murphy, C., Candee, D., and Hiltunen, E. (1994). Clinical judgment: An integrated model. *Advances in Nursing Science, 16*(4):55–70.

Jackson, L. (1993). Understanding, eliciting and negotiating clients' multicultural health beliefs. *Nurse Practitioner: American Journal of Primary Health Care, 18*(4):30, 32, 37–38.

James, L. (1992). Nursing theory made practical. *Journal of Nursing Education, 31*(1):42–44.

Johannsen, J. M. (1992). Self-care assessment: Key to teaching and discharge planning. *Dimensions of Critical Care Nursing, 11*(1):48–56.

Joint Commission on Accreditation of Healthcare Organizations (1994). *Accreditation Manual for Hospitals.* Chicago: JCAHO, Nursing Services.

Kennie, D. (1993). *Preventive Care for Elderly People*. New York: Cambridge University Press.

Kozier, B., Erb, G., and Blais, K. (1992). *Concepts and Issues In Nursing Practice*. 2nd ed. Redwood City, CA: Addison-Wesley Nursing.

Kozier, B., Erb, G., and Blais, K., and Wilkinson, J. (1994). *Fundamentals of Nursing*. 5th ed. Redwood City, CA: Addison-Wesley Nursing.

Lyon, B., and Werner, J. (1987). Stress, In J. Fitzpatrick and R. Taunton, eds., *Annual Review of Nursing Research* (New York: Springer Publishing Co.), 5:3–22.

Maslow, A. H. (1970). *Motivation and Personality*. 2nd ed. New York: Harper & Row.

Minami, H. (1985). East meets west: Some ethical considerations. *International Journal of Nursing Studies, 22*(4):311–18.

Murray, R., and Zentner. (1993). *Nursing Assessment and Health Promotion: Strategies Through the Life Span*. 5th ed. Norwalk, CT: Appleton & Lange.

North American Nursing Diagnosis Association. (1986). *Classification of Nursing Diagnoses. Proceedings of the Sixth Conference*. St. Louis: C. V. Mosby.

Orem, D. E. (1991). *Nursing: Concepts of Practice*. 4th ed. St. Louis: Mosby-Year Book.

Pender, N. (1987). *Health Promotion in Nursing Practice*. 2nd ed. Norwalk, CT: Appleton & Lange.

Pinnell, N., and de Meneses, M. (1986). *The Nursing Process: Theory, Application, and Related Processes*. Norwalk, CT: Appleton-Lange.

Roy, C. (1984). *Introduction to Nursing: An Adaptation Model*. 2nd ed. Englewood Cliffs, NJ: Prentice Hall.

Roy, C., and Andrews, H. A. (1991). *The Roy Adaptation Model: The Definitive Statement*. Norwalk, CT: Appleton & Lange.

Spector, R. (1994). Strategies for multicultural nursing education: Heritage Assessment. *Issues in Action, Spring* (3):4–5 (Redwood City, CA: Addison-Wesley Nursing).

Stoll, R. (1979). Guidelines for spiritual assessment. *American Journal of Nursing*, 79:1574–77.

Tanner, E. (1991). Assessment of a health-promotive lifestyle. *Nursing Clinics of North America, 26*(4):845–54.

Tettero, I., Jackson, S., and Wilson, S. (1993). Theory to practice: Developing a Rogerian-based assessment tool. *Journal of Advanced Nursing, 18*:776–82.

Wilbraham et al. (1990). *Critical Thinking Worksheets*, a supplement of *Addison-Wesley Chemistry*. Menlo Park, CA: Addison-Wesley Publishing Company.

Ziegler, S. (1993). *Theory-Directed Nursing Practice*. New York: Springer Publishing Co., Inc.

CHAPTER 4

DIAGNOSTIC REASONING

OBJECTIVES

On completion of this chapter you should be able to do the following:
- Explain how diagnosis is related to the other steps of the nursing process.
- Describe the process of diagnostic reasoning.
- Explain what is meant by a *patient problem.*
- Given a patient problem, correctly identify its type and status.
- Describe common diagnostic errors and explain how they can be prevented by thinking critically.
- Explain why and how you should verify your nursing diagnoses.
- Compare the advantages and disadvantages of computer-aided diagnosis.
- State how nursing diagnosis can be used with critical pathways.

INTRODUCTION

This chapter will: (1) discuss diagnosis as a step of the nursing process; (2) define *patient problem* and help you begin to differentiate between a problem and other phenomena, such as symptoms; and (3) explain the diagnostic reasoning process. In this chapter you will learn to identify three kinds of health problems:

✓ *Nursing diagnoses*—problems nurses can treat independently
✓ *Collaborative problems*—problems nurses treat in collaboration with other health professionals
✓ *Medical problems*—problems for which nurses give care prescribed by physicians

This chapter will also help you to identify and describe client problems more precisely. The diagnostic process is not just a matter of choosing likely looking labels from a standardized list. The labels must accurately reflect the client's health status. Because this chapter deals with the broader concept of *problems*, not just with nursing diagnoses, it does not always use NANDA language, such as that found on the inside covers of this text.

Terminology

Diagnosis is sometimes confusing for students and practicing nurses alike. One of the difficulties is that diagnosis is both a process and a product. That is, a nurse uses a reasoning process called *nursing diagnosis* to produce a statement of health status that is also called a *nursing diagnosis.* In order to write the

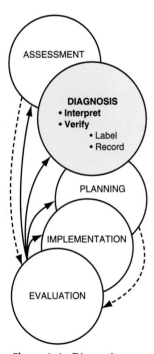

Figure 4–1. Diagnosis

statement, the nurse refers to a standardized list of terms that are sometimes called *nursing diagnoses*. You will see *diagnosis* given all these meanings in the literature. To minimize confusion, this text uses the terms as shown in Figure 4–2 (Carpenito, 1993, p. 6).

This chapter presents *diagnosis* both as a step of the nursing process and as a nursing activity, diagnostic reasoning. It will also introduce *nursing diagnosis* (the problem statement). Chapter 5 discusses nursing diagnosis in more depth and explains how to use the NANDA *diagnostic labels* to write problem statements.

DIAGNOSIS: SECOND STEP OF NURSING PROCESS

In diagnosis, the second step of the nursing process, nurses use diagnostic reasoning to analyze data and draw conclusions about the client's health status (i.e., strengths, problems, and causes of the problems). They verify these conclusions with the client, select standardized labels, and record them on the care plan. The nursing activities of the diagnosis step are shown in Figure 4–1.

Relationship to Other Nursing Process Steps

Recall from Chapter 1 that the steps of the nursing process are interdependent and overlapping. Diagnosis is a pivotal step. All activities preceding this step are directed toward formulating the nursing diagnoses. All the care-planning activities following this step are based on the nursing diagnoses (see Figure 4–3).

Diagnosis - - - - - - → 1. The second *step* of the nursing process.
2. The *reasoning process* used to interpret data in order to draw conclusions and make a

Nursing Diagnosis - - → The product: A *formal statement* of the patient's health status is written, using

Diagnostic Labels - - → The *standardized list* of diagnostic terminology approved by the North American Nursing Diagnosis Association (NANDA).

Figure 4–2. Diagnosis Terminology

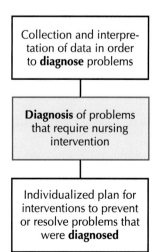

Collection and interpretation of data in order to **diagnose** problems

Diagnosis of problems that require nursing intervention

Individualized plan for interventions to prevent or resolve problems that were **diagnosed**

Figure 4–3. Diagnosis: A Pivotal Step

Diagnostic Reasoning

Diagnosis depends on the assessment phase because the quality of the data acquired during assessment affects the accuracy of the nursing diagnoses. The following example illustrates how the two stages overlap. Like most nurses, the nurse in the example begins to think of possible meanings for some of the data (diagnosis) at the same time she is collecting it (assessment).

Example: While interviewing Keisha Mandela, school nurse Julie Adkins notices that the child is speaking hesitantly and softly, giving brief answers and refusing to make eye contact. She wonders if Keisha is shy, withdrawn, anxious, or perhaps having difficulty with her self-concept. She continues to gather data to confirm or deny these possibilities. In the diagnosis step, Julie will critically examine all the data she has gathered, and draw a firmer conclusion about its meaning.

Diagnosis also affects the planning, implementation, and evaluation steps. The problems and strengths during diagnosis provide a focus for planning the patient's care (planning phase). When specifically and accurately stated, they guide the nurse in developing appropriate goals and nursing orders for the care plan.

The diagnosis and implementation steps sometimes occur almost simultaneously. For example, in an emergency situation a nurse may take action (implementation) as soon as the urgent problem is recognized—before she consciously makes a plan or identifies the rest of the problems, or even before completely analyzing the data. Diagnosis also overlaps with the evaluation phase. During evaluation, the nurse determines whether the patient's problems have changed status or been resolved. If not, they are reexamined to be sure they were diagnosed correctly and completely.

History of Nursing Diagnosis

The term *diagnosis* began to appear in the nursing literature in the 1950s. McManus (1951) used the term *nursing diagnosis* in describing the functions of a professional nurse. Fry (1953) stated that nursing diagnosis was based on the client's needs for nursing care rather than medical therapies. Until that time nursing had been conceptualized as a set of tasks, and nursing care was planned around those tasks. Nurses assisted physicians in treating diseases. They gathered data about patients, but primarily for the purpose of ensuring that doctors could make medical diagnoses, not for the purpose of planning nursing care.

In the 1960s, diagnosis was becoming an important part of the nursing process, but it was still necessary to differentiate between nursing diagnosis and medical diagnosis—to establish that diagnosis was a cognitive process that nurses could and should use and that they were not encroaching on medical territory.

In 1973, the ANA *Standards of Nursing Practice* included nursing diagnosis as an important nursing activity. This legitimized it as a function of professional nurses. In that same year the first national nursing diagnosis task force, now the North American Nursing Diagnosis Association (NANDA), met to begin working on standardizing the terminology for nursing diagnoses (Gebbie and Lavin, 1975; Gebbie, 1976). During the 1970s and 1980s, the term *nursing diagnosis* was incorporated into nearly all state nurse practice acts, making diagnosis a nursing obligation as well as a legal right. Diagnosis is now taught in most schools of nursing, commonly used in the literature, and frequently used by nurses to describe their practice.

Importance of Diagnosing

As shown in Box 4–1, diagnosing is now a standard by which professional care is measured. ANA Standard III (in Chapter 6) further states that expected client outcomes should be derived from the nursing diagnoses (ANA, 1991). Nursing diagnosis can benefit both nurses and health care consumers in the following ways:

✓ **Nursing diagnoses facilitate individualized care.** Even though clients with identical medical conditions may need similar "routine" nursing interventions, the priorities of care may differ for each (for example, refer to the box in the margin of page 92, which lists nursing diagnoses for two patients who have had myocardial infarctions). In a health care system driven by cost considerations, there is constant emphasis on standardizing care as a way to promote efficiency and decrease cost. Nursing diagnoses can be used to focus attention on client's unique needs, which may otherwise be overlooked.

✓ **Nursing diagnosis promotes professional accountability and autonomy by defining and describing the independent area of nursing practice.** According to Warren and Hoskins (1990, p. 162), "A profession must have a language that communicates its uniqueness and at the same time is understood by peers, other professionals, and consumers/clients." Nursing diagnosis language makes it clear that nurses do far more than simply carry out orders for medical treatments, and it enables them to communicate the specific nature of the health conditions they treat to legislators, consumers, and insurance providers.

✓ **Nursing diagnoses provide an effective vehicle for communication among nurses and other health care professionals.** Because a nursing diagnosis consolidates a great deal of information into a concise statement, it provides a "shorthand" means of communicating client status. For example, imagine you have collected the following data: Patient states his mouth is painful; his tongue is coated and mucous membranes are dry; there are vesicles and ulcerations in his mouth; his mouth has a strong odor. The nursing diagnosis, Altered Oral Mucous Membrane, gives you the same picture of the patient as that entire set of data.

Box 4–1. ANA Standard II: Diagnosis

The nurse analyzes the assessment data in determining diagnoses.
Measurement Criteria
1. Diagnoses are derived from the assessment data.
2. Diagnoses are validated with the client, significant others, and health care providers, when possible.
3. Diagnoses are documented in a manner that facilitates the determination of expected outcomes and plan of care.

Source: Abstracted from American Nurses Association, *Standards of Clinical Nursing Practice* (Kansas City, MO: ANA, 1991), p. 10. Used with permission.

Diagnostic Reasoning

Prioritized Nursing Diagnoses

For Mary Chinn

1. Risk for Fluid Volume Deficit related to nausea and vomiting associated with pain and stress

2. Chest Pain related to reduced oxygenation of myocardium

3. Activity Intolerance related to decreased cardiac output

For Donald Schulz

1. Anxiety related to anticipation of financial difficulties because of being away from his business

2. Ineffective Breathing Patterns related to depressant effects of medications

3. Constipation related to decreased mobility, narcotics, and fear that straining will cause another heart attack

---

✓ **Nursing diagnoses help determine assessment parameters.** Using the same example, once you have grasped the concept of *Altered Oral Mucous Membrane*, the term will suggest to you the presence of certain cues. When you observe one cue, you will be alert for other cues related to this diagnosis. For example, when you see that a patient is mouth breathing, you will check to see if his mucous membranes are dry and if he is drinking sufficient fluids.

✓ **Nursing diagnoses facilitate continuity of care.** For example, they guide the planning of nursing care from one shift to another in an acute care setting and when a client is transferred to a different unit (e.g., from operating room to recovery room). They are useful when a client moves from a hospital to a long-term care facility or is discharged to home still requiring nursing care (Sheppard, 1993).

Computer-Aided Diagnosis

In some agencies nurses use computers to classify and interpret assessment data. After the nurse enters the data, the software compares the cues to those that are associated with each nursing diagnosis in its data base. It then generates a list of abnormal cues or a list of possible diagnoses, and the nurse chooses which diagnoses to accept or reject or adds to the list. The advantages of computer-assisted diagnosis are that computers are consistent, systematic, and organized. They do not experience fatigue, distraction, or other human weaknesses; therefore, they are able to identify patterns the nurse might overlook. Nurses must use professional judgment in evaluating the computer-generated diagnoses, however. Because patients respond to health problems in infinite ways, it is impossible to predict all combinations of cues and all possible diagnoses. Furthermore, some nursing diagnoses have very small data bases, making accurate diagnosis difficult.

Using Nursing Diagnoses with Critical Pathways

In many organizations, a system called *managed care* is used to standardize practice for the medical diagnoses they treat most often. In this system, caregivers use *critical pathways* to predict client and family outcomes within a specified time frame (detailed information on critical pathways can be found in Chapters 7 and 9). The **critical pathway** is a preprinted, multidisciplinary plan of care that outlines crucial care to be given for all patients of a certain type (e.g., all patients undergoing cardiac catheterization). Although nursing diagnoses address patients' unique, individual needs, they are still appropriate to use with critical pathways. The remainder of this section describes how.

Nursing Diagnosis Incorporated into Critical Pathway

In managed care systems, the critical pathway replaces the traditional (nursing diagnosis) care plan for many clients. The critical path is a "standardized" plan for outcomes and care that can be predicted to occur for "all" clients. Nursing diagnoses are unique to the individual and cannot really be predicted to occur in the presence of particular diseases and treatments. However, some agencies do include the nursing diagnoses that frequently occur with the condition in their critical pathways.

Example:　When incorporating nursing diagnosis into a critical pathway for a newly diagnosed insulin-dependent diabetic, the following nursing diagnosis would be a part of the preprinted multidisciplinary care plan: Ineffective Management of Therapeutic Regimen related to limited information and limited practice of skill.

Nursing Diagnosis Used to Name Variance

Some agencies use nursing diagnoses to name variances from the predicted outcomes and time frames and to develop an individualized plan for achieving revised outcomes. A **variance** occurs when the patient does not achieve a goal in the time predicted by the critical pathway.

Example:　The critical pathway for a newly diagnosed insulin-dependent diabetic would not include a nursing diagnosis, but rather would list "teaching needs" for each day. On day 5, if the patient is unable to meet the outcome of self-injection, the nurse would identify and analyze this "variance." At that point the nurse would use a diagnosis of "Ineffective Management of Therapeutic Regimen …" to individualize the nursing care for this patient's variance from the critical pathway.

Nursing Diagnosis Used for Problems Not on the Critical Pathway

You should use a nursing diagnosis to individualize care to meet unique, individual patient needs that are not addressed by the standardized critical pathway.

Example:　Al Collins has had a myocardial infarction (heart attack). He is also blind. The critical pathway outlines care only for his heart condition. The nurse writes a separate nursing diagnosis to provide information about the amount of help Mr. Collins needs with eating, ambulating, and other activities of daily living.

RECOGNIZING PATIENT PROBLEMS

Diagnosing involves problem identification. Beginning diagnosticians often have difficulty understanding exactly what the client's problem *is*: they are not sure if it is a symptom, a complaint, a situation, a disease, or a pathophysiology. Therefore, this section will help you form the concept of *problem* before you attempt to work with nursing diagnoses, a special type of problem. A **health problem** is recognized by the following characteristics:

✓ It is a human response to a life process, event or stressor.
✓ It is a health-related condition that both the client and the nurse wish to change.
✓ It requires intervention in order to prevent or resolve illness, or to facilitate coping.
✓ It results in ineffective coping/adaptation or daily living that is unsatisfying to the client.
✓ It is an undesirable state.

Diagnostic Reasoning

Human Responses

When learning to differentiate between patient problems and other phenomena, remember that the focus for nursing diagnosis and care is in the area of human responses. Recall from Chapter 1 that **human responses** are human reactions to an event or a stressor.

Changes in:	Examples of Human Responses
Body appearance:	Posture; skin color
Body function:	Inability to move a joint; difficulty swallowing
Symptoms:	Fever; elevated white blood cell count
Knowledge:	Knowledge of foods low in salt
Skills:	Ability to change own dressing
Emotions:	Anger; sadness

Human responses occur in several *dimensions*. They can be biological (physical), psychological, interpersonal/social, or spiritual.

> ***Example:*** Consider the following ways a person might respond to the stressor of having a myocardial infarction (heart attack).

Physical response:	Pain
Psychological response:	Fear
Interpersonal/social response:	Returning to work before he is well
Spiritual response:	Praying

Human responses occur at different *levels*: cellular, systemic, organic, or whole person (organismic). A single stressor can cause multilevel responses. A cellular response occurs at the level of individual cells; for example, the ability of a cell to use glucose may change. Systemic responses occur in body systems, such as the circulatory or respiratory system (e.g., peripheral vasodilation or an increased respiratory rate). Localized skeletal muscle fatigue—in a runner's calves, for instance—is an example of organic response. Nursing occurs at and affects all levels, but nursing diagnosis is usually at the whole person or possibly the systemic level.

> ***Example:*** A person who is severely burned loses large amounts of body fluids. If the fluids are not replaced, she responds at the cellular level by losing water from the cells into the bloodstream (cellular dehydration). At the systemic level, the sympathetic nervous system responds to the trauma by decreasing the activity of the gastrointestinal system. At the whole-person level, the person may respond by perceiving pain or, later, by social isolation.

Responses to stressors can be helpful or harmful. Remember, not all human responses are problems. Human responses may be adaptive, helping to restore health; or they may be maladaptive and damaging to health. In fact, the same response can be helpful at one time and harmful at another.

> ***Example:*** Mrs. Mason has a "chest cold" and a severe cough. She feels very ill. Her psychological response is *fear* (that she may have pneumonia). The fear motivates her to see her physician for treatment—an adaptive response.

Example: At a later time, Mrs. Mason has an episode of postmenopausal bleeding. Her psychological response is again fear (that she may have cancer). This time she is overwhelmed by her fear. She avoids seeing a physician because she is afraid he will tell her she has cancer, thereby making it real. This time the fear was a maladaptive response because it immobilized her instead of motivating her to act.

Refer to Table 4-1 for some examples of stressors and various types and levels of human responses. Notice that a response can become a stressor that produces still another response (e.g., Mrs. Mason's fear produced avoidance).

Misconceptions about Patient Problems

A human response becomes a **patient problem** when it results in ineffective coping or daily living that is unsatisfying to the patient. While learning, you may confuse problems with various phenomena that are related but not the same. Table 4-2 provides examples of things that are *not* problems, but which may cause a human response that *is* a problem.

How you define and recognize patient problems depends somewhat on the nursing model you use. For example, in the Roy model (1984) you would recognize a problem as a failure to adapt. In the Gordon (1994) model, a health problem occurs when a health pattern is dysfunctional (that is, when it does not meet expected norms).

Types of Problems

Nurses analyze data to identify three kinds of problems: (1) nursing diagnoses, (2) collaborative problems, and (3) other (usually medical) problems. Nursing practice is not limited to consideration of nursing diagnoses. Although nursing

Table 4–1. Examples of Stressors and Human Responses

Stressor	Human Response	Dimension	Level	Effect
Blocked coronary artery, causing decreased O_2 to heart muscle	Damage to heart muscle (ischemia)	Physical	Cellular and organic	Maladaptive
	Pain	Psychological and physical	Whole-person (organismic)	Adaptive, if causes decreased activity, conserving O_2; maladaptive, if causes fight-or-flight response, increasing demand for O_2
	Fear of death	Psychological	Whole-person	Can be adaptive or maladaptive (see above)
Fear of death from heart attack	Increased heart rate	Physical	Systemic	Probably maladaptive
	Praying	Spiritual	Whole-person	Probably adaptive

95

Table 4–2. Misconceptions about Problems

A problem is not:	Examples (Incorrect)	The Problem (Human Response) is:
Pathology or pathophysiology	Loss of alveolar integrity Loss of elasticity in lungs	Inability to perform usual work role; loss of job; inability to care for self because of fatigue; anxiety because of difficulty breathing.

Implications for the nurse: (1) Focus on the effects of the pathology on the person's functioning. (2) Although pathophysiology is not actually a problem, it can be the *cause* of a problem. This is discussed later under "Diagnostic Reasoning."

A problem is not:	Examples (Incorrect)	The Problem (Human Response) is:
A nursing goal or a nursing problem	Urinary drainage device will be kept patent and draining freely.	Bladder distention
	Patient is noisy and disturbs other patients.	Anxiety; confusion, disorientation

Implications for the nurse: View the problem from the patient's perspective. The "problem" is the response (1) that will occur if the nurse's goal is not met, or (2) that is causing the nurse's problem.

A problem is not:	Examples (Incorrect)	The Problem (Human Response) is:
A nursing action or routine	Give emotional support. Check urinary catheter hourly for patency.	Anxiety; fear; grief; powerlessness Risk for urinary tract infection

Implications for the nurse: Get the right focus. The incorrect examples focus on *the nurse* (activities to be performed). Problems are statements of client health status—focus is on *the client*.

A problem is not:	Examples (Incorrect)	The Problem (Human Response) is:
A diagnostic test or medical treatment	Patient is having a barium enema.	Risk for constipation; embarrassment
	New colostomy	Lack of knowledge and skill in caring for the appliance; fear of social contact; impaired skin integrity around the stoma
	Must stay on salt-free diet	Lack of motivation to change eating habits; lack of knowledge of high-sodium foods

Implications for the nurse: Patients may respond in many ways to the same treatment. A list of treatments does not provide enough direction for individualizing care. Remember that the problem is the patient's *response* to the test/treatment.

Table 4–2. Misconceptions about Problems (concluded)

A problem is not:	Examples (Incorrect)	The Problem (Human Response) is:
The patient's equipment	Patient has cast on leg. Patient has new dentures.	Decreased mobility; itching Change in body image; speech distortion

Implications for the nurse: See comment above, regarding diagnostic tests and treatments.

A problem is not:	Examples (Incorrect)	The Problem (Human Response) is:
A patient need	Needs more sleep	Fatigue; sleep-pattern disturbance; depression
	Needs better nutrition	Altered nutrition: less than body requirements; loss of appetite
	Needs emotional support	Grief; poor self-concept; anxiety

Implications for the nurse: An unmet need may be the *cause* of a problem; but it is not the same thing as a problem. As a rule, do not use the word "need" in stating problems.

responsibility is different for each type, one is not more important than the other. Be careful not to force nursing diagnosis labels onto collaborative problems. Be equally careful not to overlook nursing diagnoses and attempt to fit all the patient's care under "Potential complications of …"

Recognizing Nursing Diagnoses

Recall that the phenomena of concern for nursing practice are human responses. It follows that nursing diagnosis should be applied to human responses. NANDA (1990) has adopted an official definition of **nursing diagnosis:**

> A nursing diagnosis is a clinical judgement about individual, family, or community responses to actual or potential health problems/life processes. Nursing diagnoses provide the basis for selection of nursing interventions to achieve outcomes for which the nurse is accountable. (p. 114)

A **nursing diagnosis** is a statement of an actual or potential (risk) health problem that nurses can legally identify and for which they can prescribe the primary interventions for treatment and prevention. The key term here is *primary*. Nurses may not prescribe *all* the care for a nursing diagnosis (for instance, most patients with a nursing diagnosis of Pain have medical orders for analgesics); but if it is a nursing diagnosis, the nurse can prescribe *most* of the interventions needed to prevent or resolve the problem. Usually the nurse does not need to confer with a physician about treatments for nursing diagnoses.

Because human responses vary, you cannot predict with certainty which nursing diagnoses will occur with a particular disease or treatment. As you can see from the preceding examples, any number of nursing diagnoses may or may

Nursing diagnosis:

A statement of an actual or risk health problem that nurses can

✓ Legally identify and treat
✓ Prevent or resolve primarily by independent nursing actions

Examples of Nursing Diagnoses

Impaired Skin Integrity (excoriation) related to incontinence

Risk for Infection (of abdominal incision) related to poor nutritional status

Dysfunctional Grieving related to unresolved guilt feelings

Diagnostic Reasoning

not occur with a particular medical diagnosis. You cannot assume, for example, that someone with diabetes will have Fear of Injections or Lack of Knowledge about a diabetic diet.

For a well client, a nursing diagnosis is a statement reflecting the client's healthy responses, or strengths, in areas where the nurse can intervene independently to promote growth or maintenance of the healthy response; for example, Maintenance of Positive Self-Concept, or Potential for Enhanced Self-Concept. Wellness diagnoses are discussed in more detail in Chapter 5. NANDA defines a **wellness diagnosis** as describing: "human responses to levels of wellness in an individual, family, or community that have a potential for enhancement to a higher state" (1994, p. 102).

Recognizing Collaborative Problems

Carpenito (1993, p. 30) states that **collaborative problems** are "certain physiological complications that nurses monitor, to detect their onset or changes in status. Nurses manage collaborative problems by utilizing physician-prescribed and nursing-prescribed interventions to minimize the complications of the events." Independent nursing interventions for collaborative problems focus mainly on monitoring the patient's condition and preventing the development of the complication. Definitive treatment of the condition requires both medical and nursing interventions.

Collaborative problems:

✓ Usually physiologic complications of a disease or treatment.

✓ Nurses collaborate with other health care professionals to treat and prevent.

✓ Independent nursing actions focus on prevention and monitoring for onset of problem.

Because there are a limited number of physiological complications for a given disease, the same collaborative problems tend to be present any time a particular disease or treatment is present; that is, each disease or treatment has particular complications that are always associated with it. Nursing diagnoses, on the other hand, involve human responses, which vary greatly from one person to the next. Therefore, the same set of nursing diagnoses cannot be expected to occur with a particular disease or condition; and a single nursing diagnosis may occur as a response to any number of diseases. For example, all postpartum patients have similar collaborative problems (potential complications), such as postpartum hemorrhage and thrombophlebitis. But not all new mothers have the same nursing diagnoses. Some might experience Altered Parenting (delayed bonding), but most will not. Some might have a Knowledge Deficit problem; others will not.

Appendix D is a list of collaborative problems that are commonly associated with the different body systems (Carpenito, 1993). Table 4-3 lists examples of some collaborative problems associated with various tests and treatments.

Recognizing Medical Diagnoses

Medical diagnoses are a type of patient problem. Although medical diagnoses and nursing diagnoses are both made by using a diagnostic reasoning process, they are quite different. A **medical diagnosis** identifies a disease process or pathology and is made for the purpose of treating the pathology. It does not necessarily consider the human responses to the pathology.

Example: The physician diagnoses hypertension and prescribes anti-hypertensive medications and a low-salt diet. The nurse will diagnose and treat the patient's and family's responses to the medical diagnosis. Is the patient motivated to change his diet? What changes will the family need to make to incorporate the diet change into their menu plan? Does the patient understand the importance of taking his medications, even though they may have unpleasant side effects? If the patient is hospitalized, the nurse will give the medications prescribed by the physician.

As long as the disease process is present, the medical diagnosis does not change. Nursing diagnoses, on the other hand, change as the client's responses change. In the preceding example, the nursing diagnosis might initially be "Risk for Noncompliance with medication regimen related to lack of understanding of

Table 4–3. Examples of Collaborative Problems Associated with Tests and Treatments		
Test or Treatment	**Collaborative Problem (Potential Complications)**	
Arteriogram	Allergic reaction Renal failure Hemorrhage; hematoma	Thrombosis at site Paresthesia Embolism
Bronchoscopy	Airway obstruction (bronchoconstriction)	Hemorrhage
Cardiac catheterization	Site-hemorrhage or hematoma Cardiac arrhythmias, infarction, perforation Paresthesia	Embolism, thrombus Hypervolemia Hypovolemia
Casts and traction	Misalignment of bones Bleeding Edema	Impaired circulation Neurological compromise
Chest tubes	Bleeding → hemothorax Blockage or displacement → pneumothorax	Septicemia
Foley catheter	Urinary tract infection	Bladder distention
Hemodialysis	Bleeding Air embolism Fluid shifts Electrolyte imbalance	Transfusion reactions Hepatitis B Shunt clotting; fistulas
Intravenous therapy	Infiltration	Phlebitis
Medications	Side effects Toxic effects; overdose	Allergic reactions
Nasogastric suction	Electrolyte imbalance Gastric ulceration → hemorrhage	
Tracheal suctioning	Hypoxia	Bleeding
Surgery	Excessive bleeding → shock Atelectasis Paralytic ileus	Fluid imbalance Electrolyte imbalance Infection
Assisted ventilation	Airway obstruction (tube plugged or displaced) Ineffective O_2–CO_2 exchange Tracheal necrosis	Acid-base imbalance Pneumothorax Respirator dependence

Diagnostic Reasoning

therapeutic and side effects of the drug." However, as the patient shows knowledge of the drug and takes it as ordered, this diagnosis would no longer apply. If the patient found the side effects unpleasant and continued to skip doses of the drug, the diagnosis might change to actual "Noncompliance with medication regimen . . ." Remember that clients who have the same medical diagnosis may have very different nursing diagnoses. Consider the previous example of Mary Chinn and Donald Schulz, who both have a medical diagnosis of myocardial infarction (heart attack), but who have very different nursing diagnoses.

Nurses make observations pertinent to patients' medical diagnoses and perform treatments delegated by the physician. Although nurses do not diagnose or prescribe treatments for medical problems, nursing judgment is required. Nurses must know the pathophysiology of the disease and understand why the medications or treatments are being given. See Table 4-4 for a summary comparison of the three types of patient health problems.

Status of Problems

Problems may be actual, potential, or possible. A comprehensive nursing care plan includes measures for prevention and detection of potential and possible problems, as well as treatment of actual problems.

Table 4–4. Comparison of Nursing Diagnoses with Collaborative Problems and Medical Diagnoses

Nursing Diagnoses	Collaborative Problems	Medical Diagnoses
Describe human responses of all kinds.	Involve human responses—mainly physiological complications of disease, tests, or treatments.	Do not consider human responses other than disease and pathology.
Nurses can diagnose.	Nurses can diagnose.	Physician must diagnose.
Nurse orders most interventions to prevent or treat.	Nurse collaborates with physician to prevent and treat (need medical orders).	Physician orders primary interventions to prevent or treat.
Nursing focus: treatment and prevention.	Nursing focus: prevent and monitor for onset or status of condition.	Nursing focus: monitor and implement physician's orders for treatment.
Independent nursing actions.	Some independent actions, but mostly for monitoring and preventing.	Dependent nursing actions.
Can change frequently.	Can change frequently; present when disease or situation is present.	Remains the same while disease is present.

Actual Problems

An **actual problem** is one that is actually present at the time you make the assessment. It is diagnosed by the presence of associated signs and symptoms (defining characteristics). For an actual problem, nursing care is directed toward relieving or resolving the problem.

> *Example:* The Crain family is experiencing many stressors. The parents, Todd and Dana, are caring for their son, Billy, who has leukemia; and Dana has had to quit her job. While making a family visit, the nurse observes that when Todd tries to discipline Billy, Dana interferes to protect him. In a later conversation, Todd tells the nurse, "I mostly just stay out of it. She can take care of Billy better than I can anyway." Dana confirms that Todd has withdrawn from contact with his son. The nurse diagnoses an actual problem, Ineffective Family Coping (Compromised) related to family disorganization and role changes.

Potential (Risk) Problems

A **potential** (or **risk**) **problem** is one that is likely to develop if the nurse does not intervene. Potential problems are diagnosed by the presence of risk factors that predispose a patient to developing a problem. Nursing care is directed toward preventing the problem by reducing the risk factors; or toward early detection of the problem to lessen its consequences. A potential problem can be either a nursing diagnosis or a collaborative problem. If the problem is a nursing diagnosis, it is labeled *Risk*. If it the problem is collaborative, it is labeled *Potential*. Note that *all* collaborative problems are potential in status.

> *Example:* Marianne Akiba is a single parent whose child, Janelle, has a new medical diagnosis of leukemia. The nurse knows that Marianne has only one or two people she can turn to for emotional or other support. In an interview, Marianne indicates, "I don't know anything about this disease or how to take care of my child." Although the nurse sees no signs of ineffective coping, she realizes that lack of knowledge and support place this family at risk, so she makes a *potential* nursing diagnosis of Risk for Ineffective Family Coping (Compromised) related to limited support system and lack of knowledge.

A potential (risk) nursing diagnosis should be used only for patients who have a higher than normal risk for developing a problem—those who have more risk factors than the general group to which they belong. NANDA says that a **risk nursing diagnosis**: "describes human responses to health conditions/life processes which may develop in a vulnerable individual, family or community. It is supported by risk factors that contribute to increased vulnerability" (1994, p. 102).

For those who have the same risk as the general population, a collaborative problem (potential complication) should be used. For example, *all* patients having a general anesthetic are at risk for respiratory problems. However, for those who have no risk factors in addition to the surgery, routine postoperative "turn-cough-deep breathe" treatment is adequate; their care planning could be based on the collaborative problem Potential Complications of Surgery (Respiratory). On the other hand, if a patient is a smoker and is having general anesthesia for a high abdominal incision, his respiratory status merits special

Recognizing Patient Problems

Actual Problems
✓ Problem present
✓ Signs and symptoms present

Potential (Risk) Problems
✓ Problem may develop
✓ Risk factors present

Possible Problems
✓ Unsure if problem is present
✓ Some signs/symptoms present, but not definitive
✓ Data incomplete

attention. He is at higher risk than the general population of surgery patients, so a nursing diagnosis of "Risk for Altered Respiratory Function related to high abdominal incision and smoking" should be written.

Possible Problems

A **possible problem**, similar to a physician's rule-out diagnosis, is one that you tentatively believe to exist; you have enough data to suspect a problem, but not enough to be sure. Nursing care is then directed toward gathering focus data to confirm or eliminate the diagnosis. Using possible problems can help keep you from: (1) omitting an important diagnosis and (2) making an incorrect diagnosis because of insufficient data.

Example: Still another patient who has had abdominal surgery has no history of smoking and has been adhering to the schedule of turning, coughing, and deep breathing every two hours. Still, she is slightly pale, and reports that she feels "a little short of breath." The nurse auscultates and finds no abnormal breath sounds. There are no other signs of respiratory distress, but the nurse wants to be sure the situation is carefully evaluated by other shifts. So she diagnoses a *possible* problem: Possible Ineffective Airway Clearance.

DIAGNOSTIC REASONING

Diagnosis is an intellectual activity in which nurses use critical thinking skills to identify patterns and make judgments about human responses to actual or potential health problems.

Diagnosis is an intellectual activity in which critical thinking skills are used to identify patterns and draw conclusions about data. It is the reasoning process that experts of a discipline use to draw conclusions about their phenomena of concern (that is, what they "work on"). Speech therapists diagnose speaking problems, teachers diagnose learning problems and automobile mechanics diagnose engine problems. Because human responses are the phenomena of concern for nurses, nursing diagnosis is used to identify patterns and make judgments about human responses to actual or potential health problems. Now that you can differentiate between different kinds of patient problems, this section introduces you to the intellectual processes that enable you to analyze data about a patient and identify the problems that apply to that individual. Diagnostic reasoning can be divided into three broad stages: (1) interpreting the data, (2) verifying the diagnosis, and (3) labeling (and recording) the diagnosis.

Use of Nursing Models

When you use a framework for organizing and interpreting data, its concepts help you to recognize relationships between isolated pieces of data. Concepts cause clusters to stand out for your attention. For example, the concept of *fluid volume deficit* helped Luisa Sanchez's nurse (Chapter 3, Figure 3–3) to notice that Luisa's decreased urine output, poor skin turgor, and elevated temperature were somehow related. This chapter will use Gordon's Functional Health Patterns as a framework for data analysis, continuing the example of Luisa Sanchez from Chapter 3.

Use of Critical Thinking

Diagnosis includes the cognitive processes of analysis and synthesis. You will use **analysis** when "taking apart" the data base to examine and interpret each piece of data, identify deviations from normal, and identify patterns and relationships in the data. **Synthesis** means combining parts or elements into a single new entity. You will use **synthesis** when comparing the cue patterns to various theories, concepts, and norms in order to identify strengths and generate explanations for client's symptoms.

You may use both inductive and deductive reasoning to interpret data. **Inductive reasoning** begins with a set of individual facts and uses them to draw a conclusion. Induction is used to find possible patterns in information and extend the pattern to predict new information.

> *Example:* Refer to Figure 3–3 in Chapter 3, page 56.
> *Particular Facts:* The nurse observes that Luisa Sanchez's skin is hot and pale, that her respirations are shallow, and that she has a cough productive of pink sputum. The nurse auscultates inspiratory crackles and dimished breath sounds throughout Luisa's right chest.
> *Conclusion:* Recognizing the pattern formed by these cues, the nurse concludes that a nursing diagnosis of Ineffective Airway Clearance exists.

Deductive reasoning begins with a principle, generalization, or major idea and proceeds to discover or predict the specific, individual facts based on that general idea.

> *Example:* Kathy Cole is a nurse in a long-term care facility, and she knows the effects of poor nutrition and immobility on skin integrity (principles and generalizations). Based on this knowledge and her clinical experience, she maintains a turning schedule for Mr. Randall, who is paralyzed; and she observes for redness and other signs of impaired skin integrity (the specific facts predicted by the principles).

Interpreting Data

After you have organized and recorded your assessment data, it must be analyzed and interpreted. Interpretation is the first stage of diagnostic reasoning, in which you determine what the data means.

This section presents data interpretation as a series of steps in order to help you understand the process. In reality, it is a complex process, not a rigid set of linear steps to be accomplished one at a time. Some steps, of course, must be taken before others; but you should use these steps as guidelines, realizing you will do some of them simultaneously, move back and forth among them, and perhaps even intuit portions of them, especially as you gain clinical experience.

Data interpretation occurs at three levels (see Box 4–6 on page 117). In the first level, you will identify significant cues; in the second level, you identify the problems; and in the final level, you determine the probable causes of the problems.

Level I: Identify Significant Cues
In your initial analysis you will organize the data, look for inconsistencies and missing data, and compare the data to established norms to identify significant cues (see Steps 1, 2, and 3).

Step 1: Organize the data. The first step in data analysis is to organize the data. If you have made an initial, comprehensive assessment, most of your data will already be grouped by your data collection form. The data collection

Diagnostic Reasoning

form is a part of the patient's permanent record, so you cannot mark on it. For that reason, especially while you are learning, you should rewrite the data base cues in a concise format according to your preferred framework. Summarizing data base information in this manner makes data gaps and inconsistencies more obvious, and allows you to more easily see relationships between the cues. Luisa Sanchez's admission assessment form (Figure 3–3 in Chapter 3) is organized according to body systems and specific nursing concerns (e.g., screening for falls); it does not use one particular nursing model. In Box 4–2, the Luisa Sanchez data from Figure 3–3 has been organized according to Gordon's Functional Health Patterns. As a rule, the nurse organizes the data using the same model as the data-collection tool. However, different models are provided here to demonstrate differences in organizing frameworks and to show that the nurse is not limited to the framework provided by the data collection tool.

Step 2: Identify data gaps and inconsistencies. Ideally, your data will be complete and you will have identified and validated incongruent data during the assessment step. However, the need for certain data may not become apparent until you cluster and begin to look for meaning in the data. To identify inconsistencies, check to see if information given under one pattern contradicts that given under another pattern or if your objective findings conflict with what the client has said. Has the client given you the same information (concerns, strengths, and so on) as other team members?

Step 3: Compare individual cues to standards and norms. In this step, you will use your knowledge of anatomy, physiology, psychology, developmental theory, and so on, to evaluate whether or not the cues are normal. You will compare them to such standards as norms for height and weight, lab values and nutritional requirements, social functioning, coping skills, and usual health status. Following are some examples of various kinds of significant cues:

✓ Deviation from population norms (e.g., height 5'2", weight 240 lb)
✓ Developmental delays (e.g., 2-year-old does not walk yet)
✓ Changes in the patient's usual health status (e.g., loss of appetite)
✓ Dysfunctional behavior (e.g., drug usage, withdrawal from social contact)
✓ Changes in the patient's usual behavior (e.g., poor hygiene, grooming)

It may help you to highlight, circle, or underline the significant or abnormal data, as was done for Mrs. Sanchez's data in Box 4–2.

Level II: Cluster Data and Identify Problems

Step 4: Establish patterns (cue clusters) and relationships in the data. In this level of data interpretation, each cue is interpreted in the context of the other cues. Look for *cues that are repeated* in more than one category (in the Gordon framework a category is called a *pattern*). For example, Mrs. Sanchez reports being "too tired to mess with hair and makeup" in the Self-Perception/Self-Concept pattern; and reports weakness in both the Cognitive-Perceptual and Activity-Exercise patterns as well. Therefore, weakness is probably an important diagnostic cue.

Next, begin to *group together (cluster) the cues that seem related.* Try to determine the relationship between facts. Does Mrs. Sanchez's report of decreased urinary frequency (Elimination pattern) have anything to do with her decreased skin turgor and elevated temperature (Nutritional-Metabolic pattern)? Why is she feeling weak? Is it related to her nausea (Nutritional-Metabolic

Luisa Sanchez, 28 years old, was admitted to the hospital with a productive cough and rapid, labored respirations. She stated that she has had a "chest cold" for two weeks and has been short of breath on exertion. Yesterday she began to experience a fever and "pain in my lungs."

Health Perception/Health Management
Knows her medical diagnosis
Gives thorough medical history
Complying with Synthroid regimen
Relates progression of illness in detail
Realistic expectations (to have antibiotics and
   "go home in a day or two")
States usually eats "3 meals a day"

Nutritional/Metabolic
5 ft. 2 in. (158 cm) tall; weight 125 lb (56 kg)
Usually eats 3 meals a day
"No appetite" since having "cold"
Reports nausea
Oral temp 103°F (39.4°C)
Decreased skin turgor
Mucous membranes dry and pale
Skin hot and pale, cheeks flushed
Synthroid 0.1 mg per day
History of appendectomy and partial
   thyroidectomy
Old surgical scars: anterior neck, RLQ abdomen
Has not eaten today; last fluids at noon today

Elimination
Last bowel movement yesterday: formed,
   "normal"
Urinary frequency and amount decreased
   X2 days
Abdomen soft, not distended
Diaphoretic

Activity-Exercise
No musculoskeletal impairment
States, "I feel weak"
Short of breath on exertion
Exercises daily
Respirations shallow; chest expansion <3 cm
Blood pressure 122/80 sitting
Radial pulse weak, regular, rate=92
Cough productive of pale, pink sputum
Inspiratory crackles auscultated throughout
   right upper and lower chest
Diminished breath sounds on right side

Sleep-Rest
Difficulty sleeping because of cough
"Can't breathe lying down"

Cognitive-Perceptual
No sensory deficits
Pupils 3 mm, equal, brisk reaction
Oriented to time, place, and person
Responsive, but fatigued
Responds appropriately to verbal and
   physical stimuli
Recent and remote memory intact
"I can think OK. Just weak."
States "short of breath" on exertion
"Pain in lungs," especially when coughing
Experiencing chills
Reports nausea

Roles-Relationships
Lives with husband and 3-year-old daughter
Sexual relationship "satisfactory"
Husband out of town; will be back tomorrow
Child with neighbor until husband returns
States "good" relationships with friends
   and coworkers
Working mother, attorney
Husband helps "some" at home

Self-Perception-Self-Concept
Expresses "concern" and "worry" about leaving
   daughter with neighbors until tomorrow
Well-groomed; says, "Too tired to mess
   with hair and makeup"

Coping-Stress Tolerance
Anxious: "I can't breathe"
Facial muscles tense; trembling
"I can think OK. Just weak."
Expresses concerns about work: "I'll never
   get caught up"

Value-Belief
Catholic. No special practices desired except
   last rites
Middle-class, professional orientation
No wish to see chaplain or priest at present

pattern), or her cough (Activity-Exercise pattern), or both? Or neither? As you compare data across the categories of your framework, some seemingly normal data may take on new significance. In Box 4–2, in the Roles-Relationships pattern, the fact that Mrs. Sanchez's husband is out of town is, by itself, not remarkable. However, taken with her expression of worry (in the Self-Perception/Self-Concept pattern) and her anxiety (in the Coping-Stress pattern), it seems that the Roles-Relationships comment may be significant. That is why it is underlined in Box 4–2, even though it seems normal when considered by itself.

While you are learning, it is a good idea to make a second written list at this point. This list will be much shorter than the first one because you will omit the healthy responses and list only "significant" data. The way you form your cue clusters and make your new list will depend on whether you reason deductively or inductively.

Recall that *deductive reasoning* begins with a major theory or generalization that generates the specific details and predictions. Therefore, if you use a deductive approach to group the abnormal data, you would begin by listing all the significant cues, underlined in Box 4–2, under the appropriate categories of your framework. For example, the abnormal cues from two of the categories in Box 4–2 would be listed in the following manner:

Self-Perception/Self Concept
Expresses "concern" and "worry" about leaving daughter with neighbors until tomorrow.
"Too tired to mess with hair and makeup"

Roles/Relationships
Husband out of town (back tomorrow)
Child with neighbor

The *inductive approach,* shown in Table 4–5, will be used in the remaining steps of data interpretation in this chapter. Recall that inductive reasoning begins with specific details and uses them to arrive at a conclusion or generalization. Using an inductive approach in Step 4, you would make your new list of cue clusters by grouping together all significant cues (underlined in Box 4-2) that seem to be related, regardless of the pattern in which they were collected on your assessment tool. Referring to Table 4–5, you will see that the same cue may appear in more than one grouping (e.g., "Can't breathe lying down" appears in Cluster 4 and Cluster 6). When you find a cue that seems significant, look for all the other data that may be related.

Next, *decide which framework category (pattern) is represented* by each cue cluster. Identifying the pattern in which the problem occurs helps to narrow your search for the specific problem. There may be more than one cue cluster in a pattern (e.g., both Clusters 2 and 3 represent the Nutritional-Metabolic pattern); or a cue cluster may involve more than one pattern. If so, list them all; it may be that the cue cluster represents more than one problem. Cluster 3, for example, yields two problems: a fluid volume problem and a potential oral mucous membrane problem.

Frequently, a cue cluster actually fits only one pattern, but you cannot be sure at first which one. If this occurs, list all the patterns that seem to fit (as was done in Table 4–5). You may be better able to identify the pattern after you begin to think about the relationships among the cues and define the specific problems.

Table 4–5. Luisa Sanchez Data—Related Cues Suggesting Problem Responses (Inductive Method)

Related Cues (Clusters)	Functional Health Pattern	Tentative Problem Statement (Inference)
Cluster 1 No significant cues	Health Perception/ Health Management	*Strength*: Healthy lifestyle; understanding and compliance with treatment regimens
Cluster 2 "No appetite" since having "cold" Reports nausea X2 days Has not eaten today; last fluids at noon today	Nutritional-Metabolic	*(Nursing diagnosis)* Altered Nutrition: Less than Body Requirements
Cluster 3 "No appetite" since having "cold" Reports nausea X2 days Last fluids at noon today Oral temp 103 F (39.4 C) Skin hot and pale, cheeks flushed Mucous membranes dry Poor skin turgor Decreased urinary frequency and amount X2 days Diaphoresis	Nutritional-Metabolic (includes hydration) or ~~Elimination~~	*(Nursing diagnosis)* Fluid Volume Deficit. Cues include elimination *data*, but are not an elimination *problem*. Decreased urine is a symptom of a fluid volume problem.
Cluster 4 Difficulty sleeping because of cough "Can't breathe lying down" States, "I feel weak" Short of breath on exertion	Sleep-Rest or ~~Activity-Exercise~~	*(Nursing diagnosis)* Sleep Pattern Disturbance
Cluster 5 Taking Synthroid 0.1 mg per day Old surgical scar on anterior neck	Nutritional-Metabolic	*(Medical treatment)* Not a problem as long as regimen is followed.
Cluster 6 Difficulty sleeping because of cough "Can't breathe lying down" Short of breath on exertion States, "I feel weak" Responsive but fatigued "I can think OK, just weak" Radial pulse rate 92, weak	~~Sleep-Rest~~ or Activity-Exercise or ~~Cognitive-Perceptual~~	*(Nursing diagnosis)* Activity Intolerance or Self-Care Deficit (needs help with hygiene and so on because of weakness). Cues from other patterns are contributing to the problem in the Activity-Exercise pattern.

Table 4–5. Luisa Sanchez Data—Related Cues Suggesting Problem Responses (Inductive Method) (concluded)

Related Cues (Clusters)	Functional Health Pattern	Tentative Problem Statement (Inference)
Cluster 7 Reports chills Oral temp 103 F (39.4 C) Diaphoretic	Cognitive-Perceptual or ~~Nutritional-Metabolic~~	*(Nursing diagnosis)* Problem is altered comfort (chills); elevated temp is contributing to problem.
Cluster 8 Husband out of town; will be back tomorrow Child with neighbor until husband returns	Roles-Relationships or ~~Coping-Stress~~	*(Nursing diagnosis)* Altered Family Processes because parents temporarily unavailable to care for child
Cluster 9 Husband out of town; will be back tomorrow Child with neighbor until husband returns Expresses "concern" and "worry" over leaving child with neighbors until husband returns Anxious: "I can't breathe" Facial muscles tense; trembling Concerns about work: "I'll never get caught up"	~~Roles-Relationships~~ or Self-Perception/ Self-Concept or ~~Coping/Stress~~	*(Nursing diagnosis)* Anxiety is a problem; the Roles-Relationships and Coping/Stress cues are contributing to (causing) the anxiety.
Cluster 10 "Pain in lungs" especially when coughing Cough productive of pale, pink sputum	Cognitive-Perceptual	*(Nursing diagnosis)* Chest pain
Cluster 11 Skin hot and pale Respirations shallow; chest expansion < 3 cm (1 ¼ in) Cough productive of pale, pink sputum Inspiratory crackles auscultated throughout right upper and lower chest Dimished breath sounds on right side Mucous membranes pale	Activity-Exercise (pattern includes respiratory and cardiovascular status)	*(Medical problem)* Pneumonia *(Collaborative problems:* respiratory insufficiency, septic shock) *(Nursing diagnosis)* Ineffective Airway Clearance caused by disease process

Example: The Group 3 cluster contains cues that fit in both the Nutritional-Metabolic and the Elimination patterns. It is only as you begin to decide cause and effect that it becomes clear that the problematic response occurs in the Nutritional-Metabolic pattern, and that the Elimination cues are merely symptoms of the Nutritional-Metabolic problem.

Step 5: Draw conclusions about each of the groups of cues (identify problems). In this part of the reasoning process you make the final judgments about the meaning of the cue clusters. The following discussion continues to use the inductive process; it would vary slightly if you were using a deductive approach.

First, *think of as many possible explanations (hypotheses) as you can for each of the cue clusters.* This helps keep you from drawing premature conclusions about the meaning of the data. You may rule out some hypotheses because of insufficient data and confirm others based on your knowledge and experience. In your own words, write the hypotheses that express the possibilities most accurately. For Cluster 3 in Table 4–5, two possible explanations are:

1. Mrs. Sanchez's decreased urine output could represent a urinary tract problem. She also has chills and a fever, which are symptoms of a kidney infection. However, she has already been seen by a physician and has a medical diagnosis of pneumonia; and she shows no other signs of a urinary tract problem, so this explanation is not likely.

2. Mrs. Sanchez's decreased urine output could be a result of a Nutrition-Metabolic problem. Inadequate fluid intake, combined with fluid loss from fever and diaphoresis, may mean there is scant fluid to be eliminated by her kidneys. In this explanation, her fever is the cause, rather than a symptom, of a problem.

Next, *for each of your explanations, make one of the following judgments:*

✓ There is no problem.
✓ There is an actual problem. Client data indicates a need for assistance in making a change.
✓ There is a potential (risk) problem. There are no signs and symptoms of an actual problem, but risk factors exist. A problem may occur if you do not intervene.
✓ There is a possible problem. You have reason to suspect a problem, but not enough data to confirm it.

Table 4–5 includes the inferences made about all eight cue clusters. For the explanations identified above for Cluster 3, you would probably conclude:

1. There is no Elimination problem.
2. There is an actual Nutritional-Metabolic problem (Fluid Volume Deficit).

Level III: Determine Etiologies and Problem Types
This is the third and final level of the diagnostic reasoning process.

Step 6: Determine the probable etiology of the problems. In this step you identify the most likely causes of the problems you identified in Step 5. These are the problem **etiologies**—the physiological, psychological, sociological,

Diagnostic Reasoning

spiritual, or environmental factors believed to be causing or contributing to the problem. The etiologies must be correctly identified in order for your nursing actions to be effective. To identify etiologies, ask yourself, "What is *causing* this problem?" You may find the Yura and Walsh (1988) categorization of etiologies in Box 4–3 helpful.

In the first level of data interpretation, you compared assessment data to standards and norms to see if problems existed. In the next level, you interpreted the cues in relation to other cues, identified broad problem areas, and then hypothesized more specific problems to explain the cue clusters. In this final level of data interpretation, you apply your knowledge and experience to the data in order to decide which responses are problems and which are causes. You must make inferences in this step, because you cannot actually *observe* the link between problem and cause. For example, in Cluster 3, observations that Mrs. Sanchez has dry mucous membranes, decreased urine output, hot skin, and poor skin turgor allow you to conclude that she has a problem: Fluid Volume Deficit. However, you cannot observe that the elevated temperature, diaphoresis, and limited fluid intake are the cause of this problem. You must infer this link between the problem and cause on the basis of your knowledge of the metabolic effects of a fever and the physiology of fluid balance in the body.

You will not always find the etiology within the same pattern as the problem. In the following example from Table 4–5, a problem in the Activity-Exercise pattern is caused by stressors in the Nutritional-Metabolic, Activity-Exercise, and Cognitive-Perceptual patterns.

		Functional Health Pattern
Problem:	Ineffective Airway Clearance	Activity-Exercise
Etiology:	(1) Viscous secretions because of fluid volume deficit	Nutritional-Metabolic
	(2) Shallow chest expansion because of pain, weakness, and fatigue	Cognitive-Perceptual Activity-Exercise

---

Box 4–3. Types of Etiologies

Personal and situational occurrences
Philosophic, ethical, and religious
Medical, dental, pharmacologic, and nursing therapies (commissions and omissions)
Pathophysiologic states
Psychopathologic states
Legal states and occurrences
Physiologic miscalculation and/or nonacceptance
Congenital alterations (reparable and irreparable)
Political impacts and impositions

Communication alterations
Environmental affronts/impositions
Social and economic affronts
Education, information, or knowledge deficits
Heredity and genetic impacts
Cultural imposition
Geographic and climate affronts
Functional role structure and impact

Adapted with permission from Yura and Walsh, *The Nursing Process,* 5th ed. (Norwalk, CT: Appleton & Lange, 1988), pp. 129–30.

Different clients may have the same problem, but different etiologies. For example, failure to comply with the prescribed medication regimen (Noncompliance) may be caused by denial of illness in Patient A and by forgetfulness in Patient B. Furthermore, a problem can have any number of etiologies. For example, Patient C may fail to comply with the prescribed medication regimen *both* because he is denying his illness and because he is forgetful. When possible, you should focus on those contributing factors that can be influenced by independent nursing interventions.

Step 7: Determine the problem type: nursing diagnosis, collaborative problem, or other.   All of Luisa Sanchez's problems are nursing diagnoses, except three. The nurse can order the definitive actions to prevent or treat all except these three problems. Cluster 5 represents a medical problem: hypothyroidism as a result of having had a thyroidectomy. This problem is being controlled by the Synthroid, prescribed by a physician. Cluster 11 reflects the medical diagnosis of pneumonia, which had already been made by a physician. It will be managed medically and need not be included on a nursing care plan. Mrs. Sanchez does have some collaborative problems (e.g., Potential Complications: Respiratory Insufficiency and Septic Shock) that are not apparent from the cue clusters in Table 4–5. They are identified from the fact that she has pneumonia, and would be included in the care plan for any patient with pneumonia.

Step 8: For each problem, make the final decision about which pattern of your framework it represents.   Relating problems to framework patterns (see Table 4–5, center column) will help you to choose a label when you begin to write your diagnostic statements. You need a good understanding of your theoretical framework to select the appropriate patterns. For instance, you must know something about the functional health patterns in order to know what cues and problems are associated with the patterns, Nutritional-Metabolic and Activity-Exercise. It may help you to look back at the discussion of nursing frameworks in Chapter 3. For the cue clusters in Table 4–5, you might ask yourself questions such as: Is this problem one of:

✓ Nutrition or metabolism? Does it involve food and fluid consumption? relative to metabolic need? Does it involve systemic or local nutrient supply?
✓ Elimination? Does it involve patterns of excretory function (bowel, bladder, and skin)?
✓ Cognitive or perception? Does it involve thinking, hearing, seeing, smelling, tasting, or touching? Does it involve language and communication, or perceptions or pain?

As previously discussed, Cluster 3 at first appeared to involve both the Nutritional-Metabolic and Elimination patterns. However, the most reasonable explanation of the cues is that Mrs. Sanchez's fluid volume deficit (Nutritional-Metabolic) is causing her decreased urine output (Elimination). Her fluid volume deficit is the problem—the human response that needs to be changed. In this step, you are categorizing the problem, not the etiology; so Cluster 3 fits best in the Nutritional-Metabolic pattern. When you write your formal diagnoses (in a later step) you will look first at the diagnostic labels in the Nutritional-Metabolic pattern. Follow this same process for each group of cues until you have listed and identified the appropriate pattern for all the patient's problems (see "Tentative Problem" column of Table 4–5).

Diagnostic Reasoning

Step 9: Identify patient and family strengths. The client's strengths should be integrated in the plan of care. Examine your original list of cues (see Box 4–2), and ask the client and family how they have coped successfully with past problems and what they see as their strengths. Strengths are those areas of normal, healthy functioning that will help the client in preventing or resolving problems. The following are some of Mrs. Sanchez's strengths:

Pattern	Strength
Health Perception/ Health Management	Shows healthy lifestyle, understanding of and compliance with treatment regimen
Nutritional-Metabolic	Normal weight for height
Activity-Exercise	No musculoskeletal impairment. Normal energy level is satisfactory. Exercises regularly.
Roles-Relationships	Husband supportive; neighbors available and willing to help

Verifying the Diagnosis

After tentatively identifying the client's problems and strengths, you should verify your conclusions. A diagnosis is your interpretation of the meaning of the data; and interpretation is not the same as fact. You can never be certain that an interpretation is correct, even after verifying it. There is always some risk that it is less accurate than it should be. Try not to think of diagnoses as right or wrong, but as being on a continuum of more or less accurate. Make your diagnoses as accurate as possible but remain open to changing them as you get new data or insights.

Ideally, you should verify the problems and strengths with the patient to be sure her perception of the situation is the same as yours. If the client is unable to participate in the decision making you may be able to verify your diagnoses with significant others.

Example: You might say to Mrs. Sanchez, "It seems to me that you are worried about getting behind in your work, but that your main worry is about leaving your daughter with your neighbors. Does this seem accurate to you?"

If the patient confirms your hypothesis, you will include the problem on her care plan. If the patient does not agree with the problems you have hypothesized, you will clarify and restate them until they accurately reflect her health status. You may occasionally include a problem in a care plan even though the patient does not verify it. It may be a problem the patient is not aware of (as in the case of an unconscious patient) or one she is denying.

Example: A client may not perceive that she has Low Self-Esteem. Yet, because your data strongly suggest it, you may wish to continue to assess for this problem and use nursing interventions to promote self-esteem. If you want to assure that other nurses will also do this, you must include the problem in the care plan as a possible problem.

> **Box 4–4. Criteria for Validating Diagnoses**
>
> ✓ The data base is complete and accurate.
> ✓ The data analysis is based on a nursing framework.
> ✓ The cue clusters demonstrate existence of a pattern.
> ✓ The cues are truly characteristic of the problems hypothesized.
> ✓ There are enough cues present to demonstrate existence of the problem.
> ✓ The tentative cause-and-effect relationship is based on scientific nursing knowledge and clinical experience.

You should further validate each tentative diagnosis by comparing it to the criteria in Box 4–4. If the client verifies it, and it meets the criteria, your diagnosis should be high on the accuracy continuum.

Labeling and Recording Diagnoses

After selecting and verifying the client's problems and strengths, the final step is to state them formally. To determine the labels for the nursing diagnoses, you simply compare the cue clusters to the definitions and defining characteristics of the NANDA **diagnostic labels** in your *Nursing Diagnosis Guide* (purple pages). The process of selecting labels and writing diagnostic statements for nursing diagnoses and collaborative problems is covered in detail in Chapter 5.

Thinking Errors in Diagnostic Reasoning

Although you can never be absolutely certain a diagnosis is correct, it is important that your diagnoses be highly accurate. The following errors keep you from noticing important cues or from thinking of certain explanations for the data. Recognizing some common diagnostic errors may help you avoid them by applying the appropriate critical thinking skills.

Premature Data Interpretation
This occurs when you make a judgment based on only one or two cues instead of looking for patterns. Critical thinkers do not usually make this error because they make it a habit to be sure they have all the evidence, and they suspend judgment when evidence is incomplete. In the following example, the nurse should have gathered more data before interpreting the patient's cues to mean Pain.

Example: The nurse, making a routine, hourly postoperative observation, sees that Ms. Foley is crying. The nurse says, "Oh, I'm sorry. I'll be right back with your pain medication," and leaves the room. On checking the medication record, the nurse discovers that Mrs. Foley has already received her analgesic. She was actually crying because her physician had just told her that the surgery was not as successful as they had hoped it would be.

Personal Bias
Bias is the tendency to slant one's judgment in a particular way. A biased conclusion is based on personal theories and stereotypes more than on reason. We all have ideas about what people are like and what causes them to behave

in certain ways, and even why they become ill. Many of these ideas are based on life experience and may or may not be accurate. Some people, for example, believe they will catch a cold if they get their feet wet or go outside with wet hair; other people believe that illness is punishment for wrongdoing. If you feel strongly that people are responsible for good health practices, for example, then you may be less open-minded about a lung-cancer patient who has a 40-year smoking history or an emphysema patient who asks to be taken off the ventilator so he can have a cigarette. This personal theory may likewise affect data interpretation for patients with AIDS or other sexually transmitted diseases.

Stereotypes

Stereotypes are expectations about a person based on beliefs about his group (physicians, elderly people, nurses, Americans, and so on.) *Fat people are jolly, men avoid commitment,* and *women are emotional* are examples of stereotypes. A negative stereotype (e.g., *adolescent males are violent*) is a **prejudice**. Stereotypes are formed by our culture and based more on hearsay than on fact or experience. The nurse who relies on stereotypes instead of patient data will not recognize the uniqueness of each individual. One common example of this is referring to patients by their medical diagnosis or their room number (e.g., "the hysterectomy patient in 220").

Forming Premature Conclusions Based on Context

Nurses sometimes make judgments before they even meet the client, based on information about the client's medical diagnosis, the type of setting, the client's record, or what others say about the client. Such information can help you to hypothesize nursing diagnoses, but be careful not to let it bias your thinking.

> ***Example:*** Janet Thomas, RN, has read about the relationship between loss of a body part and grieving. She also recognizes the theory that childbearing is an important aspect of a woman's identity. She therefore expects that her hysterectomy patients will grieve over the loss of childbearing ability. This nurse fails to see her clients as individuals and is quick to develop a Grieving diagnosis at the first sign of crying, sadness, or other emotional upset, based upon what she "knows."

Patients become upset for many reasons, and Nurse Thomas's inference of grief is highly inaccurate for some of them.

Relying Too Much on Past Experience

Basing conclusions on past experience with similar situations is a common and legitimate practice. This is different from stereotyping, since stereotypes are formed based on little or no experience. Generalizing from experience can help you to formulate tentative diagnoses, but it can also lead to error unless you validate your assumptions. Although many patients behave similarly in similar situations, it is an error to assume that they all will.

> ***Example:*** Suppose Nurse Thomas, in the earlier example, had not read about loss of body parts, grief, or female identity. Suppose instead that she had taken care of several hysterectomy patients, all of whom *did* experience grief. In this case, Nurse Thomas's expectations of grief would be based on her experience. She would have used the specific cases she experienced to generalize a rule about *all* cases.

Relying Too Much on Authority

Experienced nurses, teachers, the nursing literature, and textbooks are all good sources of ideas about the meaning of client data. However, you should critically examine even this information and remain open to new information and ideas. The patient problems you formulate with the help of an authority must be verified the same as other problems.

Empathizing/Identifying with the Patient

Empathy is the ability to imagine intellectually what another person might be experiencing or feeling. It is an important and valued aspect of therapeutic relationships. Because you know that people share certain basic human needs, behaviors, and feelings (e.g., need for food, feelings of fear and love), you can predict a patient's behavior, to some extent, on the basis of what your own would be in the same situation. The more similar you are to the patient, the more likely your predictions are to be accurate. The danger, of course, is in failing to recognize the uniqueness of individual responses—in assuming, without verifying, that the patient feels as you would.

> ***Example:*** Liam Duggan has always felt, "I can handle anything, no matter how bad, if I just know what it is. It is the unknown and the unexpected that I can't cope with." On the basis of this feeling, Liam was always careful to explain in detail what his patients could expect when sending them for diagnostic tests or treatments. Imagine his surprise when he began to teach a patient about a bone marrow aspiration and the patient stopped him, saying, "If you don't mind, I'd really rather not hear about it now. I would rather just have them tell me what to do right when it needs doing. If I start to think about things like that ahead of time I worry and get worked up into a state before it even happens."

Thinking Critically to Avoid Errors

Except for forming premature conclusions, most sources of error are also legitimate sources of hypotheses about the meaning of patient data; they cause problems only when you rely too heavily on them. The following suggestions may help you to avoid diagnostic errors. Also see Box 4–5.

Keep your mind open to all possible explanations of the data clusters. Don't jump to conclusions based in just a few cues, on the word of an authority, or on your past experiences with similar patients.

Examine your beliefs. Our beliefs are not usually acquired rationally, and they are sometimes misleading. We come to believe what those around us believe, what we are rewarded for believing, what serves our own interests, and what makes us comfortable. Examine your beliefs, keeping the ones that are supported by good reasons and evidence. This will help you avoid the errors of stereotyping and bias.

Verify. Remember that all diagnoses are only tentative until they are verified. Begin and end the diagnostic process by talking with the client and family. When you are collecting data, ask them what their health problems are and what they believe the causes to be. At the end of the process, ask them to verify your diagnoses.

**Diagnostic
Reasoning**

Build a good knowledge base and acquire clinical experience. You will need to apply knowledge from many different areas in order to recognize significant cues and patterns and generate hypotheses about the data. For example, nurses use principles from chemistry, anatomy, physiology, disease processes, communication, teaching, growth and development, and pharmacology—to name a few. Each subject helps you to understand patient data in a different way, and improves the accuracy of your diagnoses.

Develop cultural sensitivity. Health beliefs and values are acquired from our culture and environment. A situation may be considered a problem in one culture but not another. For example, in the dominant American culture, it is acceptable to bottle-feed a baby. However, some traditional Navajo people believe that breastfeeding promotes respect and obedience, while bottle-feeding does not (Clark, 1981). From that cultural perspective, bottle-feeding would be considered a problem or a symptom of a problem. The key is to understand that personal and cultural meaning is attached to a group of cues.

Be sure you have a working knowledge of what is normal. You need to know what is normal for most people for such things as vital signs, lab tests, motor skills and speech development, skin color, breath sounds, and so on. In addition, you must determine what is normal for a particular individual, taking into account age, physical makeup, lifestyle, culture, and the person's own perception of what is normal. For example, normal blood pressure for adults is in the range of 110/60–140/80. However, you may obtain a blood pressure of 90/50 that is perfectly normal for a particular individual. For another person with long-standing hypertension, 150/90 may be normal. Compare findings to the patient's baseline data when possible.

Base your diagnosis on patterns—that is, on behavior over time—rather than on an isolated incident. For example, you would not diagnose Altered Family Processes for Luisa Sanchez (Table 4–5, Cluster 8) on the basis of the two

---

Box 4–5. Thinking Critically About Your Diagnostic Reasoning

Diagnosticians should ask themselves these questions when identifying problems:
✓ What are the different possibilities for clustering the cues?
✓ How have I clustered these cues in the past?
✓ Have I distinguished relevant from irrelevant cues?
✓ What are the diagnostic hypotheses I am making based on these clusters?
✓ Are the hypotheses within the domain of nursing practice?
✓ Do I have enough evidence to support the hypotheses?
✓ Is this the best hypothesis for the cue cluster?

Diagnosticians should ask themselves these questions when determining etiologies:
✓ Which is the problem and which is the etiology?
✓ What is the probability that this etiology is influencing the problem?
✓ What evidence supports (or does not support) the link between problem and etiology?
✓ How does this problem-etiology link compare with my past clinical experience?

Adapted from Pesut and Herman (1992), Metacognitive skills in diagnostic reasoning: Making the implicit explicit, *Nursing Diagnosis*, 3(4):148–154.

cues obtained in the admission interview. There are no data to show that the family has ever been disrupted before or will ever be again. You would need to see if the situation persists or if other data are found to support such a hypothesis.

Finally, ***develop your critical thinking skills*** by applying them to every area of your life: the music you hear, the newspapers you read, and the conversations you have with your friends. Be aware of, and avoid, errors in thinking such as: overgeneralizing or stereotyping, making unwarranted assumptions, oversimplifying, and drawing premature conclusions. Review Chapter 2 as often as you need to; and do the critical thinking activities at the end of the other chapters in this text.

Many thinking errors can be avoided by being aware of them, consciously trying to keep an open mind, being sure data is complete, verifying data, and validating your conclusions with the client. You should be able to make more accurate diagnoses if you understand how the diagnostic reasoning process works. The steps of the diagnostic process, including data interpretation, are summarized in Box 4–6.

Diagnostic Reasoning

Box 4–6. Steps of the Diagnostic Reasoning Process

Interpret the data

Level One—Identify significant cues

1. Organize entire data base in concise format, according to your chosen framework.
2. Identify and remedy any remaining data gaps or inconsistencies.
3. Identify significant cues by comparing individual cues to standards and norms. Circle these cues.

Level Two—Cluster cues; identify problems

4. Identify patterns and relationships among the significant cues. Make a new list in which you cluster the related significant cues.
5. Using your knowledge of the framework, decide which category or pattern each cue cluster represents. A cluster may involve more than one framework pattern.
6. Identify the problems. Think of as many explanations as possible for each cue cluster. Then decide which hypothesis best explains the cue cluster. (Note: You may sometimes identify both problems and etiologies in this step.)
7. Determine the status of each problem: Actual, potential (risk), possible, or no problem.

Level Three—Determine etiologies and problem type

8. Determine the etiologies of the problems.
9. Identify problem type: nursing diagnosis, collaborative problem, medical problem, or other.
10. Identify client strengths and supports.

Verify the data

11. Verify problems and strengths with client, family, and other professionals or references.
12. Decide in which pattern of the framework the problem occurs.

Label the data

13. Label the problem. Write the formal problem statements, both nursing diagnoses and collaborative problems.
14. Prioritize the problems.

Record the data

15. Record the nursing diagnoses and collaborative problems on the appropriate documents: patient care plan, chart, and so forth.

**Diagnostic
Reasoning**

SUMMARY

The diagnostic process is summarized in Box 4–6 on page 117.

Diagnosis
- ✓ is a pivotal step in the nursing process.
- ✓ focuses on human responses to disease and other stressors in the area of health.
- ✓ is the process of *interpreting data, verifying* hypotheses about the data (with the client or other professionals), *labeling* the problems, and *recording* the diagnoses.
- ✓ may identify nursing diagnoses or collaborative or other health problems.
- ✓ may identify actual, risk, or possible problems.
- ✓ requires critical thinking, *not* making premature judgments or relying on experience or empathy.

A nursing diagnosis
- ✓ involves human responses to disease and other stressors.
- ✓ is a problem that nurses can independently treat or prevent.

We think some things are true because we have direct evidence. For instance, you might see your dog standing outside the door. You know that she is there because you can see her. We also believe things are true even when we do not have such clear evidence. Suppose you are in your house and you hear a scratching noise coming from the front door. Just as before, you might believe that your dog is standing at the door, but this time the evidence is different. You don't actually see your dog, but the sound you hear makes you think she is at the door. This is the best explanation you can think of for the noise. We call this process *making an inference.* An **inference** is something we believe to be true based on careful consideration of the evidence.

We cannot be totally sure of the truth of our inferences. Obviously, however, some inferences are supported by more evidence than others. In the preceding example, if you hear your dog's chain

Practice in Critical Thinking: Making Inferences

rattling and hear her barking and scratching, you can be pretty sure that she is outside the door. If, on the other hand, all you heard was some scratching you would be less sure about your inference. It could be you heard some other animal, like a raccoon.

Sometimes we get so used to making a particular inference that we do not even realize we are inferring. If every time you hear scratching at the door you go and find your dog, then you assume that the scratching always means your dog is out there because you have tested your inference many times. Many of the so-called "facts" of science are really inferences that we make so often that we do not stop to consider that we are making an inference. It is important to remember, though, that things like problems and etiologies are really inferences from evidence. In many cases they have never been observed directly.

Learning the Skill
Practice thinking about inferences by answering the following questions.

1. While sitting in a sunlit room, you notice that the direct sunlight has stopped coming through the window. List several things you might infer.

2. A few minutes after the sunlight stopped coming through the window, you observed drops of water falling from the sky. Does this provide any additional evidence for one of your inferences? Explain.

3. Can you be sure that what you have inferred is true?

Applying the Skill

In nursing diagnosis, we use the patient's signs and symptoms (cues) as evidence to support our inferences about the patient's problems and their etiologies. Some problems can be directly observed (e.g., Altered Skin Integrity), but others must be inferred (e.g., Low Self-Esteem). We can never, however, directly observe the link between the problem and the etiology; the cause of the problem is always inferred.

1. State whether the following are cues or inferences.

_____	The nurse's interpretation of the data
_____	Weight 250 lb
_____	Obesity
_____	Temperature 100° F
_____	Anxiety

2. In the following case, circle the cues.

Maria Gutierrez had a routine surgery and an uneventful recovery-room period. She was returned to her room at 4:00 P.M., still drowsy, but responding to her name. A Foley catheter was in place, draining clear, pale yellow urine. Her IV was patent; 1000 mL of D_5LR was running at 75 mL per hour. Her skin turgor was good. Her vital signs were B/P 124/76–130/82, pulse 72–86, and respirations 12–20 throughout the evening. At 8:00 P.M. she was helped to sit on the side of the bed for about 15 minutes. She moved slowly and complained of incisional pain, which she rated 10 on a scale of 1 to 10 (10 being the worst). She administered her own morphine by use of a PCA pump, and rated her pain as "about 5" when she was lying still. Her abdominal dressing was dry and intact throughout the night, as was her vaginal pad. At 9:00 P.M. she had sips of a carbonated drink. At 9:20 she complained of nausea.

3. In the preceding case, the nurse made several inferences. Write the cues that led the nurse to make each of the following inferences (use the cues you circled above).

   a. Ms. Gutierrez was drowsy from the anesthetic.

   b. There was no problem with Ms. Gutierrez's urinary system.

   c. Ms. Gutierrez was adequately hydrated.

   d. Ms. Gutierrez was experiencing acute incisional pain.

   e. The morphine was effective in relieving her incisional pain.

   f. Ms. Gutierrez became nauseated because her GI motility had not fully returned after her anesthesia.

4. Do all of these inferences have an equal amount of supporting evidence? Which ones do you think need more evidence?

5. Examine the explanations for each cue cluster. Circle the parts that are inferred and underline the parts that have direct evidence to support them.

   a. *Cues:* Your patient has just had general anesthetic. Bowel sounds are absent to auscultation. Patient drank 100 mL of fluid and immediately vomited. Patient complains of nausea.

   Explanation: Nausea and vomiting caused by decreased gastrointestinal activity secondary to general anesthetic.

   b. *Cues:* Your patient has just been admitted to the hospital. He is pale and trembling. His palms are cool and damp. He speaks rapidly.

   Explanation: Anxiety related to being in a strange environment.

   c. *Cues:* Your patient is unable to drink anything. He is vomiting and experiencing severe diarrhea. In fact, his output for the past 12 hours has been 500 mL greater than his intake. His skin turgor is poor; his mucous membranes are dry.

   Explanation: Fluid Volume Deficit caused by being unable to drink and by diarrhea and vomiting.

6. Now, for each inference in item 5, write whether you think the evidence is adequate or inadequate. If it is inadequate, what else do you need to know in order to make that inference?

Adapted from *Critical Thinking Worksheets,* a Supplement of *Addison-Wesley Chemistry,* by Wilbraham et al. (Menlo Park, CA: Addison-Wesley Publishing Company, 1990).

1. You are head nurse on a hospital unit, and your job is to encourage the staff nurses to begin using nursing diagnoses on their care plans and in their charting. One nurse says, "I didn't learn that when I went to school, and I've done just fine without it all these years. I can't see any reason to do all that extra work." What would you say to persuade her that nursing diagnosis is important to her practice?

2. Place a check mark (✔) beside the words or phrases that are patient problems.

   a. ___ Appendicitis

   b. ___ Catheter obstruction

   c. ___ Decreased peripheral circulation

   d. ___ Asthma

   e. ___ Delayed parent-infant bonding

   f. ___ Having bowel resection surgery

   g. ___ NPO (nothing by mouth)

   h. ___ Constipation

   i. ___ Activity intolerance

   j. ___ Needs skin care

   k. ___ Low white-blood-cell count

   l. ___ Uncooperative

   m. ___ Needs constant attention

3. In the following situation, circle the stressors, and underline the responses.

   Ms. Sato developed a blood clot in her right thigh. Her thigh was swollen and warm to the touch. It was also slightly red. An intravenous catheter was inserted in her right forearm, and she was started on a Heparin drip. She was placed on complete bedrest. That evening, she rang for the nurse several times, asking to have her leg checked and requesting pain medication. She was observed reading her Bible each time the nurse entered the room. Twenty-four hours later, when her clotting time returned to normal, the Heparin was discontinued.

123

4. Now list Ms. Sato's *responses* (from Question 3) below. Write whether each occurred at the cellular, systemic, organic, or whole-person *level*. Also indicate whether it was in the physical, psychological, interpersonal, or spiritual *dimension*. The first one is done for you.

Response	Level	Dimension
Thigh swollen	Organic	Physical

5. Complete the following nursing diagnoses by adding etiologies to the problems given. Remember that a problem can be caused by any number of different etiologies. Use your knowledge of the medical condition to suggest appropriate etiologies.

For a client with a medical diagnosis of	Problem	r/t Etiology
Fractured femur	**a.** Acute Pain	
	b. Risk for Impaired Skin Integrity: pressure sores or excoriation	
Pneumonia	**a.** Ineffective Breathing Pattern	
	b. Activity Intolerance	

6. Match the terms to the correct statements.

N—Nursing diagnosis

C—Collaborative problem

a. ___ Deals mainly with physiological complications.

b. ___ A two-part or three-part statement about a client response to a situation or health problem.

c. ___ A physiological complication resulting from pathophysiology or disease process.

d. ___ Independent nursing interventions are mainly to monitor for symptoms and prevent condition.

e. ___ Nurse can order definitive treatment.

f. ___ Requires medical intervention.

g. ___ Can be expected to be present any time the disease or treatment is present.

h. ___ Can be a physiological, psychosocial, spiritual, or interpersonal problem.

7. Fill in the blanks with the status of each of the following problems.

A—Actual problem   **Pot**—Potential (risk) problem   **Pos**—Possible problem

a. ___ A client states he is experiencing stomach pain.

b. ___ A blind client is at risk for falls in an unfamiliar environment.

c. ___ The problem is likely to occur if certain preventive nursing actions are not begun.

d. ___ Risk factors are the etiology for the problem.

e. ___ Data not sufficient to confirm or rule out the diagnosis. More data needed.

f. ___ Client has a group of related signs and symptoms.

g. ___ Similar to a physician's "rule-out" diagnosis.

h. ___ Nurse prescribes interventions to prevent by reducing risk factors and/or monitoring status and onset of the problem.

i. ___ Nurse prescribes interventions to treat the problem, as well as monitor status.

j. ___ Problem is identified mainly to assure additional data collection.

k. ___ The patient has arthritis. Her knee is red and swollen. She states that it is very painful. She has a/an _____ problem of Pain.

l. ___ The patient has arthritis. Her knee is red and swollen. The status of her Pain diagnosis is _____ .

m. ___ The patient has arthritis. Her knee is red and swollen. You see she is limping. The status of her Pain diagnosis is _____ .

8. Place an *N* beside the problem statements that are nursing diagnoses. Some have etiologies and some do not. Circle the part (or parts) of the statements that the nurse can independently treat or prevent.

a. ___ Potential Arrhythmia r/t myocardial infarction

b. ___ Low Self Esteem r/t perceived sexual inadequacy

c. ___ Risk for Skin Breakdown

d. ___ Perineal Rash and Excoriation r/t urinary incontinence

e. ___ Confusion and Disorientation r/t inadequate cerebral oxygenation 2° CVA.

9. Using the NANDA framework, group the following cues *inductively* into the correct patterns of the framework. The Unitary Person patterns are Exchanging, Communicating, Relating, Valuing, Choosing, Moving, Perceiving, Knowing, and Feeling. Decide the NANDA pattern in which the *problem* occurs. (You will probably have two or three cue clusters.) Refer to Chapter 3 for a review of this framework.

Cues: Ms. Petersen's blood pressure is 190/100. She says she hasn't been taking her "blood-pressure pills" because "they don't make me feel any better." She says she also has trouble remembering to take them. She is 50 pounds overweight. She says she works long hours and doesn't have time to cook—tends to eat fast food and snacks a lot. Her job is sedentary, and she does not engage in any physical exercise. For fun, she likes to "eat at a nice restaurant."

Cue Clusters	NANDA Pattern in Which Problem Occurs

10. Now look at the problems and etiologies you have identified for the cue clusters in Exercise 9. Write nursing diagnoses for the cue clusters (Problem r/t etiology). Use NANDA terminology if you wish, or simply state the problem and its etiology in your own words. You should have two nursing diagnoses.

11. In your own words, write the most likely explanation for each of the following cue clusters.

    a. An elderly client with left-side paralysis has a red, broken area of skin over his sacrum.

    b. Larry VanHuff has had severe diarrhea for two days. Today he has been vomiting each time he takes fluids by mouth. He does not yet have symptoms such as poor skin turgor or dry, sticky mucous membranes in his mouth.

12. Match the diagnostic error with the case illustrating it.

    a. ___ Mike Skarda actually hears very well; but because he is elderly, his new nurse speaks loudly when talking to him.

    b. ___ Sharon Weiss feels it is cruel to prolong life by using heroic technology. When Mr. Ivanov's family will not agree to a "Do not resuscitate" order, Sharon fails to identify their guilt feelings and need for support.

    c. ___ All the cesarean birth moms Susan Stone has cared for have been ambulatory by 24 hours post-op. Her nursing text indicates that this is the norm. When Susan asks her patient to walk to the chair so she can make her bed, the patient says, "You will need to help me." Assuming the patient is being overly anxious, Susan says, "You can do it. Just go slow." However, this particular mom cannot walk without her cane and leg braces.

    d. ___ When a young woman with long, blond hair is brought to the emergency room in critical condition, the nurse (herself a young woman) becomes immobilized, thinking "Poor thing. That could be me!"

1. Premature data interpretation
2. Personal bias
3. Stereotyping
4. Generalizing from past experience
5. Relying on authority
6. Empathy

REFERENCES

American Nurses Association. (1991). *Standards of Clinical Nursing Practice.* Kansas City, MO: ANA.

American Nurses Association. (1973). *Standards of Nursing Practice.* Kansas City, MO.

Brackstone, A., and Cooper-Page, L. (1993). Rekindling the nursing diagnosis flame. *The Canadian Nurse, 89*(4):23–25.

Bradburn, C., Zeleznikow, J., and Adams, A. (1993). FLORENCE: Synthesis of case-based and model-based reasoning in a nursing care planning system. *Computers in Nursing, 11*(1):20–24.

Briody, M., Carpenito, L., Jones, D., and Fitzpatrick, J. (1992). Toward further understanding of nursing diagnosis: An interpretation. *Nursing Diagnosis, 3*(3):124–128.

Carpenito, L. (1993). *Nursing Diagnosis.* 5th ed. Philadelphia: J. B. Lippincott.

Chang, B., and Hirsch, M. (1994). Nursing diagnosis research: Computer-aided research in nursing. *Nursing Diagnosis, 5*(1):6–13.

Clark, A. (1981). *Culture and Childrearing.* Philadelphia: F.A. Davis.

Fry, V. (1953). The creative approach to nursing. *American Journal of Nursing, 53*(3): 301–302.

Gebbie, K. (1976). Development of a taxonomy of nursing diagnosis. In Walter, J., et al., *Dynamics of Problem-Oriented Approaches: Patient Care and Documentation.* Philadelphia: J. B. Lippincott.

Gebbie, K., and Lavin, M. (1975). *Classification of Nursing Diagnoses: Proceedings of the First National Conference.* St. Louis: C. V. Mosby.

Gordon, M. (1994). *Nursing Diagnosis: Process and Application.* 3rd ed. St. Louis: Mosby.

Gordon, M., Murphy, C., Candee, D., and Hiltunen, E. (1994). Clinical judgment: An integrated model. *Advances in Nursing Science, 16*(4):55–70.

Hampton, D. (1993). Implementing a managed care framework through care maps. *Journal of Nursing Administration, 23*(5):21–27.

Harvey, R. (1993). Nursing diagnosis by computers: An application of neural networks. *Nursing Diagnosis, 4*(1):26–34.

Hirsch, M., Chang, B., and Jensen, K. (1993). Concurrent validity of a rule-based system. *Computers in Nursing, 11*(3):134–139.

Hughes, K., and Young, W. (1992). Decision making: Stability of clinical decisions. *Nurse Educator, 17*(3):12–16.

Hurst, K., Dean, A., and Trickey, S. (1991). The recognition and non-recognition of problem-solving stages in nursing practice. *Journal of Advanced Nursing, 16*:1444–1455.

Kelly, M. (1991). What's happening in nursing diagnosis?: NANDA on the move. *South Carolina Nurse, 6*(4):20–21.

Koch, B., and McGovern, J. (1993). EXTEND: A prototype expert system for teaching nursing diagnosis. *Computers in Nursing, 11*(1):35–41.

McGinty, M., Andreoni, V., and Quigley, M. (1993). Building a managed care approach. *Nursing Management, 24*(5):34–35.

McManus, L. (1951). Assumption of functions of nursing. In *Regional Planning for Nursing and Nursing Education.* New York: Teachers College Press.

North American Nursing Diagnosis Association. (1990). *Taxonomy I—Revised 1990.* St. Louis: NANDA.

North American Nursing Diagnosis Association. (1994). *NANDA Nursing Diagnoses: Definitions & Classification, 1995–1996.* Philadelphia: NANDA.

Pesut, D., and Herman, J. (1992). Metacognitive skills in diagnostic reasoning: Making the implicit explicit. *Nursing Diagnosis, 3*(4):148–154.

Roy, Sr. C. (1984). *Introduction to Nursing: An Adaptation Model.* Englewood Cliffs, NJ: Prentice Hall.

Sheppard, K. (1993). The relationship among nursing diagnoses in discharge planning for patients with lung cancer. *Nursing Diagnosis, 4*(4):148–155.

Thomas, N., and Newsome, G. (1992). Factors affecting the use of nursing diagnosis. *Nursing Outlook, 40*(4):182–186.

Warren, J., and Hoskins, L. (1990). The development of NANDA's nursing diagnosis taxonomy. *Nursing Diagnosis, 1*(4):162–68.

White, J., Nativio, D., Kobert, S., and Engberg, S. (1992). Content and process in clinical decision-making by nurse practitioners. *Image: Journal of Nursing Scholarship, 24*(2):153–158.

Woolridge, J., Brown, O., and Herman, J. (1993). Nursing diagnosis: The central theme in nursing knowledge. *Nursing Diagnosis, 4*(2):50–55.

Yura, H., and Walsh, M. (1988). *The Nursing Process,* 5th ed. Norwalk, CT: Appleton & Lange.

Ziegler, S. (1993). *Theory-Directed Nursing Practice.* New York: Springer Publishing Company, Inc.

CHAPTER 5

WRITING DIAGNOSTIC STATEMENTS

OBJECTIVES

On completing this chapter, you should be able to do the following:
- Briefly describe the history of the nursing diagnosis movement in North America.
- Use NANDA diagnostic labels to write precise, concise, and accurate nursing diagnoses for individuals, families, and communities.
- Write collaborative problem statements in correct format.
- Describe the ethical issues involved in writing diagnostic statements.
- Write diagnostic statements describing wellness states.
- Prioritize client problems using a basic needs or a preservation of life framework.
- Recognize the cultural implications inherent in many nursing diagnoses.
- Write nursing diagnoses to describe human responses in the spiritual dimension.

INTRODUCTION

In Chapter 4 you learned to analyze data in order to identify and verify nursing diagnoses, collaborative problems, and patient strengths. This chapter explains how to use the NANDA standardized terminology to write nursing diagnoses, describes formats for various kinds of problem statements, and presents frameworks for prioritizing a patient's problems. Figure 5–1 highlights the aspects of the diagnosis step that are emphasized in this chapter.

THE NORTH AMERICAN NURSING DIAGNOSIS ASSOCIATION

In the 1950s and 1960s the need for consistency in the profession was recognized. During this period, several studies were done to identify patient problems requiring nursing intervention. These evolved into lists of *nursing problems* (Abdellah , 1957) and *client needs* that might require basic nursing care (Henderson, 1964). While neither of these was actually a list of patient problems, they did demonstrate that nursing care focuses on something other than disease processes.

In 1973, the American Nurses Association published the *Standards of Nursing Practice*, which identified nursing diagnosis as an important function of the professional nurse. During that same year, nursing faculty members at St. Louis University, led by Kristine Gebbie and Mary Ann Lavin, initiated a project to identify and categorize problems that should be considered *nursing diagnoses*.

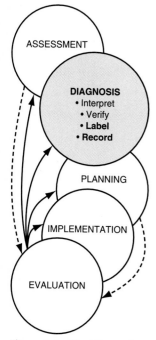

Figure 5–1. The Diagnosis Step in the Nursing Process

A national task force was formed to implement the project. One hundred nurses attended the First Conference on Nursing Diagnosis in 1973 (Gebbie, 1976). This group continued to meet every two years and, at the Fifth Conference in 1982 (Kim et al., 1984), formally became the North American Nursing Diagnosis Association (NANDA). NANDA membership consists of nurses from education, practice, research, and administration, as well as from all nursing specialty areas (e.g., intensive care, maternal-child, home health). This diversity assures input from a variety of perspectives.

The North American Nursing Diagnosis Association

The major function of the early groups was to generate, name, and implement diagnostic categories. Diagnostic titles were rapidly generated and accepted until the Fifth Conference. At the Ninth Conference, in 1990, only two new titles were accepted, bringing the total number of approved labels to 100. By the Fifth Conference, in 1982, emphasis had shifted from generating new diagnosis labels to clarifying existing labels and developing etiologies and defining characteristics. Other important issues began to emerge: the need for a classification system (taxonomy) and the need for a theoretical framework on which to base the taxonomy. These priorities still exist, along with others, such as promoting research to validate the diagnostic labels and encouraging nurses to use standardized labeling in their practice.

Review and refinement of diagnostic labels is ongoing. New and modified labels are discussed at each biannual conference, but new labels are no longer voted on at the conference. Since 1994, nurses submit diagnoses to the Diagnostic Review Committee for review. The committee "stages" the diagnosis according to how well developed and supported it is. Diagnoses on the official NANDA list are not finished products, but are approved for clinical use and further study. Many on the list have been studied only minimally. For example, the "diagnoses in progress," added in 1994, are still in the very early stages of development (see Appendix E). For that reason, they were not included in any of the NANDA lists in this text, and they are not presented in the *Nursing Diagnosis Guide*. NANDA reports ongoing work in its official journal, *Nursing Diagnosis.*

The Taxonomy of Nursing Diagnoses

A **taxonomy** is a system for identifying and classifying objects on the basis of their relationships. Any number of ordering principles can be used to classify things (e.g., size, weight, or color).

The first NANDA taxonomy was alphabetical and nonhierarchical (as in the list inside the front cover of this text). In 1986, the group accepted the nine Human Response Patterns (see Table 3–8 in Chapter 3 on page 69) as the organizing framework for classifying diagnoses (McLane, 1987). The taxonomy has undergone revisions, but still uses the same organizing framework. The current taxonomy is a hierarchical system in which each of the labels is a subcategory of one of the Human Response Patterns. Each of the Human Response Patterns is a Level I concept—the most abstract. The most useful concepts occur at Levels IV and V, which are more concrete and specific; however, a few of the approved labels occur at Levels II and III (e.g., Social Isolation and Altered Family Processes). This can be seen in Box 5–1, which is a section of the taxonomy that has been provided to illustrate how the diagnoses are categorized by NANDA.

**Writing Diagnostic
Statements**

Box 5–1. Excerpt from Taxonomy I (1994)

1.5   *[Altered Oxygenation]*
    1.5.1 *[Respiration]*
       1.5.1.1 Impaired Gas Exchange
       1.5.1.2 Ineffective Airway Clearance
       1.5.1.3 Ineffective Breathing Pattern
           1.5.1.3.1 Inability to Sustain Spontaneous Ventilation
           1.5.1.3.2 Dysfunctional Ventilatory Weaning
                 Response (DVWR)
1.6   *[Altered Physical Integrity]*
    1.6.1 Risk for Injury
       1.6.1.1 Risk for Suffocation
       1.6.1.2 Risk for Poisoning
       1.6.1.3 Risk for Trauma
       1.6.1.4 Risk for Aspiration
       1.6.1.5 Risk for Disuse Syndrome
  *1.6.2 Altered Protection
       1.6.2.1 Impaired Tissue Integrity
           1.6.2.1.1. Altered Oral Mucous Membrane
               1.6.2.1.2.1 Impaired Skin Integrity
               1.6.2.1.2.2 Risk for Impaired Skin Integrity

2. COMMUNICATION
2.1   *Altered Communication*
    2.1.1 Verbal
       2.1.1.1 Impaired Verbal Communication

3. RELATING
3.1   *[Altered Socialization]*
    3.1.1 Impaired Social Interaction
    3.1.2 Social Isolation
3.2   *[Altered role]*
    3.2.1 Altered Role Performance
       3.2.1.1 Altered Parenting
           3.2.1.1.1 Actual
           3.2.1.1.2 Risk
       3.2.1.2 Sexual
           3.2.1.2.1 Dysfunction
    3.2.2 Altered Family Processes
       3.2.2.1 Caregiver Role Strain
    3.2.3 [Role Conflict]
       3.2.3.1 Parental Role Conflict
3.3   *Altered Sexuality Patterns*

4. VALUING
4.1   *[Altered Spiritual State]*
    4.1.1 Spiritual Distress

5. CHOOSING
5.1   *Altered Coping*
    5.1.1 Individual Coping
       5.1.1.1 Ineffective Individual Coping
           5.1.1.1.1 Impaired Adjustment
           5.1.1.1.2 Defensive Coping
           5.1.1.1.3 Ineffective Denial
    5.1.2 Family Coping
       5.1.2.1 Ineffective Family Coping
           5.1.2.1.1 Disabling
           5.1.2.1.2 Compromised
       5.1.2.2 Potential for Growth

Adapted from *NANDA Nursing Diagnosis: Definitions and Classification 1995–1996*, pp. 9–10.
Used by permission.

NANDA and the ANA have worked together to adapt *Taxonomy I* for possible inclusion in the World Health Organization's 10th revision of the *International Classification of Diseases (ICD–10)*. Some changes in terminology and numbering were made to accommodate the WHO numbering system. Inclusion of nursing diagnoses in the *ICD* would be a step toward (1) developing an international nursing data base and (2) documenting nursing care for third-party payment.

Issues Associated with the NANDA Classification System

There are various criticisms of the taxonomy and of individual diagnostic labels: too broad, too abstract, too medical, and so on. These problems will probably be corrected as the system evolves and individual diagnoses are refined. Meanwhile, if you disagree with a diagnostic label, you do not have to use it, or you can add words to make it more specific and concrete. You should not reject the idea of standardized diagnostic terminology just because of a few unwieldy diagnoses. The system is evolving, as do all classification systems. In the medical diagnosis taxonomy, only in recent years was *toxemia of pregnancy* changed to *preeclampsia/eclampsia,* and only recently has *AIDS* become a medical diagnosis.

The more serious issues involve the whole system rather than individual diagnoses. We may be expecting too much from nursing diagnosis in terms of what it can do for the profession and for patients. Does it truly define nursing? And if so, will that make any difference in the long run? Nursing is changing rapidly and being shaped in part by events outside the profession (e.g., technology, the economy, military engagements). In our enthusiasm for this relatively new idea, we must remember that nursing diagnosis is simply an important *part* of nursing. It cannot be expected to singlehandedly remedy such problems as lack of autonomy and third-party pay; other measures will be necessary.

Some believe that choosing a diagnosis from a list of ready-made labels actually causes nurses to miss creative inferences they would otherwise make. Others believe that a step-by-step, scientific approach inhibits intuitive problem solving and prevents a holistic perspective (Kobert and Folan, 1990). Certainly we have all seen examples of the dehumanizing effects of science and technology. However, this does not have to be the case. Kritek (1985) says that "naming our phenomena of concern does not narrow our perception of clients, but broadens it. . . . When a child weeps, you work hard to discover why. You try to solve the problem. But of course, you always comfort the entire child, not just the problem. Nursing will retain its fidelity to holism if it chooses to do so" (p. 396). Using a common language and logical thinking should actually help nurses to identify and communicate unique aspects of patients that they might otherwise miss.

CHOOSING A LABEL

As a science emerges, a language develops to describe everyday observations. The NANDA diagnostic labels provide a common language for all nurses to use in describing health problems for any type of client and in any health care setting. You must understand the meaning of the NANDA labels if your written statements are to accurately reflect your clinical judgments.

**Writing Diagnostic
Statements**

Components of a NANDA Diagnosis

Each NANDA diagnosis has four components: label, definition, defining characteristics, and either related factors or risk factors.

Label

Also referred to as the *title* or *name*, the **label** is a concise phrase or term describing the client's health. Labels can be used as either the problem or the etiology in a diagnostic statement. Many labels include qualifying terms such as *Actual, Risk, Ineffective, Impaired,* or *Increased.* NANDA has provided a list of definitions for these qualifiers (see Table 5–1).

Notice that many of the labels are very general; you cannot know what a diagnostic concept includes by looking at the label alone. For example, what do you think Activity Intolerance means? Does it mean the patient tires easily when playing football, or that he has chest pain when he walks up the stairs? What is the difference between the labels Activity Intolerance and Fatigue? The other components of a NANDA diagnosis help to clarify these questions.

Table 5–1. Qualifiers for Diagnosis	
Qualifier	**Definition**
(Suggested/not limited to the following)	
Acute	Severe but short of duration
Altered	A change from baseline
Chronic	Lasting a long time; recurring; habitual; constant
Decreased	Lessened, lesser in size, amount, or degree
Deficient	Inadequate in amount, quality, or degree; defective; not sufficient; incomplete
Depleted	Emptied wholly or in part; exhausted of
Disturbed	Agitated; interrupted, interfered with
Dysfunctional	Abnormal, incomplete functioning
Excessive	Characterized by an amount or quantity that is greater than is necessary, desirable, or useful
Increased	Greater in size, amount, or degree
Impaired	Made worse, weakened; damaged, reduced; deteriorated
Ineffective	Not producing the desired effect
Intermittent	Stopping or starting again at intervals; periodic; cyclic
Potential for Enhanced	(for use with wellness diagnoses) Made greater, to increase in quality, or more desired

Source: *North American Nursing Diagnosis Association* (1994). *NANDA Nursing Diagnoses: Definitions and Classification 1995–1996.* Philadelphia: NANDA.

Definition

The **definition** expresses clearly and precisely the essential nature of the diagnostic label; it differentiates the label from all others. For example, the definitions for Activity Intolerance and Fatigue indicate that Fatigue is characterized by a sense of exhaustion; however, exhaustion is only a part of Activity Intolerance, in which heart changes, discomfort, and dyspnea may also be present.

***Choosing
A Label***

Defining Characteristics

Defining characteristics are the *cues* (the subjective and objective data) that indicate the presence of the diagnostic label. For actual diagnoses, the defining characteristics are the patient's *signs and symptoms;* for risk diagnoses, they are *risk factors.* It is not necessary for all the defining characteristics to be present in order to use a label; usually the presence of two or three confirms a diagnosis. The defining characteristics for many labels are classified as *critical, major,* and *minor.* Newer labels specify *major* or *minor;* the earlier labels specified which characteristics were *critical.*

Cues

Defining   Risk
Characteristics Factors
↓   ↓
Actual   Risk
Diagnosis   Diagnosis

Critical defining characteristics are symptoms that are almost always present when the problem is present and absent when the problem is absent. If critical defining characteristics are identified for a label, they *must* be present in order to make the diagnosis.

> ***Example:*** "Verbal report of fatigue or weakness" is a critical defining characteristic for Activity Intolerance. Even if the patient experiences *b, c,* and *d* (below), you cannot diagnose Activity Intolerance unless *a* is present. You could, however, make the diagnosis if *only a* is present.
>
> **a.** Verbal report of fatigue or weakness (*critical*)
> **b.** Abnormal heart rate or blood-pressure response to activity
> **c.** Exertional discomfort or dyspnea
> **d.** EKG changes reflecting arrhythmias or ischemia

Major defining characteristics are those that appear to be present in all clients who have the diagnosis. NANDA defines *all* as "present in 80%–100% of those having the diagnosis" (1990). This means that as many as 20% of the clients with a diagnosis may *not* have these signs and symptoms. However, you should be skeptical about making a diagnosis if none of the major defining characteristics is present. Note that they do not *all* have to be present.

> ***Example:*** You could diagnose Colonic Constipation if only one or two of the following major defining characteristics were present:
>
> **a.** Decreased frequency   **d.** Painful defecation
> **b.** Hard, dry stool   **e.** Abdominal distention
> **c.** Straining at stool   **f.** Palpable mass

It is easy to see that a client with a diagnosis of Colonic Constipation might experience one or more of these symptoms in various combinations. A palpable mass is present in at least 80% of clients who have Colonic Constipation, but some clients might not have a palpable mass. Furthermore, you would probably diagnose Colonic Constipation for a client who had only symptoms *b* and *c,* but you would not make that diagnosis for a client who had only symptoms *e* and *f.*

Writing Diagnostic Statements

Minor defining characteristics are those that are present in many (at least half) of the clients experiencing the diagnosis. Since these signs and symptoms are not present in all clients with the diagnosis, you can make a diagnosis even if your client does not have any of the minor defining characteristics. However, the more signs and symptoms you see that fit the picture, the more sure you can be that your diagnosis is valid.

> *Example:* If the client has the major defining characteristics, you could diagnose Colonic Constipation even if none of the following minor defining characteristics is present:
>
> **a.** Rectal pressure   **c.** Appetite impairment
> **b.** Headache   **d.** Abdominal pain

Even if *all* of these symptoms are present, though, you could not diagnose Colonic Constipation unless one of the major defining characteristics (such as straining at stool) is present. However if rectal pressure, headache, and appetite impairment are present *in addition to* one or two of the major defining characteristics, you would be even more certain that a diagnosis of Colonic Constipation is valid.

Related or Risk Factors

Related or **risk factors** are the conditions or situations that are associated with the problem in some way. They may, for instance, be conditions that precede, influence, cause, or contribute to the problem. They can be biological, psychological, social, developmental, treatment-related, situational, and so on. Each diagnostic label lists the related factors seen most often; however do not interpret this as a complete list of factors that *could* be associated with the label. Imagine, for example, the variety of situations/factors that could contribute in some way to Anxiety; it would be impossible to list them all.

Related factors are often, but not always, the etiologies of the diagnostic statement. A related factor may be a part of the etiology for several problems, or a single problem may have several related factors as its etiology.

> *Examples:*
>
> | Problem | Etiology |
> |---|---|
> | Altered Patterns of Sexuality | |
> | Constipation | Lack of privacy |
> | Sleep-Pattern Disturbance | |
>
> | Problem | Etiology |
> |---|---|
> | | Lack of privacy |
> | Constipation | Inadequate fiber intake |
> | | Inadequate fluid intake |

For potential nursing diagnoses, such as Risk for Fluid Volume Deficit, risk factors are similar to defining characteristics: they are the cues that must be present in order to make the diagnosis. Some risk nursing diagnoses list both risk factors and related factors. Risk factors are nearly always at least a part of the etiology of the risk diagnostic statement.

Example: Using the factors below, you might write the following diagnosis for a patient: "Risk for Fluid Volume Deficit related to increased urinary output secondary to diuretic medications."

Risk factors for the label Risk for Fluid Volume Deficit are: increased output, urinary frequency, thirst, altered intake

Related factors for the label Risk for Fluid Volume Deficit are: extremes of age, excessive losses through normal routes (e.g., diarrhea), medications (e.g., diuretics)

How to Choose the Correct Label

To choose the correct label, you simply match cue clusters with the definitions and defining characteristics of one of the NANDA labels. These are found in the *Nursing Diagnosis Guide* in the back of your text. Remember, though, that there are about 100 different labels, so random searching is not practical. Actually, by the time you are ready to choose a label, you should already have narrowed the possibilities. Recall that during data interpretation you identified the most likely explanation (problem and etiology) for each cluster of cues and decided which of your framework patterns fit it best. Finding labels on the list that appear to have the same meaning as your hypothesized explanation should then be a simple matter.

Refer again to Table 4–5 on page 107 in Chapter 4, the clustered abnormal cues for Luisa Sanchez. Cluster 11 is shown as follows:

Cluster 11 from Table 4–5   *Functional Health Pattern*
1. Cough productive of pale, pink sputum   Activity-Exercise (pattern
2. Respirations shallow   includes respiratory status)
3. Chest expansion < 3 cm
4. Inspiratory crackles through right chest
5. Mucous membranes pale
6. Diminished breath sounds on right side
7. Skin hot and pale

The nurse hypothesized the following explanation for Cluster 11:

Cues 1 through 4 are defining characteristics for the problem Ineffective Airway Clearance. This problem may be causing inadequate oxygenation, resulting in Cue 5. Cues 1, 6, and 7 are indicators of pneumonia, the medical problem that is creating the Ineffective Airway Clearance. Other problems are contributing as well: Fluid Volume Deficit is probably causing her mucus to be thick and hard to bring up (Cues 4 and 6); Pain and weakness are contributing to Cues 2 and 3.

The nurse concluded that this explanation represented an actual problem, and that the problem is a nursing diagnosis (not a collaborative or medical problem). Her informal problem statement was Ineffective Airway Clearance.

To find the appropriate NANDA label for this problem, you could simply look at an alphabetized list (such as the one inside the front cover of this text) for labels that seem related in some way to the explanation. You would, in this case, look for labels with words like *airway, breathing,* or *respiration.* Next, find the labels in your *Nursing Diagnosis Guide* and compare them to your cluster of cues.

Writing Diagnostic Statements

It is more efficient, though, to organize your list of diagnostic labels according to a theoretical framework (the same one you used to organize your data), so that related diagnoses are listed together. Since Luisa Sanchez's data analysis employed the Gordon Functional Health Patterns, you would look for your labels under the Activity-Exercise pattern in that table (see inside back cover). There are quite a few titles under this pattern, but certainly fewer than the 100 listed in the alphabetical table. Of the labels under Activity-Exercise, the only ones with possible connections (and some are remote, indeed) to Cluster 11 are the following:

Ineffective Airway Clearance   Impaired Gas Exchange
Ineffective Breathing Pattern

Next, look up the most likely sounding label in the *Nursing Diagnosis Guide*. Does the definition for Ineffective Airway Clearance match the nurse's explanation of the cues (Cluster 11)? Do the cues match the defining characteristics of that label? How about Ineffective Breathing Pattern? Does that fit better?

For Mrs. Sanchez, Ineffective Airway Clearance is the best-fitting label. She does not have enough of the defining characteristics for Impaired Gas Exchange or Ineffective Breathing Pattern. Notice, too, that one of Mrs. Sanchez's cues is found in the related factors listed for Ineffective Airway Clearance: decreased energy/fatigue. The complete nursing diagnosis for Mrs. Sanchez would be: Ineffective Airway Clearance related to thick secretions and shallow chest expansion secondary to pain, fluid volume deficit, and fatigue.

The diagnostic statements for Mrs. Sanchez's other cue clusters are given below. Compare the cue clusters in Table 4–5, on page 107, to the definitions and defining characteristics in your *Nursing Diagnosis Guide*. Notice that NANDA labels can be used for both problems and etiologies. Review information on human responses in Chapters 1 and 4 as needed. Recall that responses occur on many levels, and that a response can function as a stimulus that produces another response.

Cluster 1   No problem. Strengths are healthy lifestyle and understanding of and compliance with treatment regimens.

Cluster 2   Altered Nutrition: Less than Body Requirements related to decreased appetite and nausea, and increased metabolism secondary to disease process. (Note that this is a short-term problem that will be corrected primarily by medical treatment of her pneumonia. Meanwhile, though, she will need nutritional assessment and support.)

Cluster 3   Fluid Volume Deficit related to intake insufficient to replace fluid loss secondary to fever, diaphoresis, and nausea.

Cluster 4   Sleep Pattern Disturbance related to cough, pain, orthopnea, fever, and diaphoresis.

Cluster 5   No problem as long as medical regimen is followed.

Cluster 6   Self-Care Deficit (Level 2) related to Activity Intolerance secondary to Ineffective Airway Clearance and Sleep Pattern Disturbance.

Cluster 7   Altered Comfort: Chills related to fever and diaphoresis.

Cluster 8   Risk for Altered Family Processes related to mother's illness and temporary unavailability of father to provide child care. (Note that the defining characteristics for this diagnosis are not present in Cluster 8; however, there are risk factors.)

Cluster 9   Anxiety related to difficulty breathing and concerns over work and parenting roles.

Cluster 10 Chest Pain related to cough secondary to pneumonia.

Cluster 11 (See discussion on pages 102 to 103.)

The following collaborative problems (potential complications) complete the list of problems for Mrs. Sanchez:

Potential complications of pneumonia:

1. Respiratory insufficiency
2. Septic shock

Potential complications of intravenous therapy:

1. Inflammation
2. Phlebitis
3. Infiltration

Potential complications of antibiotic therapy:

1. Allergic reactions
2. Gastrointestinal upset
3. Other side effects, depending on specific medication

The potential complications do not require collaboration unless they develop into actual problems. The nurse independently monitors for all three; and the nurse can take independent action to prevent the potential complications of intravenous therapy. Because Mrs. Sanchez is not at higher risk than the usual population of pneumonia patients, individualized nursing diagnoses (such as Risk for Infection) are not written for these problems. They are prevented by the usual routines and standards of nursing care and will require no special interventions. This will be explained further in Chapter 9, "Creating a Patient-Care Plan."

FORMAT FOR WRITING THE DIAGNOSTIC STATEMENT

As shown in Box 5–2, ANA Standards of Care require diagnosis as a nursing function and specifically address format and content of diagnostic statements. NANDA provides the following definition of a nursing diagnosis, the product of diagnosing:

Writing Diagnostic Statements

A clinical judgment about individual, family, or community responses to actual and potential health problems/life processes. Nursing diagnoses provide the basis for selection of nursing interventions to achieve outcomes for which the nurse is accountable. (1994, p. 7)

As you have already learned, a diagnostic statement describes the patient's problem and the related or risk factors. This basic *Problem + Etiology* format varies slightly depending on whether you are writing a nursing diagnosis or a collaborative problem, and depending on problem status (actual, risk, or possible). Briefly, the *basic* components of a diagnostic statement are the following:

1. **Problem.** The problem part of the statement describes the client's health state clearly and concisely. Remember that it identifies what should be changed about the client's health status, so it should suggest client goals. Use the list of NANDA labels for this part of your statement when possible.

2. **Etiology.** The etiology describes factors causing or contributing to actual problems. For potential problems, it describes the risk factors that are present. NANDA does not use the term *etiology*; however, the factors causing or contributing to a problem are not limited to those listed in the NANDA related factors for a diagnostic label. The etiology may be a NANDA label, some of the defining characteristics, a NANDA risk factor or related factor, or something entirely outside the NANDA standardized language. The etiology enables you to individualize nursing care for a client. Even though the problem is the same, Impaired Verbal Communication related to *inability to speak English* would suggest different interventions than Impaired Verbal Communication secondary to *tracheostomy*.

3. ***Related to (r/t).*** This phrase connects the two parts of the statement. The phrase *due to* is not used because it implies a direct cause-and-effect relationship, which does not always hold for etiological factors in a nursing diagnosis.

Actual Nursing Diagnoses

When a client's signs and symptoms match the defining characteristics of a label, an actual diagnosis is present. Note that the word *actual* is assumed and not written in the diagnostic statement.

Box 5–2. ANA Standard II: Diagnosis, Criterion 3

Diagnoses are documented in a manner that facilitates the determination of expected outcomes and plan of care.

Source: Abstracted from American Nurses Association, *Standards of Clinical Nursing Practice* (Kansas City, MO: ANA, 1991), p. 9. Used with permission.

Basic Format: Two-Part Statement

The basic format for an actual nursing diagnosis consists of two parts: the problem and the etiology.

Problem	r/t	Etiology
↓		↓
(NANDA label)	r/t	(Related factors)
↓		↓
Self Esteem Disturbance	r/t	Being rejected by husband

Some NANDA labels contain the word *Specify.* For these you need to add words to indicate more specifically what the problem is.

Actual Nursing Diagnosis
Problem r/t Etiology

> ***Example:*** Noncompliance (*specify*)
> Noncompliance (*diabetic diet*) r/t unresolved anger about having diabetes

The NANDA labels in most listings are arranged with the qualifiers after the main word (Infection, Risk for) for ease of alphabetizing. Do not write your diagnoses in that manner; write them as you would say them in normal conversation.

> ***Example:*** *Incorrect:* Airway Clearance, Ineffective r/t weak cough reflex
> *Correct:* Ineffective Airway Clearance r/t weak cough reflex

P.E.S. Format

Besides Problem + Etiology, you may wish to include the defining characteristics as a part of your diagnostic statement. This is called the *P.E.S. format,* for "problem, etiology, and symptom." This method makes the statement more descriptive and adds the concept of validation to the diagnosis. The P.E.S. format is especially recommended when you are first learning to write nursing diagnoses. If you use this method, simply add *as manifested by (A.M.B.),* followed by the signs and symptoms that led you to make the diagnosis. Use the following format:

Problem	(r/t)	Etiology	(A.M.B.)	Symptoms
↓	↓	↓	↓	↓
(NANDA label)		(Related factors)		(Defining characteristics)
↓	↓	↓	↓	↓
Self-Esteem Disturbance	r/t	Being rejected by husband	A.M.B.	Hypersensitive to criticism; states, "I don't know if I can manage by myself." Rejects positive feedback.

Another example of the P.E.S. format follows. Notice that this method creates a very long statement.

P.E.S. Format
Problem r/t Etiology
A.M.B. *Symptoms*

> ***Example:*** Noncompliance (diabetic diet) r/t unresolved anger about diagnosis A.M.B. elevated blood pressure, 10-lb weight gain, and statements: "forget to take my pills," and "can't live without salt on my food."

Writing Diagnostic Statements

The signs and symptoms are often helpful in planning interventions for the nursing diagnosis, so it is important that they be easily accessible. If they result in a statement that is too long, you can record them in the nursing progress notes when you first make the diagnosis. This works especially well in a problem-oriented charting system. Another possibility, recommended for students, is to record the signs and symptoms *below* the nursing diagnosis, grouping the subjective and objective data.

> **Example:** Noncompliance (diabetic diet) r/t unresolved anger about diagnosis.
> S–"I forget to take my pills."
>   "I can't live without salt on my food."
> O–Weight 215 (gain of 10 lb)
>   B/P 190/100

A common error among beginning diagnosticians who use the P.E.S. format is to write a vague, nonspecific problem and etiology, hoping that the client's health status will be explained by listing the signs and symptoms. Guard against this tendency by making the Problem + Etiology as specific and descriptive as possible before adding the signs and symptoms. Your diagnostic statement should present a clear picture of your client's health status even without the listing of symptoms.

Variations on the Basic Format

There are several variations of the basic Problem + Etiology format. For any of these, you can add signs and symptoms (A.M.B.) as in the preceding example.

One-Part Statements   A few diagnostic statements can be made using the NANDA label (problem) without an etiology. As the diagnostic labels are refined, they tend to become more specific, so that the nursing interventions can be derived from the problem as well as from the etiology. Eventually all the labels may become so descriptive that it will not be necessary to include the etiology in the diagnostic statement. One label is already that specific: Rape-Trauma Syndrome.

For the following labels, it is difficult to think of an etiology other than a medical diagnosis, or if an etiology is written, it is somewhat redundant: Reflex Incontinence, Effective Breastfeeding, Post-Trauma Response, Defensive Coping. Reflex Incontinence, for instance, is fully described by its definition. The related factor is *neurological impairment* (e.g., spinal cord lesion that interferes with conduction of cerebral messages above the level of the reflex arc). As an etiology, this does not suggest nursing actions, nor does it really add to your understanding of the problem label, Reflex Incontinence. Similarly, the nursing interventions for Post-Trauma Response would be much the same regardless of whether the etiology is *related to war* or *related to earthquake.*

NANDA has specified that any new wellness diagnoses that are developed will be one-part diagnoses (for example, Potential for Enhanced Parenting).

Secondary to   Sometimes the diagnostic statement is clearer if the etiology is divided into two parts with the words *secondary to* (2°). The part following *secondary to* is often a pathophysiology or a disease process, as in "Risk for Impaired Skin Integrity r/t decreased peripheral circulation *2° diabetes.*"

Unknown Etiology   You can make a diagnosis when the defining characteristics are present, even if you do not know the cause or contributing factors. For instance, you might write, "Noncompliance (medication regimen) r/t unknown etiology."

Format for One Part Diagnosis

Problem (no etiology)

Format, Secondary to

Problem r/t Etiology 2°
pathophysiology

Format, Unkown Etiology

Problem r/t unknown Etiology

142

If you have reason to suspect an etiology, but still need more data to confirm it, use the phrase *possibly related to.* When you have confirming data you can rewrite the diagnosis more positively. You might say, for example, "Noncompliance (medication regimen) *possibly r/t* unresolved anger about diagnosis."

Complex Etiology   Occasionally there are too many etiological factors, or they are too complex to be stated in a brief phrase. The actual causes of Decisional Conflict or Chronic Low Self Esteem, for instance, may be long-term and complex. In such unusual cases, you can omit the etiology and replace it with the phrase *complex factors* (e.g., Chronic Low Self Esteem *r/t complex factors*).

Three-Part Statements   Some diagnostic labels consist of two parts: the first indicates a general response, and the second makes it more specific. Adding an etiology to these labels creates a three-part diagnosis; adding *secondary to* makes it four parts.

> **Examples:** Labels: Ineffective Family Coping: Disabling
>   Altered Nutrition: Less than Body
>   Requirements
>   Feeding Self Care Deficit (Level 3)
>
>   Nursing Diagnosis: Altered Nutrition: Less than Body
>   Requirements r/t nausea 2°
>   chemotherapy

You may need to add a third part to other NANDA labels as well. Diagnostic statements must precisely describe the client's health concern because general concepts and categorizations are ineffective for planning nursing care. Not all NANDA labels provide this level of precision. You can sometimes make them more descriptive by using the P.E.S. format or by using a two-part etiology with *secondary to,* as in the preceding example. However, this is not always a satisfactory solution. In order to make the labels more specific, you may need to add a colon and third part, using your own words. Notice that the following example does not indicate the *degree* of mobility, even though the etiology is very descriptive. Can the patient turn herself in bed? Can she transfer to the chair unassisted? Or can she not move her legs at all? In some cases, the label definition makes the problem more specific, but in this instance it does not offer much help.

> **Example:**   Impaired Physical Mobility r/t knee-joint stiffness and pain
>   secondary to muscle atrophy.
>
>   *Label Definition:* A state in which the individual experiences a limitation of
>   ability of independent physical movement.

To make the nursing diagnosis more specific, you should add a third part (descriptor):

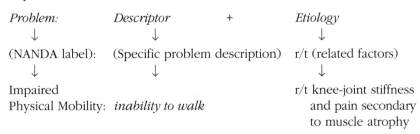

Problem:	*Descriptor*	+	*Etiology*
↓	↓		↓
(NANDA label):	(Specific problem description)		r/t (related factors)
↓	↓		↓
Impaired Physical Mobility:	*inability to walk*		r/t knee-joint stiffness and pain secondary to muscle atrophy

Format, Compex Etiology

Problem r/t complex factors

3-Part Statements

General Problem: Description r/t etiology

4-Part Statements

General Problem: Description r/t etiology 2° pathophysiology

Writing Diagnostic Statements

In the Impaired Physical Mobility example, using the P.E.S. format does not help, because the signs and symptoms are the same as the etiology: inability to walk. The statement can be improved by adding *secondary to* to the etiology: *2° muscle atrophy*. However, inability to walk is really a *type* of mobility problem rather than the *cause* of a mobility problem; therefore, it should not be used on the right side of the diagnostic statement in the etiology phrase. The most logical way to write the diagnosis is to add a colon and a more specific description to the general problem of Impaired Physical Mobility.

> ***Example:*** Impaired Physical Mobility r/t inability to walk
>
> *P.E.S.:* Impaired Physical Mobility r/t inability to walk A.M.B. inability to walk
>
> *Better:* Impaired Physical Mobility r/t inability to walk r/t muscle atrophy
>
> *Best:* Impaired Physical Mobility: Inability to walk 2° muscle atrophy
>
> *Format:* **General Problem: (Specific Descriptor) r/t Etiology**

Pain is another label that often needs an added third-part descriptor. Even when considered with its etiology and definition, it does not always fully specify the client's problem. In the example below, you cannot tell how severe the pain is or where it is located. In the *Better* example, words are added to make the diagnosis thoroughly descriptive and specific to the client. Notice that in the *Better* example, the NANDA label describes the general area of the problem, and the descriptor describes the specific type of problem in that area.

> ***Example:*** Pain related to fear of addiction to narcotics
>
> *Better:* Pain: Severe Headache r/t fear of addiction to narcotics

You may see this diagnosis written as "Pain r/t severe headache." However, headache is a *type* of pain, not the *cause* of pain; the second part of the statement is supposed to consist of etiological factors, not problems. Furthermore, while this statement clarifies the location and severity of the pain, it does not indicate the cause.

Risk for Infection and Altered Family Processes are other labels that may need a third part added to make them more specific. Risk for Infection can often be made more specific by adding *secondary to*. However, in the following example, the first statement does not indicate whether the client is at risk for systemic infection or a localized infection of a wound or incision.

> ***Example:*** Risk for Infection r/t susceptibility to pathogens 2° compromised immune system
>
> *Better:* Risk for Infection: Systemic r/t susceptibility to pathogens 2° compromised immune system, or
>
> Risk for Infection: Abdominal Incision r/t susceptibility to pathogens 2° compromised immune system

Remember that the diagnostic statement must thoroughly and specifically describe the problem and its causes (or risk factors). This is what dictates your format. In order to be fully descriptive, you will use *secondary to,* the P.E.S. format, qualifying words, a third-part descriptor, or a combination of these as needed.

Potential (Risk) Nursing Diagnoses

A potential (risk) nursing diagnosis is one that is likely to develop if the nurse does not intervene to prevent it. It is diagnosed by the presence of risk factors rather than defining characteristics. Risk nursing diagnoses have the same Problem + Etiology format as actual diagnoses—the client's risk factors form the etiology.

> ***Example:*** Risk for Impaired Skin Integrity (pressure sores) r/t *immobility 2° casts and traction*

Risk diagnoses may have most of the previously mentioned variations in format (e.g., one-part statement, three-part statement, multiple etiology). Of course the P.E.S. format cannot be used because the patient does not have signs and symptoms of the diagnosis—if signs and symptoms are present, the diagnosis is actual, not risk.

Possible Nursing Diagnoses

When you do not have enough data to confirm a diagnosis that you suspect is present, or when you can confirm the problem but not the etiology, write a *possible* nursing diagnosis. The word *possible* can be used in either the problem or the etiology. As in other kinds of diagnoses, the etiology may be multiple, complex, or unknown.

> ***Examples:*** *Possible Situational Low Self Esteem* related to loss of job and rejection by family
>
> Altered Thought Processes *possibly related to unfamiliar surroundings*
>
> *Possible Low Self Esteem* related to unknown etiology

Use *r/t unknown etiology* if you do not know the etiology; use *possibly r/t* if you suspect but cannot confirm the etiology. Remember, though, that etiologies are inferred, so you can never be *100%* certain an etiology is correct.

Collaborative Problems

Collaborative problems are complications of a disease, test, or treatment that nurses cannot treat independently. Nurses focus mainly on monitoring and preventing such problems. The etiologies of collaborative problems are likely to be diseases, treatments, or pathologies. Notice in the following example that with the usual Problem + Etiology format, the etiology does not suggest nursing interventions.

> ***Example:*** (Incorrect) Potential for Increased Intracranial Pressure r/t head injury

Carpenito (1993) suggests using the phrase *potential complication* to describe collaborative problems. The diagnostic statement should include both the possible complication you are monitoring for and the disease, treatment, or other factors that produce it. In the following example, you would monitor for signs and symptoms of increased intracranial pressure that might result from the patient's head injury.

Format for Writing the Diagnostic Statement

Risk Problems

Risk Problem (r/t) Risk Factors

Possible Problems

Possible Problem (r/t) Actual or Possible Etiology

145

Writing Diagnostic Statements

> *Example:* Potential Complication of Head Injury: Increased Intracranial Pressure

Sometimes you will be monitoring for a *group* of complications associated with a disease or pathology. In that case, state the disease and follow it with a list of the complications.

> *Example:* Potential Complications of Pregnancy-Induced Hypertension:
>
> | | |
> |---|---|
> | Seizures | Hepatic or renal failure |
> | Fetal distress | Premature labor |
> | Pulmonary edema | CNS hemorrhage |

The P.E.S. format is not used for collaborative diagnoses because they are usually potential problems. The patient does not have the signs and symptoms—you are monitoring to see if they occur.

For some collaborative problems an etiology can be helpful in planning interventions; for example, the complication may be caused by something more specific than a disease process. While you are a student, you should write the etiology, as in the following examples, (1) when it clarifies your statement, (2) when it can be concisely stated, or (3) when it helps to suggest nursing actions.

Collaborative Problems

Potential Complication of disease or treatment: (Specify Complication)

> *Example:*
>
> | Disease/Situation | Complication | r/t Etiology |
> |---|---|---|
> | ↓ | ↓ | ↓ |
> | Potential complication of *childbirth:* | Hemorrhage | r/t 1. uterine atony 2. retained placental fragments 3. bladder distention |
> | ↓ | ↓ | ↓ |
> | Potential complication of *diuretic therapy:* | Arrhythmias | r/t low serum potassium |

EVALUATING THE QUALITY OF THE DIAGNOSTIC STATEMENT

In addition to using the correct format for your diagnostic statements, you must consider the quality of their content. They should, for example, be accurate, concise, descriptive, and specific.

Relationship of Nursing Diagnoses to Outcomes and Nursing Orders

The first part of the diagnostic statement (the problem) states what needs to change, thus it determines the goals needed to measure this change. In the example below, the goal would be to relieve the anxiety.

> *Example:* Anxiety r/t lack of knowledge of scheduled venogram
> ↓
> **Goals** (Outcomes)

The second part of the diagnostic statement (the etiology) identifies factors causing or contributing to the actual problem, or the risk factors for a risk problem. In many cases the etiology serves to direct the nursing interventions. In the preceding example, the etiology suggests a nursing order for patient teaching. In addition to teaching the patient about the venogram, though, the nurse would probably intervene more directly to relieve the anxiety—for instance, by helping the patient to recognize and express his anxiety. As you can see, nursing interventions can be directed by either part of the diagnostic statement.

> ***Example:*** Anxiety   r/t   Lack of knowledge of scheduled venogram
>   ↓   ↓
>   **Nursing**   **Nursing**
>   **Orders**   **Orders**

Like Anxiety, a few other problem labels call for particular nursing interventions regardless of the cause of the problem, for example: Decisional Conflict, Fear, Hopelessness, Ineffective Denial, and Risk for Violence.

As the NANDA labels become more specific, you will probably discover more instances in which the etiology cannot be treated by independent nursing actions, and both the goals and nursing orders will be determined by the problem. In the example below, the nurse cannot treat a spinal cord lesion. Both the goals and nursing orders are suggested by "Reflex Incontinence."

> ***Example:*** Reflex Incontinence   r/t   spinal cord lesion
>   ↙   ↘
>   **Goals & Nursing Orders**

When possible, you should rewrite the etiology so that it will provide direction for nursing intervention. Usually this means replacing a disease or medical condition with a principle or pathophysiology. This is not necessary for experienced nurses.

> ***Example:*** Risk for Infection r/t *surgical incision*
>
> *Rewritten:* Risk for Infection r/t *portal of entry for pathogens* 2° surgical incision

In every case, the nurse should be able to prescribe definitive prevention and treatment for at least one side of the nursing diagnosis.

Thinking Critically about the Content of the Diagnostic Statement

After writing your diagnostic statements, judge them against the following criteria.

1. **The statement is precise and clear.** It uses terminology generally understood by other professionals and avoids jargon or abbreviations.

> ***Example:***
>
> *Incorrect:* Toileting Self Care Deficit r/t inability to get *OOB w/o* help
>
> *Correct:* Toileting Self Care Deficit r/t inability to get *out of bed without* help

Writing Diagnostic Statements

2. The statement is accurate and valid. Nurses sometimes err by associating certain diagnoses with a particular patient condition, regardless of whether the defining characteristics are present. For example, a common error is to diagnose Fluid Volume Deficit or Altered Nutrition: Less Than Body Requirements for a patient simply because the patient has a medical order of "nothing by mouth." (See *Nursing Diagnosis Guide* for discussion of this practice.) Statements are accurate and valid when they meet the following criteria:

a. Patient's signs and symptoms match NANDA defining characteristics.

b. For risk problems, patient's risk factors match NANDA risk factors.

c. The patient has validated the diagnosis.

3. The statement is concise. Using NANDA labels helps to keep the problem statement brief.

a. If etiological factors are wordy and involved, use *r/t complex etiology.*

b. If P.E.S. format produces a long statement, list the signs and symptoms under the diagnostic statement.

Example: Self Esteem Disturbance related to longstanding feelings of failure aggravated by recently being rejected by her husband as manifested by being hypersensitive to criticism, stating, "I don't know if I can manage by myself," rejecting positive feedback, and not making eye contact

> *Better:* Self Esteem Disturbance r/t complex factors
> S—"I don't know if I can manage by myself."
> O—Hypersensitive to criticism, rejects positive feedback, no eye contact.

4. The statement is descriptive and specific. The diagnostic statement should *fully* describe the client's problem. This criterion should be met even if it makes the statement longer than you would like. The NANDA label alone is usually very general (e.g., Parental Role Conflict); it is made more specific by

a. knowledge of the label definition. (Check the NANDA definition to see if it makes the label more specific.)

b. adding the etiology to make the complete problem statement.

c. adding the patient's defining characteristics (P.E.S. format).

If the statement is still not descriptive enough, make it more specific by

d. adding qualifying words (e.g., *mild, moderate, intermittent*).

e. adding *secondary to* in the etiology.

f. adding a third part (a colon and a more specific problem).

Example: Pain related to fear of addiction to narcotics.

> *Better:* Pain: *Severe headache* r/t fear of addiction to narcotics

5. Cause and effect are correctly stated; that is, the etiology causes the problem, or the etiology puts the client at risk for the potential problem. Consider the following example, comparing correct and incorrect diagnoses.

Example:

Correct: Altered Oral Mucous Membrane r/t fluid volume deficit A.M.B. xerostomia and oral leisions

Incorrect: Fluid Volume Deficit r/t altered oral mucous membrane A.M.B. xerostomia and oral lesions

To check this, insert the parts of your diagnostic statement in this sentence format (reading your statement backwards):

"(Etiology) causes (Problem)."

Example: Dysfunctional Grieving r/t inability to accept death of spouse

Read Backwards:

Inability to accept death of spouse *causes* Dysfunctional Grieving

    ↑   ↑   ↑

  (Etiology)   *causes*   *(Problem)*

Example: Risk for Infection r/t interruption of body's first line of defense 2° abdominal incision

Read Backwards:

Abd. incision *causes* break in 1st line of defense, *which causes* Risk for Infection

  ↑   ↑   ↑   ↑   ↑

(Secondary) *causes* *(Etiology)*   *which then causes*   *(Problem)*

If cause and effect are correctly stated, the sentence will make sense when read backwards.

6. **At least one side of the statement provides direction for nursing actions.** If you cannot prescribe the interventions to change either the problem or the etiology, then you should reevaluate the diagnosis. Perhaps what you have identified as the "problem," is actually the stimulus for other problematic human responses. In the following example, the nurse cannot change what was first identified as a "hearing problem." However, the hearing problem produced a social interaction problem, which the nurse *can* address.

   a. Nursing diagnoses suggest independent nursing actions to treat or prevent.

   Example:

   Incorrect: Sensory/Perceptual Alteration (Auditory) r/t progressive hearing loss 2° nerve degeneration

   Correct: Impaired Social Interaction r/t embarrassment at being unable to follow conversations r/t progressive hearing loss 2° nerve degeneration

   b. Collaborative problems suggest independent nursing interventions to detect and prevent.

7. **The statement uses nonjudgmental language.**

   Example: *Incorrect:* Risk for Injury: Falls r/t *poor housekeeping*

                  Better: Risk for Injury: Falls r/t *cluttered floors*

8. **The statement uses legally advisable language.** It should not affix blame or refer negatively to aspects of patient care.

   Example:

Incorrect	*Correct*
Impaired Skin Integrity: Pressure Sores r/t *not being turned frequently enough*	Impaired Skin Integrity: Pressure Sores r/t *inability to turn self*

9. **The problem side of the statement contains only one diagnostic label.**

   Example:

Incorrect	*Correct*
Risk for Fluid Volume Deficit and Constipation related to inadequate fluid intake	Constipation related to inadequate fluid intake.

10. **The etiology is not merely a rewording of the problem.**

    Example:

Incorrect	*Correct*
Chronic Pain r/t headache	Chronic Pain (Headache) r/t unknown etiology

11. **The complete list of nursing diagnoses and collaborative problems reflects the client's health status.** Although collaborative problems are not always written on the nursing care plan, the master problem list for the client should include all the client's collaborative problems, as well as the actual, risk, and possible nursing diagnoses. A complete list will enable you to plan all the nursing care the client requires.

12. **The statement does not include any of the errors described in Table 4–2 on page 105** (e.g., stating a patient need, nursing action, or medical diagnosis, test, or treatment instead of a problematic human response).

WELLNESS DIAGNOSES

Wellness diagnoses are especially useful for essentially healthy clients, such as school children or new parents, who require teaching for health promotion, disease prevention, and personal growth. Presently, there are a number of ways to label healthy responses. The approach you choose depends somewhat on the type of client you are working with.

Because the NANDA diagnostic labels primarily describe health problems, they do not work well for labeling healthy responses. NANDA does, however, include wellness as a nursing focus and encourages nurses to submit new wellness diagnoses for approval. Following is the NANDA definition of a wellness diagnosis.

> **Wellness diagnoses** "describe human responses to levels of wellness in an individual, family, or community that have a potential for enhancement to a higher state" (1994, p. 102).

New wellness diagnoses are preceded by the phrase *Potential for Enhanced,* and will be one-part statements (e.g., Potential for Enhanced Parenting).

Using NANDA Wellness Labels

The following wellness labels are included in the NANDA taxonomy:

Potential for Enhanced Spiritual Well-Being
Family Coping: Potential for Growth
Effective Breastfeeding
Anticipatory Grieving
Health Seeking Behaviors

The following wellness labels are included in the diagnoses in progress (see Appendix E), but are in early states of validation and should be used cautiously:

Potential for Enhanced Community Coping
Family Coping: Potential for Growth
Effective Management of Therapeutic Regimen: Individual
Potential for Enhanced Organized Infant Behavior

Health Seeking Behaviors provides a clear focus for planning interventions without indicating that a problem exists. This is a specific diagnosis, however, to be used for those with "expressed or observed desire to seek a higher level of wellness" (NANDA, 1990, p. 117). Health Seeking Behaviors—like Enhanced Family Coping and Effective Breastfeeding—is essentially for use with well clients, but these labels might be used for clients with chronic diseases who have the required defining characteristics.

Expressing NANDA Problem Labels in Positive Terms

Another way to write wellness diagnoses is to use the NANDA diagnostic labels but express them in positive terms, using *Potential for Enhanced, Maintenance of,* or other positive qualifiers (e.g., Maintenance of Positive Body Image, Potential for Enhanced Parenting, Effective Individual Coping). This works well for clients who are ill and who have only a few healthy responses; expressing all the healthy responses of a well person in this fashion would produce an unmanageable number of diagnoses.

Using this method to describe healthy responses in ill clients presents difficulties, however. Hospitalized clients usually have many nursing diagnoses and collaborative problems. From a practical standpoint, you can address only a limited number of diagnoses during the course of a workday; so you will usually prioritize a patient's diagnoses and address the high-priority ones first. Because wellness diagnoses are usually lower in priority than actual and potential health problems, they may never be addressed.

Using Patient Strengths

For ill clients, perhaps a better way to describe healthy responses is to identify strengths to use in planning interventions for the other problems you identify. Concluding that there is no problem in a pattern does not necessarily indicate the need for a diagnostic statement. It is quite acceptable to identify healthy responses as strengths rather than writing them as wellness diagnoses. Especially

Writing Diagnostic Statements

in short-term situations, it is better to label a pattern with "No problem," since there may not be time to carry out the health-promotion interventions a wellness diagnosis would suggest. Following are some examples of patient strengths:

Pattern	Strength
Communicating	Communicates adequately in dominant language
Relating	Stable family situation
	Adequate financial support (works only part-time)

Modifications of the NANDA Taxonomy

The Bureau of Community Health Nursing, Missouri Department of Health, uses the NANDA labels, but with special modifiers that reflect wellness. Box 5–3 presents this taxonomy of wellness diagnoses. The community health nurses in Multnomah County, Oregon, have also modified the NANDA taxonomy by adding wellness diagnoses based on Gordon's Functional Health Patterns (e.g., "Intake of nutrients sufficient but not in excess of metabolic need") (Multnomah County Health Services Division, 1987).

Box 5–3. Missouri Department of Health—Modified NANDA Taxonomy of Wellness Diagnoses

Activity/Rest
Adequate diversional activity
Healthy sleep pattern

Ego Integrity
Effective individual coping
Healthy self-esteem

Food/Fluid
Adequate fluid volume
Effective infant feeding pattern
Nutrition adequate to meet body requirements

Neurosensory
Appropriate sensory perception
Appropriate thought processes

Respiration
Effective airway clearance
Effective breathing pattern
Adequate gas exchange

Teaching/Learning
Compliance (specify)
Appropriate growth and development
Adequate knowledge (specify)
Effective management of therapeutic regimen (individual)

Sexuality
Adequate sexual function

Circulation
Adequate cardiac output
Adequate tissue perfusion

Elimination
Adequate bowel elimination
Adequate urinary elimination

Hygiene
Adequate self-care (specify)

Pain/Comfort
Pain free

Safety
Adequate health maintenance
Adequate home maintenance management
Adequate protection

Social Interaction
Effective family coping
Adequate family processes
Adequate parenting
Effective social interaction

Adapted by permission of Missouri Department of Health, Bureau of Community Health, "List of Nursing Diagnoses," *PHN Manual*, Subsection 200.51, pp. 6–7, 1994.

ETHICAL CONSIDERATIONS

With regard to ethics there is, first of all, the possibility of objectifying patients by overemphasizing the need to label their problems. This can be avoided if you make a conscious effort to think holistically, treating the patient rather than the problem.

The diagnostic process is not value-free. The nurse's values may lead her to emphasize or ignore certain data during assessment, affecting her choice of diagnoses. The resulting diagnoses direct the care the patient will receive and the way the patient is viewed and treated by others. Furthermore, if biased data result in missed or inaccurate diagnoses, the patient will not receive proper care.

> *Example:*   A nurse values safety over autonomy. When he cares for an elderly client, he is quick to diagnose Altered Thought Processes r/t aging A.M.B. confusion and disorientation. The nurse did not take into account that confusion is a side effect of one of the client's medications. As a result of this diagnosis, other nurses perceive the client as needing more supervision than he actually does. Gradually, the client loses his autonomy and becomes more dependent.

Even if the diagnostic process could be value-neutral, the phrasing of a statement can have ethical implications. A diagnosis that is stated in value-laden terms may influence other caregivers in their treatment of the patient. The etiology is the part of the diagnosis most likely to harbor negative or judgmental terms, because it is often complex and not stated in standardized language.

> *Examples:* Ineffective Family Coping r/t *sexual promiscuity of the mother*
>
> Anxiety r/t *unrealistic expectations of others*

The problem side of the diagnostic statement can also cause difficulty, because the NANDA diagnostic labels themselves are not entirely value-free. *Noncompliance* implies to some people that the patient is not cooperating as he should; this can negatively affect the attitude of other nurses toward that patient (Keeling, et al., 1993). Carpenito (1989, p. 42) points out that a well-written etiology can remove some of the stigma from such labels, as in the following: "Noncompliance related to the negative side effects of the drug (reduced libido, fatigue)." Geissler (1991) suggests *Nonadherence* as a less value-laden term than *Noncompliance*.

Some diagnostic labels can be perceived as negative because of the nurse's values. *Anxiety* carries a negative connotation for nurses who value strength and self-control; they may see the patient as weak or unworthy of attention. *Knowledge Deficit* may imply lack of ability or lack of motivation to learn, either of which could evoke a negative reaction from those caregivers who place a high value on learning. To diagnose in an ethical manner, you must be aware of your values and their influence on the diagnostic process. You must realize the possible effect of your diagnostic statements on other caregivers and try to phrase them in neutral, nonjudgmental language.

CULTURAL CONSIDERATIONS

Many nurses (for example, Leininger, 1990) believe that NANDA nursing diagnoses are not culturally sensitive. In a study of Impaired Verbal Communication, Impaired Social Interaction, and Noncompliance, Geissler (1992) concluded that cultural factors are not adequately represented in NANDA "related

Writing Diagnostic Statements

factors." This can lead to misdiagnosis of problem etiologies. It may help you to remember that diagnoses represent responses that clients and families find problematic from *their* perspective, cultural or otherwise. Undoubtedly, all problems and etiologies are influenced by cultural factors. However, the following labels have been specifically identified as having a strong cultural dimension (Carpenito, 1993; Heliker, 1992; McFarland and McFarlane, 1993):

Impaired Verbal Communication	Anxiety
Altered Health Maintenance	Fear
Health Seeking Behaviors	Ineffective Individual Coping
Ineffective Family Coping	Decisional Conflict
Altered Role Performance	Impaired Social Interaction
Sleep Pattern Disturbance	Altered Nutrition
Pain	Effective Breastfeeding

SPIRITUAL DIAGNOSES

Spirituality both affects and is affected by a person's health status. From a holistic perspective, then, nurses need to be able to describe problems of spirituality. The one NANDA label that relates to spiritual problems is Spiritual Distress (Distress of the Human Spirit). Potential for Enhanced Spiritual Well-Being is a diagnosis in progress that was added in 1994 (see Appendix E). O'Brien (1982, p. 81) further categorizes spiritual distress as follows:

✓ *Spiritual pain*: Difficulty accepting the loss of a loved one or intense physical or emotional suffering
✓ *Spiritual alienation*: Separation from religious or faith community
✓ *Spiritual anxiety*: Challenge to beliefs and value systems (e.g., by moral implications of therapy, such as abortion or blood transfusion)
✓ *Spiritual guilt*: Failure to abide by religious rules
✓ *Spiritual anger*: Difficulty accepting illness, loss, or suffering
✓ *Spiritual loss*: Difficulty finding comfort in religion
✓ *Spiritual despair*: Feeling that no one cares

The following diagnoses may also be helpful in describing a client's spiritual status:

Hopelessness	Fear
Powerlessness	Dysfunctional Grieving
Ineffective Individual or Family Coping	Self Esteem Disturbance
Decisional Conflict	Sleep Pattern Disturbance

LEARNING TO RECOGNIZE THE NANDA LABELS

As you become familiar with the diagnostic labels, it will be easier to recognize cue clusters in your patients—it is always easier to see something if you know what you are looking for. The best way to learn the labels is by using them; however, like most clinical skills, you need a certain degree of familiarity in order to use them. "Applying the Nursing Process," at the end of this chapter, will help you learn what the labels mean. Refer to your *Nursing Diagnosis Guide* frequently. It includes definitions and defining characteristics for each of the labels, as well as suggestions for situations in which they may or may not be useful. Detailed discussion of problematic labels is included.

Recording the Diagnoses

RECORDING THE DIAGNOSES

After validating and labeling the nursing diagnoses, you will write them in priority order in the appropriate documents: either the client's chart or the care plan. In some documentation systems, nursing diagnoses are recorded on a multidisciplinary problem list at the front of the client record (chart). In many agencies the care plan becomes a part of the client's permanent record on dismissal, so diagnoses should be written in ink. When a diagnosis is resolved or changed, you can draw a single line through it or mark over it with a highlighter pen. Some care plans include a space beside the diagnosis to write the date the diagnosis is resolved or discontinued.

Prioritizing Diagnoses

Prioritizing is sometimes considered a part of the planning step of the nursing process, but if the diagnoses are to be recorded in priority order, then prioritizing must occur in the diagnosis step. Priorities are assigned on the basis of the nurse's judgment and the client's preferences. You can rank the diagnoses from highest to lowest priority (i.e., 1, 2, 3, etc.), or you can assign each problem a high, medium, or low priority. Prioritizing problems helps to assure that care is given first for the more important problems. This does not necessarily mean that one problem must be resolved before you address another.

Example: Bathing Self Care Deficit might be a long-term problem for a patient. This does not mean you should wait until the patient can bathe himself before addressing the next highest priority, Risk for Constipation.

You should also consider risk problems when setting priorities. It is often as important to prevent a problem as it is to treat an actual one.

Example: For a poorly nourished, immobile patient, Risk for Impaired Skin Integrity is of higher priority than actual Diversional Activity Deficit.

Preservation of Life
If you use preservation of life as a criterion, you would rate the client's diagnoses high, medium, or low based on the amount of threat they pose to the client's life. Life-threatening problems would take priority over those that cause pain or discomfort. A **high-priority problem** is one that is life-threatening, such as severe fluid and electrolyte loss or respiratory obstruction. A **medium-priority problem** does not directly threaten life, but it may produce destructive physical or emotional changes (e.g., Rape-Trauma Syndrome). A **low-priority problem** is one that arises from normal developmental needs, or requires only minimal supportive nursing intervention (e.g., Altered Sexuality Patterns related to knowledge deficit). After assigning high, medium, and low priorities, you can rank the diagnoses from most to least important.

155

Writing Diagnostic Statements

Example:

Rank	Diagnosis	Priority
1	Fluid Volume Deficit related to vomiting	Medium
2	Sleep Pattern disturbance . . .	Low
3	Diversional Activity Deficit . . .	Low

Maslow's Hierarchy

Maslow's Hierarchy of Human Needs also provides a good framework for prioritizing nursing diagnoses. Recall from Chapter 3 that in Maslow's model there are five levels of human needs. Starting with the most basic (highest priority) need, they are: physiologic, safety and security, social, esteem and self-actualization. As a rule, the more basic needs must be met before the client can deal with the higher needs.

Kalish (1983) has made Maslow's system even more useful by dividing the physiological needs into survival and stimulation needs. Survival needs are the most basic; only when they are satisfied can the client be concerned about higher-level needs. When survival needs are met, the client tries to meet stimulation needs before moving up the hierarchy to safety, social, and other higher needs. Kalish's division of physiological needs includes the following:

Survival Needs: Food, air, water, temperature, elimination, rest, pain avoidance

Stimulation Needs: Sex, activity, exploration, manipulation, novelty

In this framework, diagnoses involving survival needs have priority over those involving stimulation needs.

Example: The following diagnoses are ranked from highest to lowest priority:

Need	Nursing Diagnosis
Survival	Altered Nutrition: Less Than Body Requirements related to fatigue
Stimulation	Diversional Activity Deficit related to infectious disease isolation
Esteem	Chronic Low Self Esteem related to inability to perform role functions

Patient Preference

As much as possible, patient preference should be considered in priority setting. You should give high priority to the problems the patient feels are important, as long as this does not interfere with survival needs or medical treatments. Because she is exhausted after delivery, a new mother's first priority may be to sleep. However, you must observe her closely for signs of postpartum hemorrhage, so you cannot safely follow her priorities in this situation. If you explain your priorities, you may be able to persuade the patient to agree with them.

Attending to problems that are high priorities for the patient increases the likelihood that they will be successfully resolved: the patient will cooperate most enthusiastically to solve problems she considers important. As in the following example, she may not be motivated to address other problems until her main concerns are dealt with.

Example: Pat Sams is an 18-year-old who has just had her first baby. The nurse knows she must teach Ms. Sams how to bathe her infant before she is dismissed—within 24 hours after delivery. The nurse has given highest priority to Ms. Sams' Knowledge Deficit diagnosis. However, Ms. Sams finds it difficult to concentrate on the bath demonstration. She is hoping the baby's father will come to visit, and has been washing her hair and putting on makeup. She has not heard from him since coming to the hospital, and she is worried he will not want to see her and the baby.

Summary

SUMMARY

Diagnostic statements
- ✓ use North American Nursing Diagnosis Association (NANDA) labels.
- ✓ use the format of Problem related to (r/t) Etiology (or the P.E.S.variation).
- ✓ are varied by one-part statements, use of *secondary to,* unknown and complex etiologies, and three-part statements.
- ✓ should be descriptive, accurate, and specific, using nonjudgmental, legally advisable language.
- ✓ can be used to describe the health responses of individuals, families, or communities.
- ✓ are not value-free and require nurses to be aware of their own values and the perceptions of others.
- ✓ have ethical, cultural, and spiritual dimensions.
- ✓ may describe wellness states as well as health problems.
- ✓ should be recorded on the care plan in priority order.

Scientists often make mental models to describe particular aspects of nature and to help us better understand various phenomena. For example, in the Bohr model of the atom, electrons orbit the nucleus much as moons orbit a planet. To cite a more familiar example, the nursing frameworks discussed in Chapters 3 and 4 are models that describe particular aspects of nursing. In the Roy model, for instance, nursing activity is described as promoting adaptation of the individual.

Practice in Critical Thinking: Comparing and Contrasting

You might create a model to understand something you encounter in everyday life. For instance, a model for an ideal teacher should include things like what kinds of lessons the teacher designs, what he lets students do in class, how he encourages you to think about the subject you are studying, or whether the tests are based on the stated objectives for the course. Such a model could provide a reference point to help you describe and understand a real teacher.

Here are some steps you might use when comparing real occurrences to a model:

1. List the important characteristics or behavior of the model.

2. Ask yourself if the real thing behaves like the model with regard to these same characteristics.

3. Considering the characteristics you identified in Step 2, determine what features of the real occurrence make it different from the model.

Learning the Skill
Use the three steps outlined above to compare your model of an ideal nurse with the behavior of real nurses.

1. *Use Step 1.* List the important characteristics that you think describe the ideal nurse.

2. *Use Step 2.* Considering each of the points you listed in (1), compare the behavior of someone you consider to be a typical nurse to the ideal nurse—perhaps someone you have observed during your clinical experiences.

3. *Use Step 3.* In (1) and (2) you have compared the behavior of typical and ideal nurses in a number of ways. Considering each of these points, explain why your typical nurse behaves differently from your ideal nurse.

Applying the Skill

1. This chapter presented several models of ideal diagnostic statements. The basic format of a nursing diagnosis is **Problem r/t Etiology.** List the variations of this model.

2. The chapter section "Thinking Critically about the Content of the Diagnostic Statement" provides another model of a diagnostic statement. List the qualities of an ideal diagnostic statement provided by this model.

3. Borrow a care plan from another student or copy at least six nursing diagnoses from a care plan in your clinical agency. Discuss whether or not real diagnoses are the same as the ideal diagnoses with regard to qualities listed in Steps 1 and 2 of this section.

4. If you did note a difference in Step 3, explain why a typical diagnosis might be different from the ideal diagnoses.

Adapted from *Critical Thinking Worksheets*, a Supplement of *Addison-Wesley Chemistry*, by Wilbraham et al. (Menlo Park, CA: Addison-Wesley Publishing Company, 1990).

Refer to your *Nursing Diagnosis Guide* as often as necessary when working the following exercises. Many of the exercises are designed to help you become familiar with the *Guide* and with NANDA labels.

1. Identify the underlined parts of the nursing diagnoses by writing the correct terms beneath them. Use these terms:

Label   Related factors   Qualifying term
Defining characteristics   Risk factors

    a. Risk for <u>Body Image Disturbance</u> r/t amputation of right leg

        _____

    b. Risk for Body Image Disturbance r/t <u>amputation of right leg</u>

                        _____

    c. Severe <u>Chronic Pain</u> r/t knowledge deficit (effects of exercise and rest)

        _____

    d. <u>Severe</u> Chronic Pain r/t knowledge deficit (effects of exercise and rest)

        _____

    e. Severe Chronic Pain r/t <u>knowledge deficit (effects of exercise and rest)</u>

                _____

2. Choose the most likely etiology for each of the following problems from the numbered list.

    a. Risk for Infection r/t ___
    b. Activity Intolerance r/t ___
    c. Altered Parenting r/t ___
    d. Fluid Volume Deficit r/t ___
    e. Possible Sexual Dysfunction r/t ___

    1. insufficient oxygenation for activities of daily living
    2. compromised immune system
    3. increased fluid loss secondary to vomiting
    4. delayed parent-infant contact 2° illness of infant
    5. body image disturbance 2° mastectomy

3. Place a *C* beside the correctly written nursing diagnoses.

    a. ___ Risk for Infection Transmission r/t lack of knowledge about communicable nature of the disease

    b. ___ Altered Oral Mucous Membrane r/t dry mouth

    c. ___ Elevated Temperature r/t infectious process

    d. ___ Constipation r/t inadequate fiber intake and prolonged bedrest

    e. ___ Risk for Impaired Skin Integrity r/t prescribed bedrest

    f. ___ Impaired Skin Integrity r/t prescribed bedrest

    g. ___ Rape-Trauma Syndrome

    h. ___ Acute Back Pain r/t unknown etiology

    i. ___ Impaired Skin Integrity r/t not being repositioned often enough

    j. ___ Crying r/t anxiety

4. Circle the risk factors. Underline the related factors.

    a. Fear r/t progressive loss of vision

    b. Risk for Anxiety r/t possibility of going blind

    c. Possible Fluid Volume Deficit r/t post-op NPO

    d. Pain r/t effects of surgery

    e. Grieving r/t recent loss of job

5. Write a diagnostic statement for each of the following cases. Refer to *Nursing Diagnosis Guide*.

    a. A hypertensive client states that she hasn't been taking her medication because it doesn't make her feel any better. Also, she says she has difficulty remembering to take it.

    b. An elderly patient with left-side paralysis has a red, broken area in the skin over his coccyx. The patient cannot turn himself in bed.

    c. The client is 45 pounds overweight. He states that he is in a high-stress job and doesn't have time to cook regular meals—he tends to eat fast food and snacks a lot. His job is sedentary, and he does not engage in any type of physical exercise or sport. For fun, he likes to "eat at a nice restaurant."

d. A client is two hours postoperative vaginal hysterectomy. Her blood pressure has dropped from 130/80 to 100/60, and her pulse is 90. She is slightly pale, but not cyanotic. She has a 4 cm × 4 cm spot of blood on her vaginal pad. Her abdomen is firm and tender to the touch, but not distended.

e. A client with pelvic inflammatory disease has just tested positive for gonorrhea. She states that she has unprotected sex.

6. Circle the labels that are NANDA-approved terminology.

Altered Nutrition: More Than Body Requirements

Altered Body Temperature

Diarrhea

Risk for Infection

Altered Bowel Elimination

Risk for Aspiration

Social Isolation

Anorexia

Constipation

Altered Protection

Activity Intolerance

7. Circle the labels that require additional words to make the problem more specific (e.g., Feeding Self Care Deficit, Level 3).

a. Activity Intolerance

b. Stress Incontinence

c. Sensory/Perceptual Alteration

d. Chronic Pain

e. Impaired Physical Mobility

f. Fatigue

g. Ineffective Breastfeeding

h. Colonic Constipation

8. For each of the labels you circled in item 7, write an example of words you might add to make the problem more specific.

9. Supply the label that fits the following definitions. Refer to the *Nursing Diagnosis Guide* in the back of this text as needed.

a. _____ A state in which an individual experiences a change in normal bowel habits characterized by involuntary passage of stool

b. _____ A state in which an individual experiences a change in normal bowel habits characterized by the frequent passage of loose, fluid, unformed stools

c. _____ Impairment of adaptive behaviors and problem-solving abilities of a person in meeting life's demands and roles

d. _____ The state in which an individual is at risk for entry of gastrointestinal secretions, oropharyngeal secretions, or solids or fluids into tracheobronchial passages

e. _____ A state in which an individual is unable to clear secretions or obstructions from the respiratory tract to maintain airway patency

10. Match the diagnostic label with the defining characteristics.

a. Ineffective Airway Clearance

b. Ineffective Breathing Patterns

c. Sensory/Perceptual Alterations (specify)

d. Social Isolation

e. Impaired Social Interactions

f. Impaired Swallowing

___ **1.** Abnormal breath sounds, tachypnea, ineffective cough (with or without sputum), cyanosis, dyspnea, changes in rate or depth of respiration

___ **2.** *Major:* Inaccurate interpretation of environmental stimuli
Minor: Restlessness

___ **3.** Expressed feelings of aloneness
Feels rejected; says time passes slowly

___ **4.** Changes in respiratory rate and pattern; change in pulse; orthopnea

___ **5.** Reports inability to establish stable, supportive relationships; poor impulse control

___ **6.** *Major:* Observed evidence of difficulty in swallowing (e.g., stasis of food in oral cavity, coughing/choking)

11. Write the label that fits the following cue clusters. Compare the cue clusters to the defining characteristics in the *Nursing Diagnosis Guide*. You do not need to write etiologies.

a. _____

Mr. Maier has been hospitalized with a heart attack. He has been told he needs to rest and avoid stress. He says his advertising agency cannot run without him, and he phones the office several times a day to check on things and give instructions. He tells them he will be back to work "in a few days." He says he doesn't believe this is really a heart problem; "it feels like indigestion to me." He says he does not intend to change to a low-fat diet: "I'm too old to change my ways now." He does not seem anxious: he laughs and jokes a lot.

b. _____

Althea Harper has severe, chronic arthritis in her hands. When the nurse makes a home visit, Ms. Harper meets her at the door in a robe and slippers. Her hair is uncombed. She apologizes to the nurse for her appearance, saying, "I'm sorry I'm such a mess. It's just too hard to get dressed; I can't seem to work the buttons and zippers, or even tie my shoes. It hurts even to hold a hairbrush."

c. _____

Ms. Turner has been blind in her right eye for several years. Lately, her nurse has noticed that Ms. Turner does not seem to hear him when he speaks to her while standing to her right. The aide has reported several times that Ms. Turner ate only about half the food on her tray. The nurse observes that the food remaining is on the right side of the tray. To validate his findings, he pats Ms. Turner's right shoulder; Ms. Turner does not respond.

d. _____

The client reports that she must wear a vaginal pad because she leaks urine when she laughs or lifts heavy objects.

e. _____

The client reports that he must void every 30 minutes, but only small amounts. When he feels the need to void, he must hurry to the bathroom because he cannot wait. He also reports that he gets up three or four times during the night to void.

f. _____

A 70-year-old client has a medical diagnosis of arteriosclerosis. His left foot is blue and cold to the touch. The nurse finds a weak pedal pulse. She validates the findings by elevating his leg. It becomes pale, and the color does not return when she lowers it to a dependent position. She notes that the skin is shiny on both his lower legs.

g. _____

Lorraine Richards' three-week old son has a temperature of 104°. She says he has been having diarrhea and is not nursing well. His fontanels are still firm, and his skin turgor is good.

h. _____

Mr. and Ms. Welytok have a baby with myelomeningocele. They have been attempting to care for the baby at home for the past two weeks. Ms. Welytok confides to the visiting nurse that she doesn't feel she can care for the baby adequately. "I feel guilty, but I'm afraid to touch her, much less turn her. My husband just comes home from work and goes straight to bed, so he's no help at all. I can't give the other kids the attention they need now because I have to spend all my time with Jill. I don't feel like a very good mom right now."

i. _____

Tresa Liu is twelve weeks pregnant. She is 17 years old. She says, "I want to keep the baby, but my parents won't let me. They think I need to finish school. They want me to have an abortion. I think maybe they're right, but then I've heard sometimes you can't ever get pregnant after that. But I hate to quit school and miss all the basketball games and stuff. So I want to do it and then I don't. I should have made up my mind before this, I know."

j. _____

The client has been on prolonged bedrest. While ambulating, he complains of fatigue and dyspnea; he leans on the nurse for support. When she checks his vital signs, his heart rate is 120 and irregular.

12. Circle the related factors identified by NANDA for the label Hopelessness.

Long-term stress	Loss of belief in God
Multiple caretakers	Prolonged activity restriction creating isolation
Pain	Decrease in circulation to the brain

13. Circle the correct client in each situation. Consult your *Nursing Diagnosis Guide*.

a. All clients have the appropriate defining characteristics: body weight 20% under ideal and total calorie intake less than RDA. For which client(s) should you use the problem label Altered Nutrition: Less Than Body Requirements?

Mr. Jonas, who cannot swallow because of paralysis

Ms. Petrie, who is depressed and says she is not hungry

Bobby George, who is NPO for two days after surgery

b. For which child should you diagnose Risk for Poisoning?

Billy, who is 6 months old and has a babysitter

Jana, who is an active 2-year-old

Jill, whose mother keeps her cleaning supplies under the sink

c. For which client should you diagnose Impaired Skin Integrity?

Mr. A, who has a sacral decubitus ulcer

Mr. B, who has an abdominal incision

Mr. C, who has self-inflicted razor cuts on his wrists

14. Write a diagnostic statement for each set of defining characteristics and related (or risk) factors. Focus on good format. Some of the statements are collaborative problems; others are nursing diagnoses. Use P.E.S. format only when directed to do so.

a. *Use P.E.S. format.*

Defining Characteristics — Overuse of laxatives and suppositories
Expectation of a daily bowel movement

Related Factors — Impaired thought processes

b. Defining Characteristics — Decreased frequency of bowel movement
Dry, hard stool; abdominal distention

Related Factors — There is no apparent reason for this problem.
Diagnostic tests are normal; diet appears normal.

c. Defining Characteristics — Decreased frequency of bowel movement
Dry, hard stool; abdominal distention

Related Factors — Inadequate fluid intake
Inadequate fiber intake
Inadequate physical activity

Medical Factors — Client is too weak to eat, drink, or exercise much because of advanced chronic lung disease.

d. *Use P.E.S. Format*

Defining Characteristics   Verbalizes inability to cope
Observed to be unable to solve problems

Related Factors   Related factors occupy 35 pages of history notes in the chart and show development of this problem over several years.

e. Defining Characteristics   None
Risk Factor   Intravenous therapy

f. Defining Characteristics   Possession of destructive means (gun)
Increased motor activity
(May be suicidal, but do not have adequate data to be sure)

Related Factors   Suspect toxic reaction to medications; not sure yet

g. Defining Characteristics   Expressed desire to seek higher level of wellness; has asked nurse to suggest an exercise regimen.

15. Assign high, medium, and low priorities to the following diagnoses, using a "preservation of life" criterion.

a. _____ Decreased Communication between husband and wife related to use of blaming and withdrawal

b. _____ Anxiety related to lack of knowledge of impending surgery and pre- and post-op routines

c. _____ Fluid Volume Deficit related to fever and vomiting secondary to gastroenteritis

d. _____ Fluid Volume Excess: Right Arm related to dependent position and effects of mastectomy

e. _____ Altered Nutrition: Less Than Body Requirements r/t refusal to eat secondary to dysfunctional grieving

f. _____ Risk for Injury (falls) related to weakness and decreased vision

g. _____ Nonadherance (to diabetic diet) related to unresolved anger

h. _____ Unrelieved Incisional Pain related to hesitance to "bother" nurses

i. _____ Altered Health Maintenance (breast self-exam) related to lack of knowledge of how to do the procedure, and of its importance

16. Use the Kalish/Maslow Hierarchy of Needs to prioritize the diagnoses in Exercise 15. Assign priorities as follows (1 being highest priority):

1—Survival   4—Love/Belonging
2—Stimulation   5—Esteem
3—Safety   6—Self-Actualization

REFERENCES

Abdellah, F. (1957). Methods of identifying covert aspects of nursing problems. *Nursing Research, 6*(1):4–23.

American Nurses Association. (1973). *Standards of Nursing Practice.* Kansas City, MO: ANA.

Carpenito, L. (1993). *Nursing Diagnosis: Application to Clinical Practice.* 5th ed. Philadelphia: J. B. Lippincott.

Carpenito, L. (1989). *Nursing Diagnosis: Application to Clinical Practice.* 3rd ed. Philadelphia: J. B. Lippincott.

Etheridge, S., Bos, S., and Bos, N. (1992). Staff nurse identification of nursing diagnosis from a written case study. *Nursing Diagnosis, 3*(1):30–35.

Gebbie, K. (1976). Development of a taxonomy of nursing diagnosis. In Walter, J., et al., *Dynamics of Problem-Oriented Approaches: Patient Care and Documentation.* Philadelphia: J. B. Lippincott.

Geissler, E. (1992). Nursing diagnoses: A study of cultural relevance. *Journal of Professional Nursing, 8*(5):301–307.

Geissler, E. (1991). Transcultural nursing and nursing diagnoses. *Nursing & Health Care, 12*(4):190–92, 203.

Heliker, D. (1992). Reevaluation of a nursing diagnosis: Spiritual distress. *Nursing Forum, 27*(4):15–20.

Henderson, V. (1964). The nature of nursing. *American Journal of Nursing, 64*(8):62–68.

Hoskins, L., et al. (1992). Axes: Focus of Taxonomy II. *Nursing Diagnosis, 3*(3):117–123.

Kalish, R. (1983). *The Psychology of Human Behavior.* 5th ed. Monterey, CA: Brooks/Cole.

Keeling, A., Utz, S., Shuster, G. III, and Boyle, A. (1993). Noncompliance revisited: A disciplinary perspective of a nursing diagnosis. *Nursing Diagnosis, 4*(3):91–98.

Kerr, M., et al. (1993). Taxonomic validation: An overview. *Nursing Diagnosis, 4*(1):6–14.

Kerr, M., et al. (1992). Development of definitions for Taxonomy II. *Nursing Diagnosis, 3*(2):65–71.

Kim, M., McFarland, G., and McLane, A. (1984). *Proceedings of the Fifth National Conference.* North American Nursing Diagnosis Association. St. Louis: C. V. Mosby.

Kobert, L., and Folan, M. (1990). Coming of age in rethinking the philosophies behind holism and nursing process. *Nursing and Health Care, 11*(6):308–12.

Kritek, P. (1985). Nursing diagnosis: Theoretical foundations. *Occupational Health Nursing,* (August):393–96.

Leininger, M. (1990). Issues, questions, and concerns related to the nursing diagnosis cultural movement from a transcultural nursing perspective. *Journal of Transcultural Nursing,* 2:23–32.

Lutjens, L. (1993). The nature and use of nursing diagnosis in hospitals. *Nursing Diagnosis, 4*(3):17–113.

McFarland, G., and McFarlane, E. (1993). *Nursing Diagnosis and Intervention: Planning for Patient Care.* 2nd ed. St. Louis: C. V. Mosby.

McLane, A., ed. (1987). *Classification of Nursing Diagnoses: Proceedings of the Seventh Conference.* North American Nursing Diagnosis Association. St. Louis, MO: C. V. Mosby.

Multnomah County Health Services Division. (1987). *Nursing Diagnosis Classification Codes.* Portland, OR: Multnomah County.

North American Nursing Diagnosis Association. (1994). *Nursing Diagnoses: Definitions and Classification 1995–1996.* Philadelphia, PA: NANDA.

North American Nursing Diagnosis Association. (1990). *Taxonomy I—Revised, 1990.* St. Louis, MO: NANDA.

O'Brien, M. (1982). The need for spiritual integrity. In Yura, H., and Walsh, M., ed. *Human Needs and the Nursing Process.* Norwalk, CT: Appleton-Century-Crofts, pp. 81–115.

CHAPTER 6

PLANNING

OBJECTIVES

On completing this chapter, you should be able to do the following:
- Describe the nursing activities that occur in the planning step of the nursing process.
- Explain the relationship between planning and the other steps of the nursing process.
- Discuss the importance of initial, ongoing, and discharge planning.
- Explain how to derive measurable, observable, individualized client goals/ outcomes from nursing diagnoses.
- Discuss the purpose of an outcome statement.
- Explain the process of developing and selecting nursing interventions.
- Identify the different types of nursing orders (i.e., observation, prevention, treatment, health promotion).
- Develop client goals and nursing orders for wellness diagnoses.
- Discuss the ethical and legal considerations involved in developing client goals and nursing orders.
- Write outcomes and interventions to address clients' spiritual needs.
- Give examples of culture-specific outcomes and interventions.

PLANNING: THE THIRD STEP OF NURSING PROCESS

This chapter discusses planning as a step of the nursing process, compares various types of planning, and explains how to write individualized goals and nursing orders. Figure 6–1 presents an overview of the planning step. The American Nurses Association supports planning as a professional nursing responsibility (see Box 6–1).

In the planning step the nurse, with patient and family input, derives goals from the diagnostic statements and identifies nursing activities to achieve those goals. The purpose and end product of this step is a written, holistic plan of care tailored to the patient's problems and strengths. The planning step ends when this plan has been created.

During planning, the nurse engages in the following activities:

1. Deciding which problems need individually developed plans and which can be addressed by standards of care, policies and procedures, and other forms of preplanned, routine care.

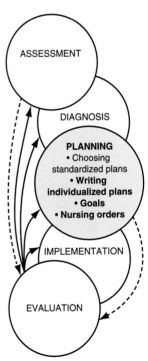

Figure 6-1. The Planning Step in the Nursing Process

Planning

2. Choosing and adapting standardized, preprinted interventions and care plans where appropriate. (This activity is explained in detail in Chapter 9, "Creating a Patient-Care Plan.")

3. Writing individualized goals and nursing orders for problems that require nursing attention beyond preplanned, routine care.

Relationship to Other Nursing Process Steps

Remember that the nursing process steps are interdependent and overlapping. The planning step is no exception. Its effectiveness depends directly on the assessment and diagnosis phases. If assessment data (assessment step) are complete and accurate and the diagnostic statements are correct (diagnosis step), the goals and nursing orders flow logically (planning step) and are likely to be effective. In the same way, implementation and evaluation depend on the planning phase. The goals and nursing orders written during planning serve to guide the nurse's actions during implementation. Furthermore, the goals developed during planning are the criteria used in evaluating whether patient care has had the desired effects (more about this in Chapter 8).

The steps overlap when nurses do **informal planning** while carrying out the activities of the other steps. For example, while listening to a patient's lung sounds (assessment), the nurse may be making a mental note (planning) to

---

Box 6–1. ANA Standards for Planning

Standard III. Outcome Identification
The nurse identifies expected outcomes individualized to the client.
Measurement Criteria
1. Outcomes are derived from the diagnoses.
2. Outcomes are documented as measurable goals.
3. Outcomes are mutually formulated with the client and health care providers, when possible.
4. Outcomes are realistic in relation to the client's present and potential capabilities.
5. Outcomes are attainable in relation to resources available to the client.
6. Outcomes include a time estimate for attainment.
7. Outcomes provide direction for continuity of care.

Standard IV. Planning
The nurse develops a plan of care that prescribes interventions to attain expected outcomes.
Measurement Criteria
1. The plan is individualized to the client's condition or needs.
2. The plan is developed with the client, significant others, and health care providers, when appropriate.
3. The plan reflects current nursing practice.
4. The plan is documented.
5. The plan provides for continuity of care.

From American Nurses Association. *Standards of Clinical Nursing Practice.* 1991. (Kansas City, MO: ANA, p. 10).

notify the physician of her findings. Although planning can be informal, this chapter emphasizes **formal planning,** which is a conscious, deliberate activity involving decision making, critical thinking, and creativity.

Types of Planning

Planning begins with the first patient contact and continues until the nurse-patient relationship is ended, usually when the patient is discharged from the health care agency. In addition to the planning involved in creating a nursing care plan, nurses use **time-sequenced planning** when they plan a patient's care for a shift or for a 24-hour period. For instance, you would use it

1. to plan the timing and order of your nursing activities for a patient (for example, giving pain medication before a painful dressing change).
2. to coordinate the timing of your nursing care with the actions of other health team members, visits from family and friends, and the patient's circadian rhythms.
3. to plan your daily work schedule. In addition to planning care for *each* patient, you must structure your own time so that you can give care to *all* the patients assigned to you for that shift.

Initial Planning

The nurse who performs the admission assessment should develop the initial comprehensive care plan. She has the benefit of the client's body language and some intuitive kinds of information that are not available from the written data base alone; thus, she is best qualified to plan the care and has that responsibility in most institutions.

Planning should be initiated soon after the assessment is done, especially with the trend toward shorter hospital stays. Even a partially developed plan can be helpful in the early nurse-client contacts. Because of time constraints or the client's condition, the initial data base is sometimes incomplete. In such situations, you should develop a preliminary plan with the information available, and refine it as you are able to gather the missing data.

Ongoing Planning

Ongoing planning can be done by any nurse who works with the client. It is carried out as new information is obtained and as the client's responses to care are evaluated. The initial care plan can be individualized even more as the nurses get to know the client better. Nurses who are not familiar with the client might not recognize the significance of new data, and important data could be lost.

Ongoing planning also occurs as you plan your nursing care at the beginning of each day. In your daily planning, you will use ongoing assessment data to do the following:

1. Determine whether the client's health status has changed.

2. Set today's priorities for the client's care.

3. Decide which problems to focus on during this shift.

4. Coordinate your activities so that you can address more than one problem at each client contact.

Planning

Discharge Planning

Discharge planning concerns the process of preparing the client to leave the health care agency. It includes preparing the client for self-care as well as providing for continuity of care between present caregivers and those who will care for the client after discharge. As with the rest of the care plan, the nurse who prepares the initial data base is in the best position to address discharge planning needs.

As a by-product of nationwide efforts to limit the cost of health care, an increasing number and variety of surgeries and treatments are being done in outpatient settings. Clients admitted to acute-care hospitals are being discharged earlier, often still in need of skilled nursing care. They may be placed in an intermediate-care facility, nursing home, or other continued-care setting, or they may be sent home to continue complicated treatments and therapies such as apnea monitors, intravenous therapies, and even mechanical ventilation. Clients and their families must also learn to manage basic hygiene and comfort needs and arrange for in-home professional help as necessary. Nursing research (for example, Naylor 1990; Schneider et al., 1993) indicates that discharge planning can reduce complications and readmissions. Standards of professional practice specify that discharge planning is an essential part of every plan of care (ANA, 1975, 1991; JCAHO, 1992).

Effective discharge planning begins with admission and continues until discharge from the agency. As home care expands, home health nurses must also emphasize discharge planning as a part of their role (Cosnotti and Sprinkel, 1993; Tirk, 1992). Nurses make referrals for home care and to other community agencies, but a physician's order may be necessary in order to obtain third-party reimbursement (e.g., Medicare or private insurance). Box 6–2 contains priorities to consider when discharging a client to home care. In addition, Tuazon (1992) has suggested using the word *MODEL* as a mnemonic device to help you concentrate on discharge planning basics:

M Make a written plan.
O Offer resources (e.g., social worker).
D Devise ways to increase compliance.
E Evaluate your teaching with immediate feedback.
L Legal implications: Document.

Critical Thinking in the Planning Step

After deciding which of the client's problems can be addressed by routine interventions contained in standards of care and model care plans, the nurse uses critical thinking to develop goals and nursing orders for the problems that require an individualized approach. The goals developed in the planning step serve later as criteria for evaluating patient progress. Outcome projection is an aspect of therapeutic judgment, in which the nurse forecasts what is possible to achieve based on human, material, and economic resources (Gordon et. al., 1994).

When generating nursing interventions, nurses use the skills of generalizing, explaining, and predicting, as well as the ability to make interdisciplinary connections and use insights from subjects such as physiology and psychology. Generating nursing interventions is similar to generating hypotheses in the scientific method. Nurses use therapeutic judgment to determine which interventions have a high probability of achieving the desired outcomes (Gordon et. al., 1994).

WRITING CLIENT GOALS/OUTCOMES

A **goal** is the desired result of a nursing intervention. On a care plan, the goals describe, in terms of observable client responses, what you hope to achieve by implementing the nursing orders. The terms *goal, outcome, expected outcome, outcome criterion,* and *predicted outcome* are used interchangeably by many nurses and in this book. You should be aware, however, that some literature does differentiate between the terms, defining *goals* as broad statements about the desired effects of the nursing activities, and *expected outcomes, predicted outcomes,* or *outcome criteria* as the more specific, measurable criteria used to evaluate whether the goal has been met.

> *Example:*
>
> | Broad Statements (Goals) | Specific Outcome Criteria |
> |---|---|
> | Improve nutritional status $\longrightarrow$ | Will gain 5 lb by April 25. |
> | Decrease pain $\longrightarrow$ | Will rate pain as less than 3 on a 1–10 scale. |
> | Increase self-care abilities $\longrightarrow$ | Will be able to feed self by end of the week. |

When goals are defined broadly, as in the above examples, the patient-care plan must include *both* goals and outcomes. In fact, they are sometimes combined into one statement; the broad goal is stated first, followed by *as evidenced by,* and then a list of the observable responses that demonstrate achievement of the goal. Do not confuse *as evidenced by* with the phrase *as manifested by,* used in writing nursing diagnoses.

Box 6–2. Discharge Planning Priorities

1. **How will the following affect the patient's self-care ability?**
   - ✓ Patient's age
   - ✓ Medical condition
   - ✓ Personal limitations (e.g., secondary condition such as blindness)
   - ✓ Nutritional status (e.g., special dietary needs)
   - ✓ Primary caregiver
2. **Is there a need for:**
   - ✓ Referral to community agencies?
   - ✓ Someone to coordinate with the insurance company?
3. **Home care teaching:**
   - ✓ Begin when patient is receptive.
   - ✓ Include family members.
   - ✓ Notify home-care agency of teaching done.
4. **At discharge, check to see that all plans are in place. For example, have arrangements been made for:**
   - ✓ Medical supplies at home?
   - ✓ A nurse or home health aide?
   - ✓ Any medically equipped (or other) transportation needed?

Source: Adapted from Tirk. (1992). Determining discharge priorities. *Nursing92, 22*(7):55.

Planning

Example:

Correct	Incorrect
Nutritional status will improve *as evidenced by* Weight gain of 5 lb by 4/25	Nutritional status will improve *as manifested by* Weight gain of 5 lb by 4/25

While you are learning, writing the broad, general goal first may help you to think of the specific outcomes that are needed. Remember, though, that while broad goals can be a starting point for planning, the specific, measurable outcomes *must* be written on the care plan.

Purpose of the Outcome Statement

Outcome statements guide the planning and evaluation of patient care and serve as motivators for both nurse and patient. Planning proceeds more easily if the outcomes state precisely and clearly what you wish to achieve; ideas for nursing actions will then flow logically from the outcomes, and it will be relatively easy to select nursing orders to achieve the desired changes in client responses.

Although predicted outcomes are developed in the planning step, they serve an important function in the evaluation step as the criteria used to evaluate the effectiveness of the nursing orders. Because the criteria are stated in terms of desired client responses, you simply look for those responses to know whether your nursing actions have been effective.

Outcome statements also provide a sense of achievement for both the client and the nurse and motivate them in their efforts to improve health status.

Example: Kay Stein has essential hypertension. She has a demanding career and family life, and she needs to lose 50 pounds. Even though she takes her antihypertensive medication faithfully, follows her low-calorie diet, and tries to decrease her stress, she still does not feel any better. In fact, she feels worse because the medication gives her a headache. However, she and her nurse have set measurable, achievable goals, such as "Loses 2 lb this week" and "B/P will be 130/80 by end of the week." When Kay's blood pressure reading is 120/80, and the scales show she has lost 4 pounds, she has proof that her efforts are really accomplishing something. This helps motivate her to continue making lifestyle changes that she finds very difficult.

Deriving Outcomes from Nursing Diagnoses

Diagnostic statements describe human responses that are problems for the patient. This suggests that the opposite response is preferred and is what you will try to achieve. The nursing diagnosis "Colonic Constipation r/t inactivity and inadequate fluid intake" indicates that the client's elimination status needs to change. An improvement in elimination status would be evidenced by an opposite (normal) response—that is, a regular, formed, soft bowel movement.

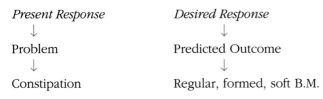

Present Response	*Desired Response*
↓	↓
Problem	Predicted Outcome
↓	↓
Constipation	Regular, formed, soft B.M.

Process

When developing outcome statements, look at the problem and think what the alternative healthy response would be. To help describe the response in terms of specific behaviors, ask yourself the following:

1. If the problem is solved (or prevented), how will the client look or behave? What will I be able to see, hear, palpate, smell, or otherwise observe with my senses?

2. What must the client do to show that the goal is achieved? How well must he do it?

Example: The nursing diagnosis is "Fluid Volume Deficit r/t insufficient fluid intake." The unhealthy response is *fluid volume deficit*; the alternative healthy response would be *adequate fluid volume*.

1. If the problem is solved (fluid volume is adequate), how will the client look or behave? One observable response you could see and palpate is *elastic skin turgor*.

2. What must the client do to demonstrate goal achievement? A possible answer to this is that he must *drink more fluids than he excretes*. Also, you might specify that he would drink *a minimum amount of fluids*, perhaps 100 mL/hour.

Therefore, your goal statement might be

Will have adequate fluid volume, as evidenced by
a. elastic skin turgor
b. Intake = Output
c. drinks at least 100 mL/hour.

Goals, like nursing diagnoses, are concerned with a variety of human responses, including appearance, body functions, symptoms, knowledge, interpersonal functioning, and emotions (see Table 6–1). Because goals are derived directly from the nursing diagnoses, they will be appropriate only if you have stated the nursing diagnosis correctly.

Example: Vincent Aarusa is highly anxious about the surgery he is to have. He does not have a good understanding of the procedure, nor of its risks and benefits. Worse, his father died after having a similar surgery 20 years ago. His admitting nurse failed to perceive the severity of his anxiety and wrote a nursing diagnosis of "Knowledge Deficit (Surgical Procedure) r/t no prior experience or teaching." The goal for this problem was stated as follows: "Will describe surgical procedure in general terms and discuss risks and benefits prior to surgery." When

Mr. Aarusa was able to perform these behaviors, the nurse on the next shift discontinued the Knowledge Deficit problem, and no further discussion of his surgery was attempted by the nursing staff. Mr. Aarusa was sent to surgery with adequate information, but with no relief of his anxiety.

Relationship to Nursing Diagnosis Clauses

The first clause (problem) of a nursing diagnosis contains the unhealthy response. This tells you what should change. The *essential* patient goals are derived from the problem clause. The second clause sometimes suggests some goals as well.

Problem + Etiology
↓

Goals/Outcomes

Goals derived from the etiology are different from those derived from the problem. Their achievement may help to resolve the problem, but they might also be achieved *without* resolving the problem. In that case, the care plan might be terminated because the goals had been met, but the client would still have the problem.

Table 6–1. Examples of Alternative Healthy Responses		
Nursing Diagnosis	**Human Response**	**Outcome**
Ineffective Airway Clearance r/t poor cough effort 2° incisional pain & fear of "breaking stitches loose"	Appearance	Within 24 hours after surgery, will have no skin pallor or cyanosis during post-op period.
	Body functioning	Lungs clear to auscultation during entire post-op period.
	Symptoms	Within 48 hours after surgery, states having no shortness of breath when ambulating to chair.
	Knowledge	After reteaching, states rationale for turn, cough, deep breathing after surgery.
	Emotions	Within 48 hours after surgery, states he is no longer afraid to cough.

Example:

	Problem		*Etiology*
Nursing Diagnosis:	Altered Nutrition: Less Than Body Requirements for Calories	r/t	Lack of appetite 2° depression
	↓		↓
Goals/ Outcomes:	**1.** Will gain 5 lb by 12/14. **2.** Will consume at least 2,000 calories per day.		**3.** Will state his appetite is better within 3 days. **4.** Will be hungry at mealtimes by 12/1. **5.** By 12/1, will be less depressed, as evidenced by **a.** no more than one crying spell per day. **b.** participation in unit activities.

Every nursing diagnosis must have at least one outcome that demonstrates resolution of the problem response.

Achieving goals No. 1 and 2 would actually show problem resolution. If the client gains 5 lb and consumes 2,000 calories per day, then he cannot have "less than body requirements for calories." This is not true for goals No. 3, 4, and 5. The client's depression might lift, and he might regain his appetite but still continue to lose weight. If you discontinued the nutritional problem after measuring only objectives No. 3, 4, and 5, you would do the client a disservice. Therefore, for every nursing diagnosis you must write at least one goal that, when achieved, shows direct resolution of the problem.

Components of an Outcome Statement

Every specific, measurable goal statement should contain a subject, an action verb, performance criteria, and a target time. A component for special conditions may also be necessary. See Table 6–2 for examples of goal statement components.

Table 6–2. Components of Goal/Outcome Statements

Subject	Verb	Special Conditions	Performance Criteria	Target Time
Patient	will list	(after attending nutrition class)	two low-fat foods from each of the Food Guide Pyramid groups	before discharge.
Patient's lungs	will be	—	clear to auscultation	within 24 hours.
Client	will walk	(using walker)	to bathroom and back without shortness of breath	within 3 days.

Planning

Subject

The subject of the goal is a noun. It is the client, any part of the client, or a property or characteristic of the client.

> **Examples:** Client
> Ms. Atwell
> Lung sounds
> Mucous membranes
> Vaginal discharge

The subject is the client unless otherwise stated. Think, "Client will . . ." as you begin the goal statement, but do not write "Client will."

> **Example:**
>
> *Incorrect:* *Client will* describe pain as < 3 on a scale of 1–10.
>
> *Correct:* *Will* describe pain as < 3 on a scale of 1–10.
> *Describes* pain as < 3 on a scale of 1–10.

Action Verb

The verb describes the desired client action (for example, what the client is to learn or do). Using actions that can be seen, heard, smelled, felt, or measured will help make your outcomes specific and observable. Action verbs create a picture of the desired client condition or performance. Each goal should describe only one desired client condition; therefore, each goal should contain only one action verb.

> **Example:**
>
> *Correct:* Will *describe* the food groups in the Food Guide Pyramid . . .
>
> *Incorrect:* Will *describe* the food groups in the Food Guide Pyramid and *choose* a balanced diet . . .

Performance Criteria

Performance criteria are the standards used to evaluate the quality of the client's performance. They describe the *extent* to which the client is expected to perform the behavior. The performance criteria suggest nursing orders for meeting the goal and indicate what should be measured in evaluating goal achievement. Performance criteria may specify amount, quality, speed, distance, accuracy, and so forth—they tell *how, what, when, or where*.

> **Examples:**

		What	**When**
Amount	Will lose	5 lb	during the first week.

		How	**What**
Accuracy	Will draw up	correct amount	of insulin.

Examples of Action Verbs

Apply
Breathe
Choose
Communicate
Define
Demonstrate
Describe
Design
Drink
Explain
Express
Identify
Inject
List
Move
Prepare
Report
Share
Sit
Sleep
Talk
Transfer
Turn
Use
Verbalize
Walk

		What	**How**
Quality	Will inject	insulin	using sterile technique.

		Where	**When**
Distance and Amount	Will walk	to the end of the hall	three times a day.

Target Time

Each goal should specify the time by which you realistically expect a change in patient response (e.g., by discharge, by April 2, prior to surgery, within 12 hours, at all times). The target time helps to pace the patient's care and motivates both the patient and the nurse by focusing on the future. It also provides a deadline for evaluating patient progress.

Example: Will name the food groups in the Food Guide Pyramid *within 24 hours* after receiving pamphlet.

The target time is a type of performance criterion, since it specifies the speed with which a goal is to be accomplished. In the example above, the client's progress would not be satisfactory if he took longer than 24 hours to learn the food groups.

Nursing knowledge and experience are needed for setting realistic target times. You will need to know the usual rate of progress for clients with the identified medical and nursing diagnoses and consider the client's particular capabilities and resources.

Example: Esther Brady has just had an abdominal hysterectomy. Review of usual progress after this surgery indicates that most patients require intravenous or intramuscular narcotic analgesics for 24 hours and are then able to obtain relief from milder, oral analgesics. However, Ms. Brady is very anxious and has a history of poor pain tolerance. It would not be realistic to set a target time of 24 hours for resolution of her Pain diagnosis. A more achievable goal might be "Will obtain adequate pain relief from p.o. analgesics within 48 hours post-op, as evidenced by patient's statement that pain is < 3 on a 1–10 scale."

Potential (Risk) Problems   Predicted outcomes for risk problems do not need target times. The broad goal is to prevent the problem from occurring, so in a sense the target time is *at all times.*

Example:

Nursing Diagnosis: Risk for Impaired Skin Integrity r/t immobility . . .
Predicted Outcome: Skin will remain intact, with no redness over bony
prominences.
(Target time: At all times)
(Evaluate plan: Daily)

In the example above, the target time is assumed, so you would not need to write it on the care plan. However, you may wish to schedule times for evaluating the predicted outcomes and the accompanying plan of care.

181

Planning

Special Conditions

If it is important to describe the conditions under which a client is to perform a behavior, you may need to add modifiers to the performance criteria. **Modifiers** describe the amount of assistance the client will need, available resources, environmental conditions, or experiences the client should have before being expected to perform the behavior. Like performance criteria, modifiers describe *how, when, where,* and *how much.*

> ### Examples:
>
> *Type of assistance*
>
> **How**   Will walk to the end of the hall three times a day, using a walker, by April 8.
>
> *Prior experience*
>
> **When**   Will list foods high in cholesterol   after consulting with dietitian.
>
> *Environmental conditions*
>
> **Where** In one-to-one session, will express fear of abandonment by Friday.

Not all goals need special conditions; they are included only if they are important. If the performance criteria clearly specify the expected performance, special conditions are not necessary.

Short-Term and Long-Term Goals/Outcomes

Short-term goals identify outcomes that can be achieved within a few days or a few hours. Goals dealing with survival needs may even be stated in terms of minutes. For this reason, short-term goals are useful in acute-care settings, such as hospitals, where nurses often focus on the client's more immediate needs. Also, the client may be discharged before the nurse can evaluate progress toward long-term goals. Some examples of short-term goals follow:

> ### Examples:
>
> Voids within 6 hours after delivery of infant.
> States relief of pain within one hour after receiving p.o. oxycodone.
> Walks to end of hall and back, unassisted, by day 2 post-op.

Short-term goals must usually be accomplished before the client can achieve long-term goals, and they are often used to measure the client's progress toward long-term goals. Achieving several short-term goals also provides frequent reinforcement for the client, encouraging him to keep working on the problem. The long-term goal for Constipation might be "Will have daily B.M. without use of laxatives within two months." The nurse would not want to wait for two months to determine whether the client's problem was improving, so a series of short-term goals should be used.

Example:

Long-Term Outcome	Will have daily B.M. without use of laxatives *within two months.*
Short-Term Outcome	After administration of enema will have bowel movement *within 4 hours.*
	Will have next B.M. *within 36 hours* without aid of p.o. laxatives.
	Will use chemical or mechanical stimulation for B.M. not more than two times *this week.*
	Immediately, diet changes include prune juice and oatmeal (or other high-fiber cereal) for breakfast, and substituting whole grain for white bread.
	Within one week reports he is eating at least one good source of fiber at every meal.

As a student, you will probably care for a patient for only a few hours at a time. You should write short-term goals to measure what you can realistically accomplish while you are with the client, so that you can evaluate the results of the care you have given. In a comprehensive care plan you should also include longer-range goals that other nurses can use to evaluate patient progress when you are not there.

Long-term goals describe changes in client outcomes over a longer period—usually a week or more. The ideal long-term goal aims at restoring normal functioning in the problem area. When normal functioning cannot be restored, the long-term goal describes the maximum level of functioning that can be achieved given the client's health status and resources. Long-term goals are especially useful for clients with chronic health problems and those in home health care, rehabilitation centers, and other extended-care facilities. Some examples of long-term goals follow:

Examples:

After attending six weekly childbirth-education classes, will correctly demonstrate abdominal and shallow chest breathing.
By 12 weeks post-op, will have full range of motion of right shoulder.
Within 3 months (12/24), will feed self using fork or spoon.

Outcomes for Actual, Risk, and Possible Nursing Diagnoses

Outcomes may reflect promotion, maintenance, or restoration of health, depending on the type of nursing diagnosis (see Table 6–3). For an *actual nursing diagnosis,* goals focus on restoring healthy responses and preventing further complications. They specify patient behaviors that demonstrate resolution or reduction of the problem and that patients should be able to achieve with the aid of independent nursing activities.

Planning

Examples:

Actual Nursing Diagnosis	*Outcome Statement*
Calf Pain with Exercise r/t muscle ischemia 2° peripheral arterial disease	Reports pain is gone after 10 minutes of rest with legs dependent.
Impaired Skin Integrity: Dermal Ulcer over coccyx r/t inability to move self in bed	Ulcer will not extend to deeper tissues.
	Ulcer will not become infected, as evidenced by absence of purulent exudate.
	By 12/1 healing will be evidenced by decreased redness and appearance of granulation tissue in wound bed.

Outcomes for *risk nursing diagnoses* focus on preventing the problem; the client responses should demonstrate a problem-free level of functioning, or if that is not possible, maintenance of the present level of functioning. Achievement of these goals should mean that the problem is not occurring at the time the assessment is made.

Table 6-3. Goals/Outcomes for Different Problem Types

Type of Problem	Patient Response Demonstrates:	Nursing Focuses on:
Actual nursing diagnosis	Resolution or reduction of problem	Resolution or reduction of problem
		Prevention of further complication
Risk nursing diagnosis	Problem has not developed	Prevention and detection of problem
Possible nursing diagnosis	No patient responses	Confirming or ruling out problem
Collaborative problem	Problem has not developed	Detection and prevention of problem
Wellness diagnoses		
Health maintenance	Continuation of healthy functioning	Health maintenance
Health promotion	Achievement of a higher level of wellness	Health promotion

Examples:

Risk Nursing Diagnosis	*Outcome Statements*
Risk for Ineffective Breast-feeding r/t breast engorgement	Infant will be observed to "latch on," suck, and swallow at each feeding.
	Mother will state satisfaction with breastfeeding.
	Infant will regain birth weight within 14 days after birth.

Possible nursing diagnoses present an exception to the rule; they are *not* written in terms of desired patient response. A possible diagnosis is written when the nurse does not have enough data to know whether or not the patient has the problem. The goal for a possible nursing diagnosis is really a *nursing* goal: that the presence of the diagnosis will be confirmed or ruled out. It is not necessary to write goals for possible diagnoses. However, to help assure that follow-up assessments will be done, you may wish to set a target time for confirming or ruling out the problem. If so, you could write a nursing goal. Nursing goals should *not* be written on the care plan for actual or potential problems.

Example:

Possible Problem:	Possible Hopelessness r/t abandonment by significant other after onset of chronic illness
Nursing Goal:	Confirm or rule out Hopelessness by 6/12.

Outcomes for Collaborative Problems

Outcomes for nursing diagnoses are "nurse sensitive." That is, they can be brought about primarily by nursing interventions. For *collaborative problems,* nurses and physicians share accountability for achieving outcomes. Therefore, outcomes for these problems are usually found in the agency's standardized care plans or critical pathways. On working care plans for professional nurses, goal statements are not necessary for collaborative problems because it is understood that the broad goal is prevention or early detection of the problem. Furthermore, it may not be legally advisable to write goals that imply nursing accountability, when accountability for the problem actually is shared with other professions.

As a student, it may enhance your learning to write goals for collaborative problems. This will assure that you know precisely what symptoms you are looking for and can recognize whether or not the problem is developing. When writing such outcomes, remember that a collaborative problem is a type of potential problem, not an actual problem. Independent nursing care focuses on prevention and early detection of the complication. Outcomes for collaborative problems should describe the patient responses that will be seen as long as the problem has not developed. The goals may describe normal functioning or problem symptoms that you do *not* want to occur.

Planning

Examples:

Collaborative Problem	Outcome Statements
Potential Complication of Childbirth: Postpartum Hemorrhage	Postpartum hemorrhage will not occur, as evidenced by **1.** saturating less than 1 vag. pad per hour during first 24 hours. **2.** fundus firm and below umbilicus during first 24 hours. **3.** pulse and B/P in normal range for patient.

Outcomes for Wellness Diagnoses

Recall that wellness diagnoses describe essentially healthy responses that the client wishes to maintain or improve. Goals for these diagnoses describe client responses that demonstrate health maintenance or achievement of a higher level of healthy functioning (e.g., "Over the next year, Mrs. Jacobs will continue participating in religious activities that provide spiritual support").

Community Health

In community health settings, goals are often written for "aggregates" (groups of people). Table 6–4 is a list of health promotion and disease prevention goals that the U. S. Public Health Service has set for improving the health of the nation.

Outcomes for Patient Teaching

Some patients may need a special teaching plan to address their learning needs (see Chapter 9). **Teaching objectives** are patient outcomes that describe in behavioral terms what the patient is to learn or how he will demonstrate learning. You should write objectives to reflect whether the learning is to take place in the cognitive, psychomotor, or affective domain. **Cognitive learning** involves perception, understanding, and the storing and recall of new information. **Psychomotor learning** involves physical skills. **Affective learning** involves changes in feelings, attitudes, and values.

Examples:

Cognitive domain	Learner will *explain* the effect of weight on B/P.
Psychomotor domain	Learner will *apply* B/P cuff correctly.
Affective domain	Learner will state that he *feels* confident with his ability to obtain correct B/P readings.

As with all outcomes, choose active verbs for learning objectives; they will help you to think of teaching strategies and make it easier to evaluate whether learning takes place. Table 6–5 on page 188 provides a few suggestions for active verbs in each of the learning domains.

When writing objectives for the affective domain, keep in mind that you cannot directly observe a feeling or an attitude. Therefore, you could not write an objective such as "Learner will feel happier by May 2." You can, however, observe behaviors (cues) that *indicate* the client's feelings or moods. The following examples allow you to infer that the client is happy:

Examples: By May 2, will state that he feels happier than before.
By May 2, will be observed smiling at least twice a day.
By May 2, will resume past habit of singing in the shower.

Guidelines for Writing Outcome Statements

The following guidelines may help you to improve the quality of your outcome statements. Ask the following questions about each of the goals you write. (Guidelines 1, 2, and 3 were discussed in detail earlier in this chapter.)

1. For each actual nursing diagnosis, *does at least one outcome clearly demonstrate resolution of the problem clause?* Outcomes *b* and *c* in Figure 6–2 demonstrate this guideline.

2. *Is the outcome appropriate to the nursing diagnosis?* Achievement of the outcome should clearly demonstrate that the problem is resolved (actual problems), that healthy responses have been supported (wellness diagnoses), or that potential problems are not occurring (risk diagnoses and collaborative problems).

Writing Client Goals/ Outcomes

Table 6–4. U.S. Public Health Service Priorities for the Year 2000

Goals	Objectives
Health Promotion	1. Increase physical activity and fitness. 2. Improve nutrition. 3. Reduce use of tobacco. 4. Reduce alcohol and other drug abuse. 5. Improve family planning. 6. Improve mental health and prevent mental disorders. 7. Reduce violent and abusive behavior. 8. Enhance educational and community-based programs.
Health Protection	9. Reduce unintentional injuries. 10. Improve occupational safety and health. 11. Improve environmental health. 12. Ensure food and drug safety. 13. Improve oral health.
Preventive Services	14. Improve maternal and infant health. 15. Reduce heart disease and stroke. 16. Prevent and control cancer. 17. Reduce diabetes and chronic disabling conditions. 18. Prevent and control HIV infection. 19. Reduce sexually transmitted diseases. 20. Increase immunization and prevent infectious diseases. 21. Expand access and use of clinical preventive services.
Surveillance and Data Systems	22. Improve surveillance and data systems.

From *Healthy People 2000: National Health Promotion and Disease Prevention Objectives.* DHHS Publication No. (PHS) 91-50212. Washington, DC: U.S. Government Printing Office.

Planning

3. *Does each outcome have all the necessary components*: subject, action verb, performance criteria, special conditions (when needed) and target time (usually)?

4. *Is each outcome derived from only one nursing diagnosis?* An outcome derived from more than one nursing diagnosis is likely to include more than one client behavior, making evaluation difficult. In Outcome *a* in Figure 6–2, suppose the client had no urge incontinence but was still having pain when voiding. Would you say the outcome was met or not met?

5. *Is the outcome valued by the client and family?* The plan of care is more likely to be effective if it is designed to help the client achieve goals that he values. For example, knowing that obesity aggravates hypertension, your goal may be that the client lose 40 lb. However, if eating is the client's only pleasure, he may not share your goal; he may prefer to accept the risks of hypertension

Table 6–5. Active Verbs for Learning Objectives

Compare	Arrange	Choose
Define	Assemble	Defend
Describe	Construct	Discuss
Differentiate	Manipulate	Express
Explain	Organize	Help
Identify	Show	Justify
List	Start	Select
Name	Take	Share
State		

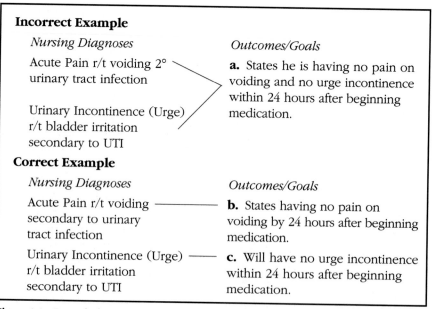

Incorrect Example

Nursing Diagnoses

Acute Pain r/t voiding 2° urinary tract infection

Urinary Incontinence (Urge) r/t bladder irritation secondary to UTI

Outcomes/Goals

a. States he is having no pain on voiding and no urge incontinence within 24 hours after beginning medication.

Correct Example

Nursing Diagnoses

Acute Pain r/t voiding secondary to urinary tract infection

Urinary Incontinence (Urge) r/t bladder irritation secondary to UTI

Outcomes/Goals

b. States having no pain on voiding by 24 hours after beginning medication.

c. Will have no urge incontinence within 24 hours after beginning medication.

Figure 6-2. Example for Guideline 1

rather than deprive himself of the pleasure of eating. If his goals do not include losing weight, then no matter how well you plan and carry out your nursing orders, the plan will probably fail.

When nurse and client goals conflict, it may help to explore the client's reasoning with him, provide a rationale for your goals, and look for alternative approaches. This has the advantage of involving the client in decisions about his care and keeping communication open.

Involve the client and family to the extent of their interest and abilities. Be sure they agree that the problem is one that requires change and that the outcome is worth achieving. This will ensure that your time and energy are spent on plans that meet the unique needs of each client and are likely to succeed.

Writing Client Goals/ Outcomes

6. *Is the outcome congruent with the total treatment plan?* The outcome "Will demonstrate correct technique for bathing baby by postpartum day 2" would not be compatible with the medical treatment plan for a mother whose newborn is too ill to be bathed.

7. *Is the outcome stated in terms of client responses, rather than nurse activities?* Thinking "Client will . . . " at the beginning of each goal may help you to focus on what the client will be able to do rather than on your own actions. However, do not actually write "Client will." Always assume that the outcome refers to the client or some part of the client.

Example:

Nurse Activity (Incorrect)	Prevent infection of incision.
Client Response (Correct)	Incision will not become infected, as evidenced by
	1. absence of redness and drainage.
	2. edges approximated.

8. *Are the predicted outcomes phrased in positive terms*—that is, in terms of what you hope will occur rather than what you hope will not occur?

Example:

Negative Wording:	Skin will not become broken or ulcerated.
Positive Wording:	Skin will remain intact.

For potential problems, it may be difficult to think of positive terms to describe your predicted outcomes. It is easier to write "No redness" than to describe exactly the color of normal skin. You cannot say, "Skin color will be normal," because *normal* is too vague. In such instances, you may use negative terms. A measurable, negatively worded outcome is actually a list of the signs and symptoms you are trying to prevent.

Example:

Problem	Risk for Infection of Surgical Incision . . .
Predicted Outcomes	Incision will not become infected, as evidenced by
	1. No redness (negative wording).
	2. No purulent drainage (negative wording).
	3. Edges approximated (positive wording).

Planning

9. *Is the outcome directly observable or measurable?* Observable, measurable outcomes use action verbs to describe what the client will be able to do and *to what extent.* This assures that other nurses can make observations to determine whether the outcome has been achieved and the problem resolved. In the following example, you cannot observe what Ms. Fretsch *knows.* However, you could observe whether Ms. Fretsch can *name* the high-sodium foods.

Example:

Incorrect   By 11/30 (Ms. Fretsch) will *know* which foods to avoid.

Correct   By 11/30 (Ms. Fretsch) will *name* the high-sodium foods to avoid in each food group.

You cannot directly observe such actions as *understands, knows, feels,* or *appreciates.* If you cannot avoid using such verbs, make them measurable by adding the phrase *as evidenced by* followed by the signs and symptoms you wish to reduce or the positive responses you wish to achieve (e.g., Will *experience* relief of pain *as evidenced by* rating of < 2 on a 10-point scale, absence of facial grimace, and walking erect).

10. *Is the outcome specific and concrete?* Other nurses reading the statement should have no doubt about the focus for nursing care. Vague, general words that can be interpreted in several ways can lead to disagreement about whether the outcome has been met. Avoid performance criteria such as *normal, adequate, sufficient, more, less,* and *increased.* Does an outcome of "increased activity tolerance" mean that the client can run a mile in four minutes or does it mean that he can ambulate from the chair to the bed with no shortness of breath? Action verbs, performance criteria, special conditions, and target times increase outcome specificity.

When possible, make outcomes more specific by individualizing them to describe the client's normal baseline measurements. The upper limit of normal blood pressure for most people is 140/90, and a goal of "B/P within normal limits" would imply this number. However, for a client who usually has a blood pressure of 90/50, the normal limit is probably too high.

Example:

Incorrect: Blood pressure will be *within normal limits.*

More specific: Blood pressure will be *less than 130/80.*

It may not be possible to write specific outcomes for an initial care plan, but as you continue to work with the patient you will gain a clearer idea of his health status and abilities. You will then be able to write more specific, individualized outcomes. Of course, you will continue to revise the outcomes as the patient's status changes. The following example shows how outcomes may be individualized and revised for a patient with a nursing diagnosis of Activity Intolerance r/t prolonged immobility.

Example:

Initial Goal/Outcome: (General)	Ability to tolerate activity will improve, as evidenced by **1.** walking progressively farther each day. **2.** increased ability to perform self-care (hygiene, feeding, etc.).
Revised Goal/Outcome: (More specific)	Ability to tolerate activity will improve, as evidenced by the following: **1.** by 5/12, walks to chair (8 ft.) without shortness of breath. **2.** by 5/12, assists with bath by washing own hands and face.
Revised Goal/Outcome: (After condition change)	Ability to tolerate activity will improve, as evidenced by the following: **1.** by 5/18, walks to bathroom (20 ft.) without shortness of breath. **2.** by 5/18, washes hands, face, and upper torso.

11. *Are the predicted outcomes realistic and achievable* in terms of the client's internal and external resources? The client's physical and mental status, coping mechanisms, support system, finances, and available community services should be considered. The outcome "Will demonstrate desire to comply with treatment by keeping all clinic appointments," may not be realistic for a client with no car and no money for cab fare. Clients are not motivated to achieve outcomes they perceive to be impossible.

Consider also whether the capabilities of the nursing staff and the resources of the agency are adequate to achieve the outcomes. "Uses individualized relaxation techniques to achieve pain relief" is not achievable unless staffing is adequate to allow time for teaching and supervised practice.

12. *Is there an adequate number of outcomes to address each nursing diagnosis?* Ask yourself, "If these predicted outcomes are achieved, will the problem be resolved?" If they are written in very specific terms, several outcomes may be needed for each diagnosis in order to determine that the problem has been resolved or prevented. For the diagnostic label of Anxiety, none of the following outcomes by itself would show that the anxiety was sufficiently relieved:

Example:

Nursing Diagnosis	Severe Anxiety r/t unresolved role conflicts (mother-wife-attorney)
Outcomes	After one-on-one interaction, will be less anxious, as evidenced by **1.** statements that she feels better. **2.** fewer than two episodes of tearfulness in the next 24 hours. **3.** smoking no more than one cigarette per hour.

Planning

13. *Is the outcome concise?* Outcomes should be stated in as few words as possible without sacrificing clarity.

> ***Example:***
>
> *Wordy* By April 15, the client will demonstrate adequate knowledge of an appropriate low-calorie diet by listing foods to avoid and foods allowed in each of the Food Guide Pyramid groups.
>
> *More Concise* By 4/15, lists for each food group foods to avoid and foods allowed on low-calorie diet.

Occasionally the goal will refer to behaviors of someone other than the client, for instance, a parent or spouse. Specify who is to perform the behavior only when it is *not* the client. You might write, for example, "By dismissal, *Ms. Rauh* will demonstrate ability to change Mr. Rauh's dressing according to the printed guidelines given to her."

14. Remember that *outcomes can be written for an individual, family,* or *community.* For example, the U.S. Public Health Service (1990) has published the following overarching goals for the health of the nation:

> Increase the span of healthy life for Americans.
> Reduce health disparities among Americans.
> Achieve access to preventive services for all Americans. (p. 43)

Box 6–3. Guidelines for Writing Goal/Outcome Statements

1. Is each outcome derived from only one nursing diagnosis?
2. For each actual nursing diagnosis, does at least one goal clearly demonstrate resolution of the problem clause?
3. Is the outcome appropriate to the nursing diagnosis?
4. Does each outcome have all the necessary components: subject, action verb, performance criteria, special conditions, target time?
5. Is the outcome valued by the client and family?
6. Is the outcome congruent with the total treatment plan?
7. Is the outcome stated in terms of client responses rather than nurse activities?
8. When possible, are the outcomes stated in positive terms?
9. Can the outcome be directly measured or observed?
10. Is the outcome specific and concrete?
11. Is the outcome realistic and achievable?
12. Is there an adequate number of outcomes to address each nursing diagnosis?
13. Is the outcome concise?
14. Does the outcome describe responses of an individual, family, or community as appropriate?

WRITING NURSING ORDERS

After writing the outcomes, the next step is to select and write nursing orders to help achieve them. **Nursing orders** (also called nursing *actions, interventions, measures,* or *strategies*) are the written, detailed instructions for performing nursing interventions. Nursing interventions are the activities and behaviors performed to change present client responses to the desired responses described in the outcomes. Nursing activities may be something you do for the client or something you help her to do for herself.

Nursing orders contain more specific, detailed instruction than physician's orders. A physician's order regarding a client's nutritional status might read "Diet as tolerated." Related nursing orders would specify how the diet is to progress, as well as assessments that need to be made.

Examples:

1. Auscultate bowel sounds q4h.
2. Observe for abdominal distention, nausea, or vomiting.
3. Limit ice chips to 1 cup per hour until bowel sounds are auscultated; then give clear liquids × 8 hours.
4. If no nausea or vomiting, progress to full liquids . . .

Purpose

Nursing orders provide specific direction and a consistent, individualized approach to the patient's care. They are written as instructions for others to follow, and other nurses are held responsible and accountable for their implementation. Since many different nurses may be involved in caring for the patient, nursing orders must be detailed enough to be interpreted correctly by all caregivers. An order to "force fluids" could be interpreted in many ways. A nurse accustomed to working with young adults might expect this to mean 200 mL per hour; a gerontology nurse might think it means 50 mL per hour; another nurse might focus on total volume rather than a consistent hourly intake. A better nursing order would be "Give fluids hourly: Day shift = 1,000 mL total; Evening shift = 1,000 mL; Night shift = 400 mL."

Nursing orders guide documentation as well as implementation of care. Using the preceding nutrition example, the nurse would know to chart the client's abdominal assessment as well as his tolerance of the fluids. For example:

> "0800—Abd. soft, not distended. Faint bowel sounds auscultated in all
>   4 quadrants. Taking 50 mL ice chips/hour with no nausea since
>   0600.
> 0830— 50 mL carbonated beverage p.o.
> 0930— Complained of nausea at 0900. 30 mL clear emesis."

When nurses use the nursing orders as a guide for documentation, the nursing process is automatically reflected in the patient's chart. This is important in meeting standards set by agencies that accredit health care institutions (e.g., Joint Commission on Accreditation of Healthcare Organizations).

Types of Nursing Orders

Interventions are identified and ordered during the planning step; however, they are actually performed during the implementation step. Nursing interventions may be dependent, interdependent, or independent.

Independent interventions are those that the nurse prescribes and performs or delegates. They include physical care, emotional support and comfort, teaching, counseling, environmental management, and making referrals to other health care professionals. Recall that nursing diagnoses are treated primarily by independent nursing interventions.

Dependent interventions are prescribed by the physician and carried out by the nurse. Medical orders commonly include orders for medications, intravenous therapy, diagnostic tests, treatments, diet, and activity. The nurse is responsible for explaining, assessing the need for, and administering the medical orders. Nursing orders may be written to individualize the medical order, based on the patient's status.

Example:

Medical Order	Progressive ambulation, as tolerated
Nursing Orders	**1.** Dangle for 5 min, 12 hr post-op.
	2. Stand at bedside 24 hr post-op; observe for pallor, dizziness, and weakness.
	3. Check pulse before and after amb. Do not progress if P >110.

Medical orders are usually transcribed to special sections of the care plan; however, you may sometimes wish to record a medical order in your individualized plan for a nursing diagnosis (see number 3 in the next example).

Example: A nursing diagnosis of Pain includes interventions for helping the client to take less medication. The nursing orders follow:
1. Coach client in using guided imagery. If ineffective,
2. Try cutaneous stimulation.
3. If pain is > 4 (on a 1–10 scale), *give Tylenol No. 3* (see Medication Record).

Interdependent interventions are the actions the nurse carries out in collaboration with other health team members, such as physical therapists, social workers, dietitians and physicians. For example, the physician might order physical therapy to teach the patient crutch-walking. As the nurse, you would be responsible for informing the physical therapy department and for coordinating the patient's care to include the P.T. sessions. You would be responsible for assisting the client to walk with his crutches when he is back on your unit, and you would also collaborate with the physical therapist to evaluate the client's progress.

Nursing Orders and Problem Status

Depending on the type of patient problem, you will write nursing orders for observation, prevention, treatment, and health promotion.

1. *Observation.* This includes observations to determine whether a complication is developing, as well as observations of the client's responses to nursing, medical, and other therapies. Observation orders should be written for every problem: actual, risk, and possible nursing diagnoses and collaborative problems.

Examples: Auscultate lungs q8h.
Observe for redness over sacrum q2h.
Assess for urinary frequency.
Intake and output, hourly.

2. *Prevention.* Prevention orders prescribe the care needed to prevent complications or reduce risk factors. They are used mainly for risk nursing diagnoses and collaborative problems, but they can also be appropriate for actual nursing diagnoses.

Examples:

Turn, cough, and deep breathe q2h.	(Prevents respiratory complication)
If fundus is boggy, massage until firm.	(Prevents postpartum hemorrhage)
Refer to county health department for measles immunizations.	(Prevents specific disease: measles)

3. *Treatment.* This includes teaching, referrals, physical, and other care needed to treat an existing problem. Treatment measures are appropriate for actual nursing diagnoses. Notice that the same nursing order may accomplish either prevention or treatment of a problem (compare examples below to the preceding examples).

Examples:

Turn, cough, deep breathe q2h.	(Treat respiratory problem)
If fundus is boggy, massage until firm.	(Treat actual postpartum hemorrhage)
Help client plan exercise regimen.	(Treat actual activity intolerance)

4. *Health Promotion.* When there are no health problems, the nurse helps the client to identify areas for improvement that will lead to a higher level of wellness. Health-promotion strategies encourage approach behaviors; that is, they help the client promote positive outcomes rather than avoid negative outcomes. Health promotion is not specific to any disease or problem, but aims to encourage activities that will actualize the client's general health potential.

Examples:

Discuss the importance of daily exercise.
Teach components of a healthy diet.
Explore infant-stimulation techniques.

Table 6–6 shows how orders for observation, prevention, and treatment are related to the status of the patient's problems.

Planning

Generating and Selecting Nursing Orders

For any given problem, several nursing interventions might be effective. You will select the ones that are most likely to achieve the desired goal, taking into consideration the patient's abilities and preferences, the capabilities of the nursing staff, the available resources, and the policies and procedures of the institution. Creativity is needed for generating new and effective interventions. One of the dangers in using preplanned (standardized) care plans is the temptation to plug in ready-made solutions rather than look for different, more effective approaches for a particular patient. Even if an intervention has been useful in the past, always rethink it to be sure it is the best way for the patient with whom you are working.

The following decision-making process will guide you in reviewing the nursing diagnosis and goals, identifying all the possible nursing orders, and selecting the best options from among the alternatives.

Review the Nursing Diagnosis

You should first review the nursing diagnosis to be sure you understand the problem and etiology. Be sure you are familiar with the factors causing or contributing to actual problems, and the risk factors that predispose the client to risk problems. You should also know the signs and symptoms associated with any risk diagnoses or collaborative problems. Try to think of nursing actions to reduce or eliminate causal, contributing, and risk factors, or to relieve problem symptoms. In the following example, the nursing orders should reduce the contributing factor, breast engorgement.

Table 6–6. Types of Nursing Orders in Relation to Diagnoses			
Actual Nursing Diagnoses	**Risk Nursing Diagnosis**	**Possible Nursing Diagnosis**	**Collaborative Problems**
Observation for improvement or complications	**Observation** for change to "actual" status	**Observation** to confirm or rule out diagnosis	**Observation** for onset of complication
			Physician Notification of problem onset
Prevention of further complications	**Prevention** Remove or reduce risk factors		**Prevention** Includes physician orders, nursing policies and procedures
			Collaborative treatments to relieve or eliminate problem
Treatment Remove causal and contributing factors Relieve symptoms			

196

Example: *Nursing Diagnosis:*   Ineffective Breastfeeding r/t breast engorgement

Nursing Orders:

1. Teach to massage breasts before feeding.
2. Use hot packs or hot shower before nursing infant.

Nursing orders are individualized primarily from the second clause (etiology) of a nursing diagnosis. The etiology describes the factors that cause or contribute to the unhealthy response, and the nursing orders would specifically target these causal and contributing factors.

Problem + Etiology

Nursing orders

Any number of factors might contribute to a problem, but it would be inefficient and probably ineffective to address them all. Individualized nursing orders address the etiological factors specific for a given client. For example, many factors could contribute to Chronic Constipation: lack of knowledge, lack of exercise, eating habits, long-term laxative use, or a schedule that causes the client to ignore the urge to defecate. A well-written nursing diagnosis states which factors are causing the client's problem suggesting nursing interventions that deal directly with those factors. The following example illustrates how different etiologies suggest different nursing orders. Notice that in both cases, the *problem* is the same.

Example:

Nursing Diagnosis   *Nursing Orders*

Chronic Constipation
r/t *long-term laxative*   →   **1.** Work with the client to develop
use   a plan for gradual withdrawal
                                   of the laxatives.

Chronic Constipation
r/t *inactivity and*   →   **1.** Help client to develop an exercise
insufficient fluid intake   regimen that he can follow at home.
                           2. Help client plan for including
                                   sufficient fluids in his diet.

You may also need to write nursing orders (especially observation orders) for the problem clause of the nursing diagnosis. For a diagnosis of Chronic Pain related to joint inflammation, nursing orders might include some pain-relief interventions that have nothing to do with relieving joint inflammation:

Observe level of pain before and after activity.
Give back rub (to promote general relaxation of tension).
Instruct client to take analgesic before pain becomes too severe.
Teach slow, rhythmic breathing as a pain control method.

197

Planning

Review the Goal/Outcome

You should also review the goals to recall the patient outcomes you wish to produce. The goals will help you to develop nursing orders that are specific to the individual patient.

Example: *Nursing Diagnosis*: Risk for Ineffective Breastfeeding r/t breast engorgement

Goals:	*Nursing orders suggested by goals*:
1. Infant will be observed to "latch on," suck, and swallow.	**1a.** Observe infant at breast for effective latching on, sucking, and swallowing.
	1b. Teach mother to make these observations.
	1c. When sucking is not long and rhythmic, institute massage of alternate areas of breast without removing infant from breast.
2. Infant will regain birth weight of 8 lb 6 oz within 14 days after birth.	**2a.** Weigh infant daily at 0600.

Identify Alternative Actions

Keeping goals and etiology in mind, think of all the nursing activities that might bring about the desired responses. Include unusual or original ideas. Don't try to predict at this point which ones would be best.

Perhaps you are wondering, "How will I be able to think of interventions to address the etiology? How will I know which actions will achieve the goals?" Principles and theories from nursing and related courses (e.g., anatomy, physiology, psychology) are good sources of ideas for nursing actions. You may also wish to consult resources such as model care plans, agency procedure manuals, nursing texts, journal articles, instructors, and practicing nurses. Remember to consult the patient and his family about the care they find to be most helpful.

To begin thinking of interventions, ask yourself two broad questions: (1) What should I watch for? and (2) What should I do? Branch out to consider all the possible activities that might address the etiology or achieve the goals. Depending upon the type of problem, include both independent and collaborative activities from the following categories, discussed previously in "Types of Nursing Orders."

Observation of patient status	Treatments
Preventive measures	Health-promotion measures

Specific nursing activities in each of those categories might include the following:

Physical care	Emotional support
Teaching	Making referrals
Counseling	Managing the environment

***Writing
Nursing Orders***

Teaching Orders Not all teaching requires a separate, formal teaching plan. Informal teaching is an intervention for many, if not most, nursing diagnoses. You may do specific teaching to enable the patient to do some of his own care (e.g., how to take his own pulse and blood pressure), and you will find that you are teaching almost constantly as you explain to clients what you are doing for them and why. Informal teaching may include such activities as explaining the expected effects and side effects of a medication you are giving, explaining why the client should not ambulate without help, or clarifying the need to remain NPO.

Teaching orders should include the teaching strategies to use in presenting the new information or skill. The appropriate strategy depends on the client's needs and the learning outcome you are working toward. Cognitive content is usually taught through discussion, lecture, printed materials, and audiovisuals. Psychomotor skills need to be demonstrated and discussed, and then reinforced with practice. Affective goals generally require role-modeling, discussion, and counseling to help the client gain insight. An example of a teaching order would be "Demonstrate technique for drawing up insulin."

Counseling and Emotional Support Orders Counseling includes the use of therapeutic communication techniques to help clients make decisions about their health care and perhaps make lifestyle changes. It also involves techniques for helping clients recognize, express, and cope with feelings such as anxiety, anger, and fear. Counseling includes emotional support—but emotional support may occur on a less complex level: it may be given simply by the nurse's touch, presence, or apparent understanding of the patient's situation. An example of a counseling order would be "Help client to recognize when she is anxious by pointing out symptoms as you observe them."

Referral Orders You should make referrals when the client needs in-depth interventions for which other professionals are specifically prepared. For instance, while the nurse may counsel an anxious patient, long-term treatment of severe anxiety would be referred to a psychotherapist or counselor. Nurses often make referrals for follow-up care after dismissal. An example of a referral order is "Refer to Social Service Department for transportation to clinic."

Environmental Management Orders Nursing orders are often created to provide for a safe, clean, therapeutic environment. Environmental management includes removing hazards for clients who are particularly at risk for injury—for instance, children, the elderly, and those with a decreased level of consciousness.

> ***Examples:*** Teach mother to check temperature of formula with back of hand.
> Remain at bedside while client is smoking.
> Keep crib rails up at all times.

Selection Grid Figure 6–3 is a grid you might use to be sure you have considered all the various types of nursing orders for a patient. First think of the observation orders that apply to the problem. If one of the orders is to auscultate the patient's lungs, you would place an *X* in the box under "Observation" and beside "Physical Care." You might wish to teach a client to assess her own blood

Planning

glucose level; if so, place an *X* in the box under "Observation" and beside "Teaching." Probably none of the other actions in the vertical column would fit under "Observation." Next consider what kind of physical care, teaching, and so on would be involved in preventive nursing orders. Continue to move across the top of the grid in this manner.

Select the Best Options

Selecting the best interventions is a matter of hypothesizing that certain actions will bring about the desired outcome. The best options are those you expect to be most effective in helping the client to achieve the goals. To determine this, ask yourself the following questions:

1. What nursing orders have been successful in solving this problem in the past?
2. Which nursing orders are especially appropriate for the client's knowledge, abilities, and resources?
3. Which actions directly address the cause of the client's problem?

Your knowledge, experience and intuition will help you make these judgments, as will the "Guidelines for Writing Nursing Orders" that conclude this section (see pages 203–204).

Even carefully selected nursing orders do not guarantee success in meeting client goals. A successful intervention for one client may not work at all for another. In fact, for the same client, an intervention may be effective at one time and not at another. Nursing research has established the probability of success for some interventions. Use nursing orders based on scientific principles and sound research, when possible, to improve the likelihood of success.

	Observation	*Prevention*	*Treatment*	*Health Promotion*
Physical Care	×			
Teaching	×			
Counseling				
Emotional Support				
Activities of Daily Living				
Environmental Management				
Referrals				

Figure 6–3. Grid for Identifying Alternative Nursing Orders

Components of a Nursing Order

After selecting the appropriate nursing interventions, write them on the nursing care plan in the form of nursing orders (see Table 6–7). A well-written nursing order contains the following components:

1. *Date the order was written.* The date will be changed to reflect review or revisions.
2. *Subject.* The subject is implied, not written. Nursing orders are written in terms of *nurse* behaviors; so the subject of the order is *the nurse.* As you learn to write nursing orders, think "The nurse will . . ." or "The nurse should . . ." at the beginning of the statement, but do not write it.

   Example:

Goals	Nursing Orders
Patient behaviors	**Nurse behaviors**
↓	↓
(Pt. will) Walk to the door with help beginning on 2/12.	*(Nurse will)* Assist pt. to ambulate to the door t.i.d.

3. *Action verb that directs what the nurse is to do.* Examples of action verbs are *offer, assist, instruct, refer, assess, auscultate, change, give, listen, demonstrate,* and *turn.*

   Examples: *Auscultate* lungs at 0800 and 1600 daily.
   Assist to chair for 30 min. t.i.d.

4. *Descriptive qualifiers.* This is the phrase that tells the nurse how, when, and where to perform the action. It may also describe the action in more detail (*what*). When one activity depends on another, the descriptive qualifier also includes the sequence in which actions are to be done.

   Examples:

   What **When**

   Give written instructions for incision care before dismissal.

   What **Sequence/When**

   Take B/P before and after ambulating.

Table 6–7. Examples of Nursing Orders

Subject	Action Verb	Descriptive Phrase	Time Frame	Date and Signature
(Nurse)	(will) Monitor	for verbalization of interest in group activities	With each patient contact	4-14-96 J. Jonas, RN
(Nurse)	(will) Instruct	to avoid drinking liquids with meals if nausea occurs	Evening shift 4/14	4-14-96 J. Jonas, RN
(Nurse)	(will) Pad	side rails	During periods of restlessness and confusion	4-14-96 J. Jonas, RN

5. *Specific times.* State when, how often, and how long the activity is to be done.

> ***Example:***   Assist to chair *for 30 minutes b.i.d.*
> Change dressing at *0800 and 1400 daily.*

When scheduling times for the nursing actions, be sure to consider the patient's usual rest, visiting hours, mealtimes, and other activities of daily living. Also coordinate the times with collaborative tests and treatments (e.g., physical therapy).

Because you must document nursing interventions, the times and frequencies written in the nursing orders actually specify when and how often you will chart information about each problem. If the documentation interval is *not* the same as the frequency of the nursing care, you should indicate both on the care plan. Some forms have a separate column in which to write the documentation interval.

6. *Signature.* The nurse who writes the order should sign it, indicating acceptance of legal and ethical accountability. A signature also allows other nurses to contact the writer for questions or feedback about the order. Nursing orders should be followed only if all components are present. You would not follow an unsigned physician's order; the same should be true of a nursing order. You would not follow an imprecise medical order such as, "Give an analgesic occasionally"; nor should you implement an imprecise nursing order such as, "Give emotional support."

Formal Teaching Plans

Nursing orders for formal teaching plans are written in the same format as other nursing orders. They contain the content to be covered by the nurse, the teaching strategy to be used, and the learner activities assigned or used in the session.

Teaching orders and strategies should be based on principles of teaching and learning. You may wish to refer to a basic nursing text for more information about various teaching strategies, such as role modeling, discussion, demonstration, and use of audiovisual materials. Teaching is likely to be more effective under the following conditions.

1. *The learner's knowledge and abilities are assessed first.* Many factors affect a client's ability to learn, including existing knowledge, previous experience, education, age, and state of health. Misconceptions and misinformation may interfere with learning new facts. Illness or sensory-perceptual deficits may make it difficult for the client to process or remember information.

2. *The learner has no unmet physical or emotional needs* that interfere with learning (e.g., pain, fatigue, hunger).

3. *Teaching proceeds from simple to complex.* This makes the content easier to understand. Learning is a sequential process, in which new information builds on previous knowledge and experience.

4. *The learner is ready and motivated to learn.* People learn best when they can see a need to learn. A client with hypertension may not be ready to learn about a low-calorie diet until he begins having symptoms of the disease. Denial is a common psychological defense mechanism for persons who develop serious illness. Clients who have not yet worked through their denial do not learn well because they cannot see the need to learn about a problem they do not yet acknowledge having. If the client is not ready, the nurse may need to direct the teaching to significant others.

5. *The learner is actively involved.* A learner who is involved in an activity learns and retains more than one who is listening passively. Encourage the client to ask questions, and periodically ask him to summarize his understanding of what you have said. Supervised practice, feedback, and positive reinforcement are other forms of active involvement that promote learning.

6. *The environment is conducive to learning.* It should be quiet, at a comfortable temperature, appropriately lighted, and free from distractions.

7. *The emotional climate is favorable.* Very little learning occurs in the presence of intense emotions such as anger, anxiety, and fear. When such emotions are present, the nurse should use therapeutic communication to help the client deal with these emotions before attempting to teach.

8. *Rapport exists between patient and nurse.* A positive relationship, in which the client trusts and perceives the nurse as caring, promotes client cooperation and learning.

9. *Repetition and reinforcement are used.* Continued practice helps the client to retain new information. Rewards may be internal (personal) or external (praise). Pride in accomplishment can be a good learning incentive.

*Writing
Nursing Orders*

Guidelines for Writing Nursing Orders

After choosing the nursing orders, evaluate them by applying the following criteria. Each nursing order should meet most, if not all, of these criteria.

The nursing orders should:	Example or Comments	
1. be written in terms of nurse behaviors.	*Incorrect*:	Wear ice collar.
	Correct:	(Nurse will) Apply ice collar prn.
2. be individualized for the client's specific needs.	*Incorrect*:	Encourage fluids
	Correct:	Offer fluids qhr. Ct. likes orange juice.
3. be specific and detailed enough to be interpreted the same by everyone.	*Incorrect*:	Encourage fluids.
	Correct:	Give 2400 mL/24 hr 7–3, 1000 mL 3–11, 800 mL 11–7, 600 mL
4. be concise.	*Incorrect*:	Complex, routine procedures written on care plan.
	Correct:	"See Unit 6 Procedure Manual for tracheal suctioning procedure."
	(*Note*: If modifications need to be made to adapt the procedure to the client, these changes *should* be noted in the nursing orders; e.g., "Use alcohol; client allergic to Betadine.")	

203

Planning

The nursing orders should:	Example or Comments
5. be consistent with standards of care.	ANA, JCAHO, the health care agency.
6. be realistic in terms of client abilities and resources.	It would be unrealistic to order "Refer to home health agency for aide," if the client could not afford this service.
7. be realistic in terms of nursing and institution resources and abilities.	"Turn hourly" may not be a realistic order on a unit that is short-staffed.
8. be congruent with the client's values, beliefs, and psychosocial background.	If a client were protein-deficient, you would not write an order to add meat to the diet if she were a vegetarian.
9. be safe.	A nursing order for range-of-motion exercises that specifies "Do not force beyond the point of resistance."
10. be compatible with medical and other therapies.	*Incorrect:* A nursing order to assist the patient with ambulation to prevent constipation, when there is a medical order for bed rest.
11. be complete. (All components present: date, signature, action verb, descriptive qualifiers, specific times.)	Who, what, where, when, how, how often, how much.
12. be moral (ethical).	A nursing order to withhold information in order to prevent emotional upset may be morally questionable because it does not respect the patient's autonomy.
13. be based on scientific rationale or research.	Research shows that axillary temperatures for newborns are accurate and safer than rectal temps.
14. address all aspects of the etiology.	Remove or decrease causal, contributing, or risk factors.
15. include independent and collaborative actions as appropriate.	
16. address observation, prevention, treatment, and health promotion as appropriate.	(See grid, Figure 6–3)
17. include a variety of approaches.	For example, teaching, counseling, referring (see grid, Figure 6–3).

Wellness Intérventions

Wellness Interventions

Nursing interventions for well clients stress self-responsibility and active client involvement. The nurse may suggest health-promotion strategies, considering the client's age, sex, lifestyle, education, sociocultural background, and other variables. However, the client is the primary decision maker; the nurse functions mainly as teacher and health counselor. Activities needed for goal achievement may be written in terms of what the nurse is to do or what the client is to do.

Nursing orders on wellness care plans may take the form of specific behavioral changes the client wishes to make (e.g., "I would like to stop smoking") and strategies for reinforcing the new behaviors. The most effective rewards are self-rewards rather than reinforcement from the nurse.

> **Example:** A moderately overweight client wishes to lose weight.
>
> | *Specific Behavioral Changes* | *Rewards* |
> | --- | --- |
> | I will walk for 45 minutes every day for the next two weeks. | I will buy myself a new jogging suit. |
> | I will not eat between meals for one week. | I will treat myself to dinner out at my favorite seafood restaurant. |

Most disease-prevention/health-promotion strategies involve lifestyle changes such as diet changes, regular exercise, stress reduction, or cessation of smoking. Motivation for change is sometimes difficult when no actual problem exists. A number of behavior-change strategies are available for helping clients to modify health behaviors, for example, self-confrontation, cognitive restructuring, modeling, and operant conditioning. Pender (1987, Chapters 9 and 10) and Schafer (1987, Chapters 8–14) may be useful if you wish to develop detailed nursing strategies to promote high-level wellness.

Nursing Interventions Classification (NIC)

Chapter 5 described the efforts of the North American Nursing Diagnosis Association to standardize the language for describing *problems* that require nursing care. A research team at the University of Iowa recognized the need for a standardized language to describe the *treatments* that nurses perform, as well. They recently pioneered the development of a classification system (taxonomy) for nursing interventions to include all direct care treatments that nurses perform on behalf of patients, whether nurse-initiated or physician-initiated (Iowa Intervention Project, 1992, p. xvii).

In the NIC taxonomy, all nursing treatments are classified into six "domains": basic physiological, complex physiological, behavioral, family, health system, and safety. **Domains** are the broadest, most abstracting grouping. **Interventions,** which are at the lowest, most concrete level, are classified into these six domains. Similar to NANDA diagnoses, each intervention includes a category label and a definition. The research team has used a multimethod process, drawing on the judgment of experts in nursing research and practice, to link the

Planning

interventions to the NANDA diagnosis labels (Iowa Intervention Project, 1993b). For example, Table 6–8 contains the NIC interventions and definitions for the NANDA diagnosis of Sleep Pattern Disturbance.

Each nursing intervention requires a series of actions or activities to carry it out. In NIC terminology, **activities** are the specific, detailed actions taken by the nurse (e.g., taking vital signs, assessing for pallor, monitoring intake and output). As you can see from Table 6–9, you would not perform all the activities listed for an intervention, but would choose those that apply to each patient. When writing nursing orders, you should use activities, not intervention labels. However, when the NIC taxonomy becomes more widely used, it may be possible to write only the intervention labels and assume that all nurses would know how to carry them out.

ETHICS IN PLANNING

Ethical issues in the planning step involve decisions about the extent to which a client should be involved in planning her own care and about whether or not she is truly able to make free and informed decisions about her care. Goals are not value-neutral—not even the goals that nurses and clients set together. Merely by stating a goal in the direction of health, the nurse and client declare that health is something they value. Most people probably do value health, but the situation is not so clear with all goals.

Table 6–8. NIC Interventions for Sleep Pattern Disturbance

Sleep Pattern Disturbance: Disruption of sleep time causes discomfort or interferes with desired lifestyle.

Intervention	Definition
Environmental Management	Manipulation of the patient's surroundings for therapeutic benefit
Environmental Management: Comfort	Manipulation of the patient's surroundings for promotion of optimal comfort
Security Enhancement	Intensifying a patient's sense of physical and psychological safety
Simple Relaxation Therapy	Use of techniques to encourage and elicit relaxation for the purpose of decreasing undesirable signs and symptoms such as pain, muscle tension, or anxiety
Sleep Enhancement	Facilitation of regular sleep/wake cycles
Touch	Providing comfort and communication through purposeful tactile contact

Adapted from: Iowa Intervention Project (1993b). Compiled by J. Daly. *NIC Interventions Linked to NANDA Diagnoses.* Iowa City, IA: Iowa Intervention Project, pp. 108, 136, 141, 142, 144.

Obligation to Inform

The first tenet of the American Nurses Association *Code for Nurses* (1985) states that "The nurse provides services with respect for human dignity and the uniqueness of the client . . ." Respect for human dignity derives from the moral principle of autonomy. An autonomous person is one who is both free and able to choose. This suggests that nurses should provide clients with information so that they can make informed choices about their care, that is, about the goals for improving their health and the means for achieving those goals (nursing interventions and treatments). Clients may not know which goals are possible for them to achieve, nor of what is required in order to achieve them.

Obligation to Respect Choices

From a practical standpoint, involving clients in goal setting increases their motivation to achieve healthy outcomes. Client involvement is also a moral obligation. Mutual goal setting and care planning demonstrate respect for clients'

Table 6–9. Nursing Activities for the NIC Intervention, Touch

Definition of touch: Providing comfort and communication through purposeful tactile contact.

Activities:

Observe cultural taboos regarding touch

Give a reassuring hug as appropriate

Put arm around patient's shoulders as appropriate

Hold patient's hand to provide emotional support

Apply gentle pressure at wrist, hand, or shoulder of seriously ill patient

Rub back in synchrony with patient's breathing as appropriate

Stroke body part in slow, rhythmic fashion as appropriate

Massage around painful area as appropriate

Elicit from parents common actions used to soothe and calm their child

Hold infant or child firmly and snugly

Encourage parents to touch newborn or ill child

Surround premature infant with blanket rolls (nesting)

Swaddle infant snugly in a blanket to keep arms and legs close to the body

Place infant on mother's body immediately after birth

Encourage mother to hold, touch, and examine the infant while umbilical cord is being severed

Encourage parents to hold infant

Encourage parents to massage infant

Demonstrate quieting techniques for infants

Provide appropriate pacifier for nonnutritional sucking in newborns

Provide oral stimulation exercises prior to tube feedings in premature infants

Source: Iowa Intervention Project. (1992). J. McCloskey and G. Bulechek, eds. *Nursing Interventions Classification (NIC)*. St. Louis: Mosby Year Book, p. 502.

Planning

values and for their dignity and worth as persons. Clients in the health care system are in a vulnerable and dependent state. They often feel that caregivers are more capable than they are to make decisions about their care, and their decision-making abilities may actually be diminished by their illness. When clients are experiencing conflict about choices, or when they are too ill to choose, it is appropriate to propose alternatives. In your eagerness to help, however, you can, without even realizing it, impose your own values on the client. Unless you are very sensitive, clients may defer to what they believe you want them to do, without making their true preferences known. Nurses must be aware of their power to influence patient decisions and make sure the choices are truly the client's.

LEGAL ISSUES

Writing an outcome and target time on a nursing care plan implies that you accept accountability for helping the client achieve the outcome. Consider this outcome: "Will be able to walk to bathroom without help by discharge (8/15)." If the client goes home without achieving this goal and falls while walking to the bathroom, you may be found negligent unless you have documented good reasons why the outcome was not achieved. For this reason, some nurses choose to write goals for collaborative problems only on multidisciplinary care plans (to be discussed in Chapter 9), and not on nursing care plans. Recall that for each client problem you identify, you must decide whether to refer the problem to another professional or start an independent plan of care. To help you decide, ask: "Is nursing responsible for initiating the plan to achieve this outcome? Can nursing care reproduce the outcome?" If not, refer the problem to the professional who is accountable. If you are unsure, consult with a more experienced nurse.

CULTURAL CONSIDERATIONS

During planning, the nurse uses information about the client's and family's cultural values, beliefs, and practices to identify interventions that will fulfill their cultural needs. For example, the nurse considers the client's food preferences and practices; identifies the person responsible for selecting and preparing foods; and then works with the family to teach them how to select and prepare cultural foods that will comply with therapeutic diet prescriptions (e.g., a low-fat diet).

When planning care activities, you should assess language barriers and consider the need for an interpreter. Sometimes culturally diverse clients require information to avoid confusion or embarrassment. For example, the position for bowel evacuation or the norm for the frequency of bowel movements may differ; or the client who is very modest may need much preparation and support before having an enema. When planning client education for clients whose primary language is not English, try to have written materials translated, use pictures to reinforce the written instructions, and have an interpreter give verbal instructions in the client's primary language.

Identify community resources available to assist clients of different cultures. And finally, try to learn from each transcultural nursing situation you encounter in order to improve the delivery of culture-specific care to future clients (Kozier et. al., 1994).

SPIRITUAL CONSIDERATIONS

Planning should be directed toward helping clients achieve the overall goals of spiritual strength, serenity, and satisfaction. A common intervention is to arrange a visit from a clergy member. Some clients may directly ask to see the hospital chaplain or their own clergyman. Others may discuss their concerns with the nurse and ask about the nurse's beliefs as a way of seeking an empathic listener. Families may wish spiritual assistance, as well. It is important to ask the client before arranging such assistance, though. Some people may profess no religious beliefs and may not wish to see a chaplain. The nurse should respect the clients' wishes in this area and not make judgments about whether they are right or wrong.

Planning in relation to a nursing diagnosis of Spiritual Distress should be designed to meet one or more of the following needs. Nursing actions should help the client:

✓ fulfill religious obligations
✓ draw on and use inner resources to meet the present situation
✓ maintain or establish a dynamic, personal relationship with a supreme being in the face of unpleasant circumstances
✓ find meaning in existence and the present situation
✓ acquire a sense of hope
✓ access spiritual resources otherwise unavailable

NIC interventions for Spiritual Distress include: anticipatory guidance, coping enhancement, counseling, crisis intervention, decision-making support, dying care, emotional support, grief work facilitation, guilt work facilitation, hope instillation, and presence (Iowa Intervention Project, 1993b, p. 111).

Critical Thinking Questions: Examining Your Own Feelings and Thoughts

Mr. Lance has emphysema. He receives oxygen therapy at home and is frequently admitted to the hospital for acute respiratory distress—at times requiring mechanical ventilation. When you make a home care visit, you smell stale cigarette smoke and see ashtrays full of ashes and cigarette stubs. Mr. Lance begins smoking a cigarette.
✓ What would your feelings be?
✓ What thoughts, perhaps about past experiences, might contribute to the feelings you are having?

Planning

SUMMARY

Planning
✓ begins when the client is admitted and continues until dismissal.
✓ provides a written framework necessary for individualized care and third-party reimbursement.

Goals/Outcomes
✓ are guides to planning and evaluation that motivate client and nurse by providing a sense of achievement.
✓ are stated in terms of observable, achievable client behaviors.
✓ are composed of subject, action verb, performance criteria, target time, and special conditions.
✓ may be short-term or long-term.
✓ can be written for groups and individuals.

Nursing orders
✓ should be culturally sensitive and specific.
✓ should include those directed toward achieving clients' spiritual goals.
✓ provide specific direction and a consistent, individualized approach to patient care.
✓ should address observation, prevention, treatment, and health promotion.
✓ are composed of date, subject, action verb, descriptive qualifiers, specific times, and signature.
✓ may address dependent or independent nursing interventions (i.e., teaching or environmental manipulation).

Ethical and Legal Considerations
✓ in planning center around the principle of autonomy, implying a moral obligation to inform and involve clients in planning their own care.
✓ require the nurse to be accountable for outcomes written on the nursing care plan.

In everyday life you often analyze complex situations. You might watch a football game and try to understand the plays. Analyzing football plays is easy for some people because they have learned to see the relevant information. They know, for instance,

that watching the quarterback just after the play starts can help them understand whether the play is a run or a pass. If you want to learn to analyze football plays you must learn how to find the relevant information.

Learning the Skill

Example A.   Recognizing football plays is a two-step process.

> *Step 1.* Learn the names used to identify the various plays. The meanings of these names help you to remember what the plays are. For instance, there are *running* plays; during a running play, what is the player doing?

> *Step 2.* Learn to focus your attention on the relevant aspects of the play—the people involved and the situation at hand. At the beginning of a football play, which player should you watch most carefully?

Example B.   Recognizing the presence of a client's nursing diagnosis uses the same two-step process.

> *Step 1.* Learn the names and definitions of the various NANDA labels.

> In the *Nursing Diagnosis Guide* you will find labels like Anxiety, Fear, and Personal Identity Disturbance. These names may be familiar to you. Which one means inability to distinguish between self and nonself?

> Which one means a vague, uneasy feeling with a nonspecific source?

> *Step 2.* Learn to focus your attention on important aspects of the nursing diagnosis—the defining characteristics or risk factors. If you do not know which signs and symptoms are associated with a particular label, you may not realize the significance of the client's signs and symptoms. In fact, if you do not know what signs and symptoms to look for, you may not even be aware of the cues, much less the existence of a problem.

> Nurses often misdiagnose Fear and Anxiety because some of the physical and emotional manifestations may be the same. If you focus only on the relevant cues, however, you can make the distinction. Use your *Nursing Diagnosis Guide* as needed.

1. For which label is the feeling one of *dread*?
   For which label is the feeling *vague and uneasy*?
   Write a rule you could use to tell these two labels apart.

2. In which label is the source of the feeling known to the client?
   In which label is the source of the feeling nonspecific or unknown to the client?

   Write another rule you could use to tell these two labels apart.

3. Which of these labels has only one defining characteristic?
   What is the defining characteristic?
   Write another rule you could use to differentiate between Anxiety and Fear.

4. In the following case study, your client is exhibiting physical and emotional signs of distress. Circle the cues that are *relevant* to a diagnosis of Fear.

   Mr. Cheng has pneumonia. His I & O record shows he has not been drinking fluids. When you auscultate his lungs, you hear bilateral crackles and rales. His temperature is 100°, and his B/P is 140/90. He says he is very weak. He states, "I just feel like something awful is going to happen to me." He is perspiring, and his hands are shaking. He has just been started on oxygen therapy, and he tells you the mask makes him feel that he is suffocating. You check his data base and find he has a history of claustrophobia.

Applying the Skill

The same process is used in identifying collaborative problems. You must know the complications that may occur with medical diagnoses and therapies and the signs and symptoms of the complications.

1. Read the following case study. Refer to a basic nursing text or a medical-surgical nursing text if you need to.

   Katie O'Hara has severe vomiting and diarrhea because of gastroenteritis. Because she needs fluids and antibiotics, her physician has prescribed intravenous therapy, which she will need for several days.

a. What are the two obvious potential complications of intravenous therapy?

b. What are the symptoms of those complications?

    (1)

    (2)

c. If you are assessing Katie for Complications of Intravenous Therapy: Infiltration and Phlebitis, which data would be relevant? (Circle the relevant data.)

> B/P 110/80, pulse 80, temperature 100° F. Katie states that she feels afraid, but "just can't put my finger on what it is." She remains NPO. Her output for the shift is 350 mL emesis, 150 mL of urine, and six unmeasured liquid stools. Her hands are warm and dry; the skin turgor is good on her forearms. Her IV is infusing at 100 mL per hour, but it is positional (i.e., it sometimes stops running when she changes the position of her arm). You have opened the roller clamp completely, but it will not run at the prescribed rate of 150 mL per hour. There is no redness at or above the insertion site. The area around the insertion site is pale and cool to touch. Katie states that it is a little tender to touch. When you hang her piggyback antibiotic, she complains that it burns her arm. Katie's data base shows no allergy to any medications.

2. Suppose you were assessing a patient for Impaired Tissue Integrity (Decubitus Ulcer). List the relevant data (i.e., what signs, symptoms, and risk factors would you look for?).

Adapted from *Critical Thinking Worksheets,* a Supplement of *Addison-Wesley Chemistry,* by Wilbraham et al. (Menlo Park, CA: Addison-Wesley Publishing Company, 1990).

1. Place a check mark beside the measurable, observable goals (for brevity, none of the goals has a target time).

   ___ Will be progressively less anxious.   ___ Rates pain as < 3 on a 1–10 scale.

   ___ Eats fruit at least 3 times/day.   ___ States less anxious than before exercise.

   ___ Skin warm and dry to touch.   ___ Will not have foul-smelling lochia.

   ___ Temp. will be < 100.1.   ___ B/P will be normal.

   ___ Explains importance of exercise.   ___ Tolerates increased activity.

   ___ Normal skin color.   ___ Experiences increased confidence.

   ___ States he feels more confident.   ___ Verbalizes understanding of home-care instructions.

2. The problem responses are given for you. Write an opposite, normal response that might be used in an outcome statement. The first one is done for you.

	Problem Response	Desired (Opposite) Response
a.	Constipation	Regular, formed, soft bowel movement
b.	Impaired Skin Integrity: Pressure Sore	
c.	Hypothermia	
d.	Dressing Self Care Deficit	
e.	Altered Oral Mucous Membrane	

3. Use the normal responses you wrote in Exercise 2 to create outcomes. Fill in the boxes with the necessary components. Since there is no actual client, target times have been omitted. The first one has been done for you.

Subject	Action Verb	Special Conditions	Performance Criteria
a. (Client)	will have	(none)	regular, soft, formed B.M.
b.			
c.			
d.			
e.			

4. Write outcomes for the following nursing diagnosis:

Back Pain r/t incision of recent spinal fusion and muscle stiffness from decreased mobility

a. An outcome derived from the *problem*:

b. An outcome derived from the *etiology*:

5. A nursing diagnosis for Ms. Jackson follows: "Risk for Impaired Skin Integrity (Pressure Ulcers) r/t long periods of lying in bed." Write outcomes and nursing orders for this diagnosis.

Goals/Predicted Outcomes	Nursing Orders

6. Place an *O* by the outcomes and an *N* by the nursing orders.

  a. ___ Will verbalize anxieties about his surgery by 12/16.

  b. ___ Will rate pain as less than 3 on a scale of 1 to 10.

  c. ___ Keep head of bed elevated to 45°.

  d. ___ Turn patient every 2 hours.

  e. ___ Force fluids up to 250 mL per hour.

  f. ___ Circulation to left foot will be improved, as evidenced by pink color, warm skin.

  g. ___ Infection will be prevented, as evidenced by temp < 100.1.

  h. ___ Wear sterile gloves for dressing change.

  i. ___ Take temperature hourly if elevated.

  j. ___ Will list foods allowed on low-fat diet by 12/16.

7. Circle the action verbs:

Apply	Improve	Be
Demonstrate	Have	Verbalize

8. Label the following objectives, *A*—Affective, *C*—Cognitive, *P*—Psychomotor

  a. ___ (Learner will) draw up the correct amount of insulin.

  b. ___ (Learner will) explain the syringe markings correctly.

  c. ___ (Learner will) discuss his fear of needles openly.

  d. ___ (Learner will) list four foods that can be used as bread exchanges.

  e. ___ (Learner will) express anger appropriately.

  f. ___ (Learner will) inject himself, using sterile technique.

  g. ___ (Learner will) state the relationship between exercise and insulin requirements.

  h. ___ (Learner will) insert needle at a 45° angle.

9. Circle the letter of the correctly written outcomes. If it is incorrectly written, state what is wrong with it (refer to Box 6.3 and "Guidelines for Writing Outcome Statements" on pages 187 to 192). Some of the predicted outcomes address potential problems, so it is not an error if no time frame is given.

	Predicted Outcome	Errors (Guideline Violated)
a.	Client will develop adequate leg strength by 9/1.	
b.	Will have no signs of hemorrhage: VS-WNL, Hct and Hbg WNL, uses < 1 vag. pad per hour.	
c.	Will state the signs and symptoms of angina by 9/1.	
d.	Will feel better by morning.	
e.	Improved appetite.	
f.	Will be able to feed self by 9/1.	
g.	(On a 30-bed unit with only 2 wheelchairs) Will spend 4 hours each day in a wheelchair.	
h.	Client will discuss expectations of hospitalization and will relate the effects of a high-carbohydrate diet on blood-sugar levels with a basic knowledge of exchange diet for diabetes.	
i.	After second teaching session, will demonstrate correct technique for testing blood for glucose.	
j.	Injects self with insulin.	
k.	Will state adequate pain relief from analgesics and will take at least 100 Ml of p.o. fluids per hour.	
l.	IV will remain patent and run at 125 ml/hr.	
m.	By 7/15 expresses a desire for social contact and interaction with others.	
n.	Reports no numbness or tingling in left hand.	
o.	Voids at least 150 Ml within 4 hr after removal of catheter.	

10. Read the following list of nursing actions. Classify them (e.g., Dependent/Independent) by writing the letters beside the appropriate category in the chart. Interventions can be classified in several ways, so most will belong in more than one category. (The first one has been done for you.)

Nursing Orders

a. Review booklet on postmastectomy exercises with Ms. Petrie on evening of 7/13.

b. Spend at least 10 minutes per shift sitting with Ms. Adkins; encourage her to express her feelings about her husband's death.

c. Give acetaminophen gr. 500, p.o. q3h if temp >101.2.

d. Remove staples from abdominal incision today.

e. Minimize environmental stimuli: dim lights, restrict visitors, speak and move slowly and quietly.

f. DO NOT take rectal temperatures.

g. Cut food for patient. Allow at least an hour for meals. Reheat food as needed.

h. Palpate uterine fundus for firmness q hr until saturating < 1 pad/hr.

i. B/P q4h unless elevated. If >150/94, take q hr.

j. Pad side rails with blankets or rubber pads.

k. Teach patient to wash hands carefully before handling infant.

l. Refer to Public Health Dept. for Rubella immunization.

m. Give pamphlets on "The Food Guide Pyramid" and "Foods for Healthy Living."

Independent: *a*   Dependent:
Observation: Treatment: *a*   Prevention: Health promotion:
Physical care: Teaching: *a*   Counseling: Referral: Environmental management:

Case Study. Exercises 11–13 pertain to this case.

Ms. Nancy Atwell is a 32-year-old, unmarried teacher who has been diagnosed as having rheumatoid arthritis for approximately 4 years. This change has made her knees painful and has limited the motion and weight-bearing ability of the knee joints themselves. Ms. Atwell's knee inflammation is aggravated by the fact that she is 75 lb overweight. Her diet history reveals that she eats when feeling depressed or stressed and that she snacks frequently on potato chips and colas.

She has recently been diagnosed as having endometriosis, and now enters the hospital to have a hysterectomy. On her previous admission for treatment of her arthritis, she had been quiet, withdrawn, and extremely concerned for her privacy. Now she seems more outgoing and less overtly concerned about privacy. When questioned, Ms. Atwell states that she has had no previous surgical experience, but denies feeling nervous about the operation.

Her preoperative orders follow:

1. NPO

2. pHisohex shower

3. Pre-op med: Demerol 50 mg. and Vistaril 25 mg. IM at 0600

The nurse has identified the following nursing diagnoses for Ms. Atwell. (*Note*: There are other appropriate nursing diagnoses; for simplicity, we consider only these four.)

   a. Risk for Low Situational Self Esteem r/t unresolved feeling about inability to bear children after hysterectomy
   b. Chronic Pain r/t inflammation of knees 2° rheumatoid arthritis
   c. Altered Nutrition: More Than Body Requirements for calories r/t excess calorie intake from "emotional eating"
   d. Risk for Noncompliance with NPO Order r/t lack of understanding of its importance for anesthesia

11. Prioritize the nursing diagnoses. Number them in order, giving #1 to the highest priority. Put an asterisk beside the ones that the nurse *must* address today.

12. Underline the portion of each of the nursing diagnoses for which you *must* write a goal.

13. On the following chart, write goals/outcomes, and nursing orders for the two top-priority nursing diagnoses. Include dependent nursing actions (e.g., medications) under nursing orders on this care plan.

Nursing Diagnoses	Goals /Outcomes	Nursing Orders

14. Refer to Figure 3–3 (Luisa Sanchez's data base in Chapter 3), page 56, and the problem list for Luisa in Chapter 5, pages 138 and 139.

One of Mrs. Sanchez's collaborative problems is Potential Complications of Intravenous Therapy: Inflammation, Phlebitis, Infiltration. Develop a care plan for this problem.

(1) List the signs and symptoms of each of the complications.

Inflammation:

Phlebitis:

Infiltration:

(2) In the columns below, write outcomes and nursing orders for each of the complications.

Goals/Outcomes	Nursing Orders
For inflammation	
For phlebitis	

Goals/Outcomes	Nursing Orders
For infiltration	

REFERENCES

American Nurses Association. (1991). *Standards of Clinical Nursing Practice*. Kansas City, MO: ANA.

American Nurses Association. (1985). *Code for Nurses with Interpretive Statements*. Kansas City, MO: ANA.

American Nurses Association. (1975). *Continuity of Care and Discharge Planning Programs in Institutions and Community Agencies. A Statement of the American Nurses Association Division on Medical Surgical Nursing Practices and the Division of Community Health Nursing Practice*. Kansas City, MO: ANA.

Bailey, D. (1988). Computer applications in nursing. *Computers in Nursing, 6*(5):199–203.

Beck, L., Miller, B., and Adams, D. (1993). Use of the Code of Ethics for accountability in discharge planning. *Nursing Forum, 28*(3):5–12.

Cosnotti, J., and Sprinkel, L. (1993). Roanoke Memorial Hospitals' Home Health Services discharge planning process. *Caring, 12*(8):70–77.

Eisenhauer, L. (1994). A typology of nursing therapeutics. *Image: Journal of Nursing Scholarship, 26*(4):261–276.

Foust, J. (1994). Creating a future for nursing through interactive planning at the bedside. *Image, Journal of Nursing Scholarship, 26*(2):129–132.

Gordon, M., et al. (1994). Clinical judgment: An integrated model. *Advances in Nursing Science, 16*(4):55–70.

Iowa Intervention Project (1995). Validation and coding of the NIC taxonomy structure. *Image: Journal of Nursing Scholarship, 27*(1):43–49.

Iowa Intervention Project (1993a). The NIC Taxonomy Structure. *Image: Journal of Nursing Scholarship, 25*(3):187–192.

Iowa Intervention Project (1993b). Compiled by J. Daly. *NIC Interventions Linked to NANDA Diagnoses*. Iowa City, IA: Iowa Intervention Project.

Iowa Intervention Project (1992). McCloskey, J., and Bulechek, G., eds. *Nursing Interventions Classification (NIC)*. St. Louis: Mosby Year Book.

Joint Commission on Accreditation of Healthcare Organizations (1992). *Accreditation Manual for Hospitals*. Vol. 1, *Standards*. Chicago: JCAHO.

Kozier, B., Erb, G., Blais, K., and Wilkinson, J. (1994). *Fundamentals of Nursing*. 5th ed. Redwood City, CA: Addison-Wesley.

Naylor, M. (1990). Comprehensive discharge planning for hospital elderly: A pilot study. *Nursing Research, 39*(3):156–161.

Pender, N. (1987). *Health Promotion in Nursing Practice*. 2nd ed. Norwalk, CT: Appleton & Lange.

Schafer, W. (1987). *Stress Management for Wellness*. New York: Holt, Rinehart, and Winston.

Schneider, J., et al. (1993). A medication discharge planning program. Measuring the effect on readmissions. *Clinical Nursing Research, 2*(1):41–53.

Tirk, J. (1992). Determining discharge priorities. *Nursing92, 22*(7):55.

Tuazon, N. (1992). Discharge teaching: Use this MODEL. *RN, 55*(4):19–22.

U.S. Department of Health and Human Services, Public Health Service. (1990). *Healthy People 2000*. DHHS Publication No. (PHS) 91-50212. Washington, DC: Superintendent of Documents, U.S. Government Printing Office.

CHAPTER 7

*I*MPLEMENTATION

OBJECTIVES

On completing this chapter, you should be able to do the following:
- Discuss the relationship of the implementation step to the other steps of the nursing process.
- Discuss preparations necessary before implementing patient-care activities.
- Follow guidelines for successful implementation of the nursing care plan.
- Compare team nursing, primary nursing, functional nursing, case management, and managed care.
- Compare and contrast four methods of writing nursing progress notes: narrative, SOAP, Focus charting©, and charting by exception.
- Observe guidelines for documenting and reporting patient care and status.
- Explain how patient dignity and privacy can be maintained during implementation.
- Explain how implementation can be done in a culturally and spiritually sensitive manner.
- Explain the relationship between critical thinking and autonomous nursing interventions.

Figure 7-1.
The Implementation Step in the Nursing Process

INTRODUCTION

Implementation is the nursing process step in which the nurse performs the activities necessary for achieving the client's health goals. Described broadly, the activities in this step are (1) doing, (2) delegating, and (3) recording (see Figure 7–1). During implementation the nurse performs or delegates the nursing orders that were developed in the planning step. The implementation step ends when nursing actions and the resulting client responses have been recorded in the client's chart.

Professional standards for nursing practice support client participation in implementation, as in all phases of the nursing process (see Box 7–1). The degree of participation in this step depends on the client's health status and resources, as well as on the type of action being considered. For example, an infant or an unconscious person cannot participate at all in implementation strategies; all interventions for such patients are carried out by nurses, significant others, or other caregivers. In the case of health-promotion strategies, the client alone might carry out the strategies.

Example: With the help of his nurse, David Mikos devised a plan for lowering his cholesterol intake. The plan is to follow a low-fat diet at home and reward himself with concert or theater tickets for each month of successful dieting. In this case, the nurse is not involved at all in the implementation step.

RELATIONSHIP OF IMPLEMENTATION TO OTHER NURSING PROCESS STEPS

Implementation depends on the first three steps of the nursing process: assessment, diagnosis, and planning. These steps provide the basis for the autonomous nursing actions performed during implementation. Without them, implementation (and nursing) would reflect only dependent functions—carrying out medical orders and institutional policies. In turn, the implementation step provides the actual interventions and client responses that are evaluated in the evaluation step.

Implementation is also interrelated to and overlaps with the other steps of the nursing process. Using data acquired during assessment, the nurse can individualize the care given during implementation, tailoring interventions to fit a specific client rather than applying them routinely to categories of patients (e.g., "All pneumonia patients . . . "). Ongoing assessment often occurs simultaneously with implementation. While implementing, you will continue to assess the patient at every contact, gathering data about her responses to the nursing actions and about any new problems that may develop. Ongoing assessment is not the *same* as implementation; it occurs *during* implementation.

Examples:

Implementation	Assessment
While bathing an elderly patient,	the nurse observes a reddened area on the patient's sacrum.
When emptying the catheter bag,	the nurse measures 200 mL and notices a strong odor.

The nurse also implements nursing orders that specifically *direct* ongoing assessment. For example, a nursing order might read, "Auscultate lungs q4h." When performing this activity, the nurse is both carrying out the nursing order and performing ongoing, focused assessment.

Box 7–1. ANA Standard V: Implementation

The nurse implements the interventions identified in the plan of care.
Measurement Criteria
1. Interventions are consistent with the established plan of care.
2. Interventions are implemented in a safe and appropriate manner.
3. Interventions are documented.

American Nurses Association. 1991. *Standards of Clinical Nursing Practice.* (Kansas City, MO. ANA, p. 71). Used by permission.

Implementation

Data obtained during implementation activities is used to identify new diagnoses, or revise existing diagnoses (diagnosis step). It also enables the nurse to revise and adapt the original goals and nursing orders (planning step) as the patient's unique needs become more apparent.

DELIVERY SYSTEMS FOR NURSING CARE

Six models commonly used for implementing nursing care are (1) functional nursing, (2) team nursing, (3) primary nursing, (4) differentiated practice, (5) case management, and (6) managed care. These systems, except for differentiated practice, differ in the way they allocate responsibilities, tasks, and authority; however, all can be used in a variety of settings (e.g., hospitals, clinics, home health).

In **functional nursing** a charge nurse (or head nurse) assigns caregivers to various tasks according to their level of knowledge and skill. For example, on a given shift, one RN might administer medications to all patients on the floor, another RN might perform the physical assessments and the patient teaching, a nursing assistant might take vital signs and make unoccupied beds for all the patients, and an LPN might bathe patients and perform some of the treatments. This system is efficient but tends to fragment care, as each patient sees several different caregivers during the course of a day.

In **team nursing** a team of registered nurses, licensed practical nurses, and nursing assistants work together to care for a group of patients during a shift. In some settings the team keeps the same group of patients from day to day. The team leader, an RN, is responsible for planning and assigning care to team members (nursing assistants, LPNs and other RNs), who function under her direction. Although the team leader plans and directs care, she does not always give care under this model. The success of this model depends greatly on communication between team members and the management abilities of the team leader.

In **primary nursing** a registered nurse is responsible for managing the care of a small group of patients 24 hours a day, 7 days a week. The primary nurse develops and implements the plan of care while she is at work and gives total, direct care to a caseload of patients. When she leaves, the plan is followed by nurse associates on the other shifts. Although the primary nurse may be assisted by other levels of staff, she is responsible for planning and coordinating all aspects of the patient's care, including medications, treatments, hygiene, comfort needs, communication with other professionals, emotional support, and so on. An advantage of this model is the continuity of care it provides; each patient has one nurse who is accountable for and well informed about his care.

Unlike the preceding delivery systems, **differentiated practice** cannot be characterized by the way it allocates responsibilities, tasks, and authority. Differentiated practice is an attempt to reorganize nursing care within an institution so that quality care can be achieved using fewer RNs. Its effect on staffing patterns and allocation of responsibilities varies from agency to agency, but it usually involves the analysis of tasks and the creation of new job descriptions. New levels of practitioners may be added, or new caregiver roles created (e.g., nurse aides may be used in new ways). Sometimes partnerships are created by permanently scheduling two caregivers to work together. **Partnering** may involve, for example, an RN and an aide, or a bachelor's degree RN and an associate degree RN. Differentiated practice tends to place the RN in a supervisory role. It is similar to functional nursing in that it distributes tasks among various levels of personnel. However, it includes careful consideration of client goals, using them as the criteria by which the system of care delivery is evaluated.

Managed Care and Case Management

Escalating health care costs and the demand for health care reform have brought about a restructuring of traditional care delivery systems and practice patterns. Two multidisciplinary clinical systems that have emerged are managed care and case management. The stated objectives of such systems include:

1. Achieving the following high-quality patient outcomes within an appropriate time frame:
   ✓ Patient wellness
   ✓ Patient/family self-care skills
   ✓ Patient/family satisfaction

2. Establishing collaborative practice and improving service coordination and continuity of care

3. Using health care resources appropriately

4. Directing the contributions of all care providers toward the achievement of patient outcomes

5. Increasing job satisfaction and job enrichment for caregivers

6. Encouraging innovation and ongoing integration of advances in health care

Managed Care

Managed care is used to standardize practice for the most common and prevalent case types in an agency. For example, case types in a cardiac care unit might be "myocardial infarction" and "cardiac catheterization." Third-party payers (e.g., insurance companies) make payments based on a client's diagnosis, or *diagnosis-related group (DRG)*, rather than on the actual number of days the client is hospitalized. Because an institution is paid only a specified amount, regardless of the time and resources a client consumes, it has become essential to achieve specific client outcomes within the length of stay allowed by the client's DRG.

Managed care systems try to facilitate achievement of predictable client and family outcomes within a specified time frame. Therefore, instead of the traditional, individualized nursing care plan, managed care systems use a form called a **critical path**. The critical path is a standardized, multidisciplinary care plan that outlines crucial activities to be performed by nurses, physicians, and other health team members at designated times. Explained very simply, creating a critical path is a matter of combining the care plans from nursing, medical, and other services and imposing a timeline on the combined plan. All outcomes, care, and treatments are shown on the plan, but they may be different each day, because the plan is organized by time.

Implementation

For a patient having an appendectomy, part of the critical pathway for pain might be as follows:

Day 1 post-op

Outcomes: Will verbalize pain appropriately to RN; will state pain is < 5 on a 1–10 scale.

Interventions: Self-controlled administration of morphine per IV pump.

Day 2 post-op

Outcomes: Will verbalize pain appropriately to RN; will state pain is < 2 on a 1–10 scale with no need for IV narcotic analgesics.

Interventions: Tylenol #3, tabs 1 p.o., as needed

A different critical pathway is created for each case type. For example, there would be one critical pathway for patients with myocardial infarction, and a different critical pathway for those having a cardiac catheterization. See Figure 9–10 on page 331 for an example of a critical pathway.

Case Management

Case management is "a form of personalized helping directed at connecting an individual to resources (internal-external) for improving their quality of community life" (Modrcin, Rapp, and Chamberlain, 1985, p. 64). Having evolved from primary nursing, this system uses health care professionals to coordinate care for high-risk, complex populations who may use a disproportionate share of health care resources. Unlike the "common" patients in managed care, case management deals with the unusual, uncommon cases seen in an agency—patients whose condition changes frequently and unpredictably, and whose complex needs cannot be addressed by a standardized critical pathway.

In this system a case manager is responsible for a caseload of clients throughout their hospitalization. Case managers are professional nurses with expertise in a particular clinical area. Their caseloads may be organized geographically by hospital unit (e.g., surgical units), by diagnosis (e.g., cardiac rehabilitation), or by physician. The case manager manages a network of services for patients and families in all settings in which the patient receives care. Some case managers act "as a service broker, linking the client to needed services, while others focus on developing consumers' skills to increase success in their selected environment" (Skinner, 1995, p. 3).

PREPARING TO ACT

Preparation for patient-care activities actually begins in the planning step of the nursing process. When you use time-sequenced planning to set your work priorities and make your daily work schedule, you are actually taking the first step in delivering care to your assigned patients. Box 7–2 is a guide you may wish to use in organizing your nursing care for a clinical day. It may be helpful, especially for students, to create a time schedule around this guide to provide structure for the day and ensure that the patient's needs are met.

During a time when many institutions are focusing on cost and efficiency, it is important that each nurse-patient encounter be fully utilized. When possible, try to implement care for several goals simultaneously. While at the bedside taking vital signs and making physical assessments, for instance, you might use that time to talk with the patient, show interest and concern, or do patient teaching.

Box 7–2. Student Guide for Organizing Clinical Activities

Client profile: Name_____ Age_____

    Admitting diagnosis_____Admit date_____

    Name client wishes to be called_____

    Significant other(s)_____

Current health status (today):

    Has the client's physical or emotional status changed since
you received your assignment?

    Do you need to modify your care plan?

Basic Care Needs:

    Hygiene _____

    Elimination _____

    Feeding _____

    Dressing _____

    Other _____

    Special safety precautions _____

Medications and IVs:

**Collaborative tests and treatments (for scheduling and
observation)**—e.g., physical therapy, X ray.

Prioritized nursing diagnoses and strategies (that you can
realistically address today):

New medical orders that need to be implemented
(e.g., discontinue IV, ambulate):

Special teaching or counseling needs:

Implementation

Preparing the Nurse

Before beginning an intervention, be sure that both you and the patient are prepared. Always review the care plan to familiarize yourself with the actions you are to take. This allows you to clarify any details and determine if you need help in performing any of the interventions. You may require assistance under the following conditions:

1. *You lack the skill or knowledge to implement a nursing order.* For example, if you have never taught a patient to crutch-walk, you should ask a colleague for help or review the written procedure before attempting the intervention.

2. *You cannot safely perform the action alone.* For example, you should obtain help when moving a large, immobile patient from a bed to a chair.

3. *Assistance would reduce the client's stress.* For example, having help in repositioning a patient who experiences pain when being moved will minimize her pain.

You are legally and ethically responsible for questioning nursing or medical orders that you believe to be inappropriate or potentially harmful. This should also be done as a part of your preparation.

Preparation includes determining points in the activity where you need to pause for feedback. The immediate feedback you obtain during an activity guides you in making on-the-spot alterations in the action. For example, when preparing to help a patient ambulate, you might plan to look for responses (feedback) after he sits on the side of the bed for a minute, after standing, after walking to a chair, and again after he has been sitting in the chair for 15 minutes.

Preparing the Client

Just before implementing, you should *reassess whether the intervention is still needed.* Never assume that an order is still necessary simply because it is written on the care plan; the situation or the client's condition may have changed. For example, a nursing diagnosis for Gayle Fischer is Sleep Pattern Disturbance related to anxiety and unfamiliar surroundings. When the nurse makes rounds, she discovers that Gayle is sleeping, so she omits the back rub that was planned as a relaxation strategy.

You should also *assess the client's readiness.* The client's behavioral cues will help you to choose a time when the activity will benefit her most. A great deal of time can be wasted in performing interventions when a client is not psychologically ready. For example, when the nurse goes to Ms. Fischer's room to teach her about diabetic foot care, she notices that Ms. Fischer has been crying. Realizing that the patient would probably not be receptive to new information at this time, the nurse decides to postpone the teaching.

Finally, *explain to the client what is to take place.* The client is entitled to an explanation of the action, the sensations he can expect, what he is expected to do, and the results the therapy or procedure is expected to produce. Preparation also includes provision for privacy, as well as any physical preparation, such as positioning.

Example: Before administering an enema to Jo Slevin, the nurse explains that this will prevent contamination of the surgical area during her bowel surgery. She shuts the door, pulls the curtain around the bed, helps Jo to assume a side-lying position, and drapes her with a bath blanket. She tells Jo she will feel pressure and perhaps some cramping as the fluid is instilled, and that she should retain the solution for 5 or 10 minutes, until she feels a strong urge to defecate.

Action: Doing or Delegating

Preparing Supplies and Equipment

Assemble all necessary equipment and materials before entering the room, so that you can proceed efficiently and with a minimum of stress to the patient. You may need supplies for dressing changes, equipment for removing staples from an incision, linen for a bath and bed change, or pamphlets for a teaching session. The following example demonstrates how inefficient and ineffective it is to stop in midprocedure because the necessary supplies are not at hand.

Example: A nurse is inserting a urinary catheter. After draping the patient, opening the sterile kit, and donning sterile gloves, the nurse breaks sterility when one of her gloves brushes against the patient's leg. Because she did not think to bring an extra pair of sterile gloves into the room, she is faced with the choice of leaving the patient draped and positioned while she goes for another pair, continuing the procedure with an unsterile glove, or going for new gloves, opening a new cath kit, and redraping the patient to be sure sterility is maintained.

Is the Patient Prepared?
- ✓ Determine whether the action is still needed.
- ✓ Assess the patient's readiness.
- ✓ Explain what is to be done and what results to expect.
- ✓ Tell the client what sensations to expect.
- ✓ Tell the client what he is expected to do.
- ✓ Provide for privacy.

ACTION: DOING OR DELEGATING

After preparations are complete, activity begins. The nurse applies a wide range of knowledge and skills in performing or delegating planned nursing strategies. The number and kind of specific nursing activities is almost unlimited. They consist of every skill, process, and procedure you have learned as a student and as a practitioner.

Critical Thinking and Levels of Autonomy

The nursing process enables nurses to identify, evaluate, and emphasize their independent activities. However, the full nursing role encompasses dependent and collaborative functions as well. Most nurses provide care for ill clients, whose comprehensive health needs include attention to their medical condition. In the implementation step, you will implement both (1) the nursing orders on the patient's care plan and (2) physician's orders for the medical care plan.

Recall that **dependent interventions** are those performed when following physician orders or agency policies. Usually they relate directly to the client's medical diagnosis or disease processes.

Example: The nurse gives IV morphine sulfate for pain relief, according to a physician's written order.

Implementation

These so-called dependent interventions are not performed mindlessly; nurses use critical thinking to make judgments about how, when, and to what extent they carry out medical orders.

The amount of time spent on dependent functions varies with the type of client, the employment setting, and the nurse's position, education, and experience. Critical-care nurses, for instance, spend more of their time on dependent functions than do home-health nurses and gerontology nurses (Guzzetta, 1987, p. 634). Some clinical nurse specialists perform few, if any, dependent interventions.

Collaborative (interdependent) interventions are performed either with other health professionals or as a result of decisions made jointly with them. Suppose, for example, that a nurse determines that a patient with a recent myocardial infarction needs concentrated teaching about his diet. She asks a dietitian to see the patient and reinforces the dietitian's instructions in her own interactions with the patient. The nurse and dietitian later use critical thinking to jointly evaluate the patient's progress toward understanding, accepting, and following diet restrictions.

Coordination of the patient's care is an important nursing activity that is related to, but not the same as, collaboration. This activity involves scheduling the client's contacts with other hospital departments (e.g., laboratory and X-ray technicians, physical and respiratory therapists) and serving as a liaison among the members of the health care team. As the professionals who are in touch with the patient 24 hours a day, nurses are in the best position to receive all the fragments of information and synthesize a holistic view of the patient. By making rounds with other professionals, reading their reports, and interpreting their findings to patients and families, the nurses assure that everyone gets the "big picture" as well as the specialized one.

Independent (autonomous) interventions are performed when carrying out the nursing orders, and often in conjunction with medical orders. Bulechek and McCloskey (1985) group independent nursing interventions into the following categories:

Category	Examples
1. Stress management	Imaging; alternate muscle-relaxation techniques
2. Lifestyle alteration	Counseling, teaching, support groups
3. Acute-care management	Preoperative teaching, surveillance
4. Self-care assistance	Bathing, assisting with ambulation, positioning
5. Communication	Discharge planning, active listening

When working with well clients, the nursing focus is to promote self-responsibility and self-care. Health-promotion and disease-prevention activities consist mainly of educating and motivating clients to maintain healthy lifestyles (Items 1, 2 and 5 above).

In addition to legally conferred autonomy, the nurse's knowledge and critical thinking determine the degree to which an action can be considered autonomous; the same activity can be independent in one situation and dependent in another.

Example: Taking vital signs can be a dependent or independent activity. Mr. Rauh has a temperature of 100.1°. The nurse realizes that many things can affect body temperature, and asks Mr. Rauh if he had anything to eat or drink before his vital signs were taken. The medical order reads, "V.S. t.i.d;" but because the temperature represents an unusual reading for Mr. Rauh, and because the nurse knows he is at risk for infection, she retakes his temperature an hour later to establish whether this is a pattern or an isolated cue.

This nurse's actions are independent. If she had been functioning in a completely dependent manner, she would have recorded Mr. Rauh's vital signs without validating their accuracy or questioning their meaning. She might have telephoned the physician for instructions, or simply passed the data on to the next shift without checking to see if Mr. Rauh's temperature remained the same, continued to rise, or returned to normal.

Accountability is an aspect of autonomy. **Autonomy** implies that the nurse is answerable for her actions and can define, explain, and evaluate the results of her decisions. The nurse in the preceding example is answerable for the decisions she made (i.e., to wait an hour and retake Mr. Rauh's temperature before calling the physician) and would have been able to provide a rationale for her actions. Critical thinking will enable you to expand the scope of your independent and collaborative functioning. Confidence in your clinical competence, knowledge, and skills, and a willingness to assume responsibility for your actions all add to the autonomous nature of your practice.

Skills Needed for Implementation

Nurses must have good cognitive, interpersonal, and technical skills in order to successfully implement the care plan. These skills are discussed individually in order to facilitate understanding; in practice, however, you will use them in various combinations and with different emphasis, depending upon the activity. For instance, when inserting a urinary catheter, you need cognitive knowledge of the principles and steps of the procedure, technical skill in draping the patient and manipulating the equipment, and interpersonal skills to inform and reassure the patient.

Cognitive (intellectual) skills include problem solving, decision making, critical thinking, and creative thinking. In the implementation step, nurses use these skills to apply theories and principles from nursing and related courses to each specific patient-care situation. When performing nursing strategies, the nurse may discover new problems that require quick identification and solution. For example, when helping a patient walk, a nurse identifies that the IV flow rate is too slow. She quickly checks to see that the tubing is not kinked and that the insertion site is in satisfactory condition. If no mechanical problems are noted, she opens the roller clamp to regulate the flow rate. If it is still a little slow, she raises the bag higher to make use of gravity.

Critical thinking is especially important in making the quick, on-the-spot decisions that are characteristic of implementation. It enables the nurse to rapidly think of alternative courses of action when the planned strategies do not work as predicted and, as in the example of Mr. Rauh's elevated temperature, to decide whether, and when, to notify a physician about a client's status.

Implementation

Nurses use **interpersonal skills** in nearly every contact with patients, families, and other health team members; for example, when they are listening actively, conveying interest, giving clear explanations, comforting, making referrals, and sharing attitudes, feelings, and knowledge. It is usually not possible for you to provide all the nursing care a client needs. You will use interpersonal skills to delegate some activities to other team members and to supervise and evaluate the performance of those interventions. The effectiveness of an intervention depends in part upon your ability to convey information to patients and other health team members so that they will know exactly what to expect and what to do.

Technical (psychomotor) skills are used during the implementation step in performing a variety of hands-on skills, such as changing dressings, giving injections, turning and positioning patients, attaching a monitor to a patient, and suctioning a tracheostomy. When procedures are done skillfully, the plan is more likely to be successful. Competent performance of technical skills also helps build rapport with the client. If, for instance, you can turn and reposition a client with minimal discomfort, the client will perceive you as someone who can help, and begin to trust you. Refer to Box 7–3 for a summary of guidelines to help you implement your nursing strategies successfully.

Delegation and Supervision

The ANA defines **delegation** as "the transfer of responsibility for the performance of an activity from one person to another while retaining accountability for the outcome," and **assignment** as "downward or lateral transfer of both the responsibility and accountability of an activity from one individual to another" (ANA, 1993, pp. 6–8). Because many hospitals now use RN extenders (e.g., licensed practical nurses, nursing assistants) to augment professional nurses, the ability to delegate patient care and assign tasks is now a vital skill. However, because it has not been emphasized in the past, many RNs are not well prepared to do it (Conger, 1994; Wiggins et al., 1990).

The nurse-delegator has two responsibilities in making work assignments: (1) *appropriate delegation* of duties (that is, within the nurse extender's scope of practice); and (2) *adequate supervision* of personnel (Barter and Furmidge, 1994). To delegate appropriately, the nurse-delegator must match the needs of the client and family with the skills and knowledge of various support personnel. This requires knowledge of the background, experience, knowledge, skills, and strengths of each person, and an understanding of which tasks are and are not within their legal scope of practice.

The RN can assign certain tasks to an unlicensed person, but cannot assign responsibility for total nursing care. The RN is responsible for adequate supervision to see that delegated tasks are performed adequately. Nurse-extenders may perform simply nursing tasks (such as measuring intake and output), but the RN always is responsible for analyzing data, planning care, and evaluating outcomes. Development of nurse-extenders is an important aspect of delegation. Because there are presently no communitywide standards for the training of unlicensed personnel, nurses must often assume responsibility for supplementing the minimal training they receive (Barter and Furmidge, 1994).

RECORDING

After doing or delegating, the nurse completes the implementation step by recording the nursing interventions and client responses. These nursing progress notes are a part of the agency's permanent record for the client. This section of the text describes different systems for organizing client records and then specifically describes nursing responsibilities for documentation.

The **client record (or chart)** is a permanent, comprehensive account of information about the client's health care. It consists of various forms on which information is recorded about all aspects of the client's care (e.g., physician's

---

Box 7–3. Guidelines for Successful Implementation

Prepare the Nurse

1. *Determine whether you need help* to perform the action safely and minimize stress to the client.

2. Be sure you *know the rationale* for the action, as well as any potential side effects or complications. When actions are based on practice wisdom, examine them critically.

3. *Question any actions you do not understand* or that seem inappropriate or potentially unsafe.

4. *Determine feedback points* and *assess the client's response* during the activity.

5. *Schedule activities* to allow adequate time for completion.

6. *Delegate tasks to other team members* in order to use your time efficiently.

7. *Improve your knowledge base* by continually seeking new knowledge.

Prepare the Client

8. *Determine that the action is still needed and appropriate.*

9. *Assess client readiness.*

10. *Inform the client* of what to expect and what is expected of him.

11. *Provide for privacy and comfort.*

Prepare Supplies and Equipment

12. *Gather and organize all necessary supplies.*

During Implementation:

13. *Adapt activities to the individual's* age, values, and health status. Remain flexible and make creative modifications as you work.

14. *Encourage the client to participate actively.*

15. *Perform actions according to professional standards* of care and agency policies and procedures.

16. *Perform actions carefully and accurately.*

17. *Supervise and evaluate delegated activities.*

Implementation

orders, results of laboratory and diagnostic tests, and progress notes written by physicians, nurses, and other caregivers). *Nursing* documentation in the permanent record is found on the following forms:

1. The initial, comprehensive nursing assessment (admission data base)
2. The individualized nursing care plan
3. Nursing progress notes
4. Flowsheets (e.g., graphic sheets, medication records)
5. The client discharge summary

Functions of Client Records

The written record *facilitates communication* among professionals from different disciplines and on different shifts, helping to coordinate care and avoid duplication of effort. Written notes about the client's progress and condition serve as a reference for nurses on other shifts who later need to refresh their memory or clarify the verbal report they received. Caregivers also refer to the chart as a reference point to help them assess new client responses.

As a *legal document*, the patient's record may be entered into court proceedings as evidence for a number of purposes (e.g., accident or injury claims by the client; malpractice charges against health professionals). The chart may be the only evidence that competent care was given. The chart itself is generally considered the property of the institution; however, courts recognize the client's right to the information contained in the record (Feutz, 1989).

Reimbursement from third-party payers (e.g., Medicare, private insurance companies) to clients and health care institutions is tied directly to documentation. The chart is examined to see that all medical orders were carried out properly, that medications were given, that equipment charged for was actually used, and so on. For instance, if a client's hospital bill included a charge for a urinary catheter, the progress notes might be examined for an entry stating that the client had been catheterized.

Of course, health team members refer to the client's chart when *planning care*. For instance, the physician may change a client's anticoagulant dosage on the basis of blood-clotting times found in the laboratory reports, or a nurse may use blood gas values and progress notes from the respiratory therapist to evaluate the effectiveness of nursing strategies for improving pulmonary ventilation.

Formal evaluations of the quality of care that clients receive in an institution are usually done after the client has been discharged. Outside groups also perform audits for accreditation purposes (e.g., Joint Commission on Accreditation of Healthcare Organizations). Therefore, written records are essential sources of data.

In addition, client records *provide educational information* for students in health disciplines, *statistical information* for institutions and government agencies, and *data for research and tracing historical trends*. Administrators involved in *financial planning* for a hospital may use nursing documentation to help them estimate nursing costs in the institution. Nursing costs represent a significant part of a hospital's budget, so it is important to estimate them accurately.

236

Client Record Systems

Two systems commonly used to keep an ongoing and permanent record of the patient's health care are (1) source-oriented records, and (2) problem-oriented records. These systems differ in the way the information is organized and/or stored.

Source-Oriented Records

In this widely used, traditional system the client's record is divided into sections according to the source of the data. Each discipline records data on its own special form. For example, physicians use an order sheet, a medical history form, and physician's progress notes; nurses record data on a nursing history form and in the nursing progress notes; and results of blood and urine tests are found on a laboratory report. Source-oriented records are convenient because each discipline can easily locate the necessary forms on which to write its entries. It is also easy for each professional to track the data of specific interest to his or her discipline.

The disadvantage is that information about a particular problem is scattered throughout various sections of the chart, so it is difficult to track a client's progress with regard to a problem. For example, if a client has diarrhea, the physician's history and physical records trace the development of the symptom; the physician's progress notes describe the client's daily elimination and hydration status and the proposed therapy; the nursing progress notes describe the number and nature of the stools and related physical status; the activity flowsheet notes that the client is too weak to bathe herself; the graphic sheet reflects an elevated pulse and total intake and output; the laboratory report shows a negative stool culture. To find data about that particular problem, you would have to search through six different forms in different sections of the chart.

Problem-Oriented Records

In problem-oriented medical records (POMR), also called *problem-oriented records (POR)*, information is organized according to the client's problems. All health professionals, regardless of discipline, record on the same forms. The entire team contributes to a master list of client problems and to the plan of care for each problem. The basic components of a POR follow:

1. *Defined data base.* The data base consists of all the *initial* information about the client's health: the nursing admission assessment, the medical history and physical examination, initial laboratory and diagnostic test results, and social and family histories if pertinent.

2. *Master problem list.* The initial problem list is developed from the data base. All health care professionals contribute to the problem list, which may contain medical, psychological, sociocultural, and spiritual problems. The master list is usually at the front of the chart, and serves as an index to numbered entries on the progress notes. Problems are listed in the order in which they are identified (see Table 7–1).

3. *Problem-oriented plan of care.* An initial plan is developed for each problem on the master list. Physicians write plans (or orders) for medical problems; nurses write orders for nursing diagnoses. Note that in this system the nursing care plan is not a separate document, but is integrated within the progress notes in the client's chart.

Implementation

Table 7–1. Master Problem List			
No.	Problem	Identified	Resolved
1	Appendicitis	1985	1985
2	Hysterectomy	12/4/96	
2A	Pain related to surgical incision	12/4/96	12/10/96
3	Grief related to loss of childbearing ability	12/4/96	

4. *Multidisciplinary progress notes.* All health professionals involved in the client's care make narrative entries in these notes, which are numbered to correspond with the problems on the master list. To follow the client's progress in resolving a problem, one simply reads all the progress notes labeled with that problem number.

The POR method promotes collaborative relationships between health professionals, who record on the same forms and work together to develop the master problem list and the plan of care. It also facilitates tracking a client's progress with regard to any particular problem and is likely to improve understanding of that problem, since each professional can observe what other disciplines have done. With all members of the health care team addressing the same problems, quality of care should be improved.

The disadvantages of this method are that (1) time and money must be committed to teaching members of all disciplines to use the POR system; (2) some disciplines may resist the use of an integrated system; (3) the care plan is scattered throughout the progress notes.

Computerized Records

As computers become more cost-effective, more and more agencies are using computerized information systems for all their records. This means that nurses use a computer to store the client's data base, add new data, create and revise care plans, and document client progress. Some institutions have a computer terminal at each client's bedside, enabling the nurse to document care immediately after it is given.

Information can be easily retrieved in a variety of forms (e.g., you could obtain the results of a blood test for a patient, a schedule of all patients on the unit having surgery today, a suggested list of interventions for a nursing diagnosis, or a printout of all the progress notes for a patient). Many systems can generate a work list for the shift, with a list of all the treatments, procedures, and medications needed by the client.

After the initial learning curve, computers make care planning and documentation relatively easy. Because computerized record keeping is fast, efficient, and thorough, nurses find it easier to plan and deliver individualized patient care. Automated speech recognition technology now allows nurses to do voice-activated documentation. One study demonstrated that this system dramatically reduced errors and decreased documentation time by 66% (Trofino, 1993).

Forms for Nursing Documentation

Recording

Institutions usually develop forms to meet their particular needs. Therefore, forms vary, and you will need to become familiar with new forms and record systems when you move to a different health care agency. Whether the system is source-, problem-, or computer-oriented, three kinds of forms are usually used to record nursing progress notes: (1) flowsheets, (2) descriptive nursing progress notes, and (3) discharge summaries. They all provide for time-sequenced documentation of assessments, interventions, and client responses.

Flowsheets

Several kinds of flowsheets are used as a quick way to record routine nursing care. A **medication record** is used to record all medications administered to the client. (Refer to a nursing fundamentals text for examples of medication records.) **Graphic flowsheets** are used to record routine measurements made at specified intervals (e.g., daily weights, vital signs). Graphic sheet data consists mainly of numbers. A **daily activity record** is a modified flowsheet for recording routine activities, especially those repeated frequently or at specified times (e.g., bath and skin care, diagnostic tests performed, activity level). In addition to daily activity flowsheets, most institutions design **special assessment flowsheets** for situations in which the same assessments are repeated routinely or frequently (e.g., hourly neurological assessments). Figure 7–2 is an example of a graphic flowsheet; it also incorporates a few basic care activities, such as the bath and oral care.

Nursing Progress Notes

Progress notes are usually a narrative description of patient progress toward goal achievement. They should include (1) assessments of client's mental and physical condition, (2) client activities, (3) nursing treatments and interventions and client responses, (4) visits by other caregivers or family members, if pertinent, and (5) treatments performed by the physician that affect nursing care. The form used and the manner of recording will vary, depending on whether the hospital's record system is source-oriented or problem-oriented. In all systems, though, nursing progress notes, written in brief phrases and sentences, are used to augment but not duplicate the data in the flowsheets.

Figure 7–3 on pages 241–242, "Patient Care Notes," is a combined record of the patient's activities and assessments of patient status (to save space, one page of this form is omitted). Instead of writing a narrative note, however, the nurse simply circles the descriptive words and phrases that apply to the client. Notice that this form is organized according to Gordon's Functional Health Patterns (1994), as is the admission assessment form for this hospital (Appendix C). Such consistent use of a nursing framework throughout the entire set of nursing records promotes thorough, efficient data collection, analysis, and recording.

Figure 7–4 on page 244 is an example of a Nursery Flow Record that is used to record assessments and care of normal newborns. This form combines a flowsheet format with space for brief narrative progress notes.

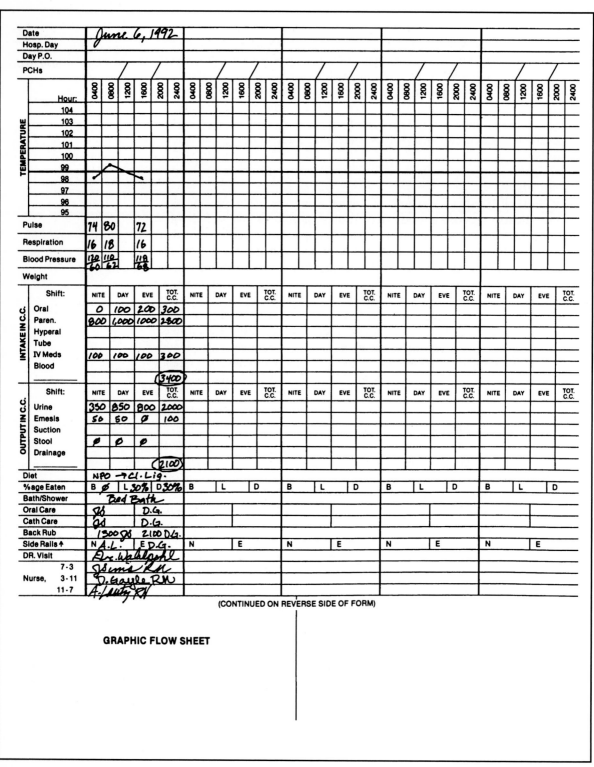

	Date	June 6, 1992												
	Hosp. Day					
	Day P.O.					
	PCHs					

Hour: 0400 0800 1200 1600 2000 2400 (repeated across)

TEMPERATURE
104, 103, 102, 101, 100, 99, 98, 97, 96, 95

Pulse	74	80		72		
Respiration	16	18		16		
Blood Pressure	120/60	110/62		110/68		
Weight						

INTAKE IN C.C.

Shift:	NITE	DAY	EVE	TOT. C.C.
Oral	0	100	200	300
Paren.	800	1,000	1000	2800
Hyperal				
Tube				
IV Meds	100	100	100	300
Blood				(3400)

OUTPUT IN C.C.

Shift:	NITE	DAY	EVE	TOT. C.C.
Urine	350	850	800	2000
Emesis	50	50	0	100
Suction				
Stool	0	0	0	
Drainage				(2100)

Diet	NPO → Cl. Liq.
%age Eaten	B Ø L 30% D 30%
Bath/Shower	Bed Bath
Oral Care	50 D.G.
Cath Care	01 D.G.
Back Rub	1300 50 2100 D.G.
Side Rails ↑	N A.L. E D.G.
DR. Visit	Dr. Wahlquist
Nurse 7-3	J. Sims RN
Nurse 3-11	D. Gayle RN
Nurse 11-7	A. Lauty RN

(CONTINUED ON REVERSE SIDE OF FORM)

GRAPHIC FLOW SHEET

Figure 7–2. Graphic Flowsheet
Courtesy of Shawnee Mission Medical Center, Merriam, KS.

PATIENT CARE NOTES

TIME:

	Column 1	Column 2	Column 3
Neuro	Alert Lethargic Unconscious Oriented X 3 Disoriented Speech: Clear Slurred Absent	Alert Lethargic Unconscious Oriented X 3 Disoriented Speech: Clear Slurred Absent	Alert Lethargic Unconscious Oriented X 3 Disoriented Speech: Clear Slurred Absent
Integument/Wound	Skin: warm ·cool dry moist color: IV location: N/A or Skin care: N/A Simple Extensive Skin breakdown: N/A or Wound Location: N/A or DSG Appearance: Dry or Wound Care: Drains: N/A or	Skin: warm cool dry moist color: IV location: N/A or Skin care: N/A Simple Extensive Skin breakdown: N/A or Wound Location: N/A or DSG Appearance: Dry or Wound Care: Drains: N/A or	Skin: warm cool dry moist color: IV location: N/A or Skin care: N/A Simple Extensive Skin breakdown: N/A or Wound Location: N/A or DSG Appearance: Dry or Wound Care: Drains: N/A or
Cardio-Vascular	Radial pulse: regular irregular Edema: N/A or _____	Radial pulse: regular irregular Edema: N/A or _____	Radial pulse: regular irregular Edema: N/A or _____
Respiratory	Resp: unlabored labored Lungs clear or Oz @ ____ per _____ Cough: nonproductive productive	Resp: unlabored labored Lungs clear or Oz @ ____ per _____ Cough: nonproductive productive	Resp: unlabored labored Lungs clear or Oz @ ____ per _____ Cough: nonproductive productive
Gastrointestinal	Abdomen: soft or Bowel Sounds: active or Nausea Vomiting Passing Flatus Stoma: N/A or Stool: None or continent incontinent x_____ Supp/enema: N/A or Results: NG: N/A or Placement Verified Suction: Irrigation: Drainage:	Abdomen: soft or Bowel Sounds: active or Nausea Vomiting Passing Flatus Stoma: N/A or Stool: None or continent incontinent x_____ Supp/enema: N/A or Results: NG: N/A or Placement Verified Suction: Irrigation: Drainage:	Abdomen: soft or Bowel Sounds: active or Nausea Vomiting Passing Flatus Stoma: N/A or Stool: None or continent incontinent x_____ Supp/enema: N/A or Results: NG: N/A or Placement Verified Suction: Irrigation: Drainage:
Genitourinary	Urine continent incontinent x_____ catheter: N/A or Irrigation: N/A or Vag ding: N/A small mod. large Color: _____	Urine continent incontinent x_____ catheter: N/A or Irrigation: N/A or Vag ding: N/A small mod. large Color: _____	Urine continent incontinent x_____ catheter: N/A or Irrigation: N/A or Vag ding: N/A small mod. large Color: _____
SIG.			

NAME _____ HOSPITAL NO. _____ DATE _____

FORM OS-328 (10/89)

Figure 7–3. Patient Care Notes © Department of Nursing, Bronson Methodist Hospital, Kalamazoo, MI. All rights reserved.

TIME:		
Psycho Social	Calm Resting Quiet Anxious Restless	Calm Resting Quiet Anxious Restless	Calm Resting Quiet Anxious Restless
Activity/ Rest	Bedrest/BRP chair ambulate Self Assist of _____ Gait: Steady Unsteady Immobility: N/A or 2⁰ _____ Slept:	Bedrest/BRP chair ambulate Self Assist of _____ Gait: Steady Unsteady Immobility: N/A or 2⁰ _____ Slept:	Bedrest/BRP chair ambulate Self Assist of _____ Gait: Steady Unsteady Immobility: N/A or 2⁰ _____ Slept:
Equipment	Eggcrate Clinitron/Kinnair _____ ⁰F warm/cool pad _____⁰F to _____ feeding pump Trapeze/frame IV Controller X ___ IV Volumetric X ___ Isolation:	Eggcrate Clinitron/Kinnair _____ ⁰F warm/cool pad _____⁰F to _____ feeding pump Trapeze/frame IV Controller X ___ IV Volumetric X ___ Isolation:	Eggcrate Clinitron/Kinnair _____ ⁰F warm/cool pad _____⁰F to _____ feeding pump Trapeze/frame IV Controller X ___ IV Volumetric X ___ Isolation:
Safety	Sensory deficit N/A or bed position: low or siderails: up down visual observation q: restraints: N/A or remove/ROM/reapply q: sitter: N/A or continuous ID Band on: Yes No Reapplied	Sensory deficit N/A or bed position: low or siderails: up down visual observation q: restraints: N/A or remove/ROM/reapply q: sitter: N/A or continuous ID Band on: Yes No Reapplied	Sensory deficit N/A or bed position: low or siderails: up down visual observation q: restraints: N/A or remove/ROM/reapply q: sitter: N/A or continuous ID Band on: Yes No Reapplied
Assessment	Time _____ Location/Type: Severity 1 2 3 4 5 6 7 8 9 10 Action/Results:	Time _____ Location/Type: Severity 1 2 3 4 5 6 7 8 9 10 Action/Results:	Time _____ Location/Type: Severity 1 2 3 4 5 6 7 8 9 10 Action/Results:
	Time _____ Location/Type: Severity 1 2 3 4 5 6 7 8 9 10 Action/Results:	Time _____ Location/Type: Severity 1 2 3 4 5 6 7 8 9 10 Action/Results:	Time _____ Location/Type: Severity 1 2 3 4 5 6 7 8 9 10 Action/Results:
Pain	Time _____ Location/Type: Severity 1 2 3 4 5 6 7 8 9 10 Action/Results:	Time _____ Location/Type: Severity 1 2 3 4 5 6 7 8 9 10 Action/Results:	Time _____ Location/Type: Severity 1 2 3 4 5 6 7 8 9 10 Action/Results:
Tests/ Procedures	Specimen: time: procedure: prep:	Specimen: time: procedure: prep:	Specimen: time: procedure: prep:
SIG.		

LABS								NUTRITION:		BREAKFAST	LUNCH	DINNER
TIME / INITIALS								DIET/SOLUTION:				
SUGAR / ACETONE								% AMT./RATE				
STOOL / HEMATEST								S—SELF A—ASSIST F-FEED TF—TUBE FEEDING				
CHEM BG												

HYGIENE: TIME: _____

    BEDBATH   SHOWER   TUB/SITZ

    SELF   ASSIST   COMPLETE

NAME _____ HOSPITAL NO. _____ DATE _____

Figure 7–3. (concluded)

NURSERY FLOW RECORD
SHAWNEE MISSION MEDICAL CENTER.

WEIGHT: Birth Weight: 7 lb. 6 g.

DELIVERY INFORMATION:
Date: 6-13-91 Wt. 7 lb. 3 g.
Date: 6-12-91 Time: 0815
Method: Vaginal
Apgar: 1 min 8 5 min 9
Comments: Fred Joseph

FEEDING:
Date: _____ Wt. _____
Date: _____ Wt. _____
Date: _____ Wt. _____

FEEDING: Breast   Bottle

KEY:

Activity:
+ + = Active
+ = Active c stim
L = Lethargic

Feeding:
FW = Feeding well
FP = Feeding poorly
FF = Fed fair
DDF = Did not feed
FTA = Feeding Tube Assist

Color:
P = Pink
W = Pale
M = Mottled
J = Jaundiced
D = Dusky
A = Acrocyanotic
C = Cyanotic

Stools:
M = Meconium
Y = Yellow
G = Green
T = Transitional

DATE	TIME	TEMP.	RESPIR.	APICAL PULSE	ACTIVITY	SKIN COLOR	DEXTRO-STIX	INTAKE TOLERANCE	URINE	STOOL	LAB WORK/ X-RAY	OTHER	OTHER	NURSING NOTES/SIGNATURE
6/13/91	0900	97²	32	124	++	A	40	FW	X1	M	serum bilirubin		✓	Cord Care: 7-3 _MB_ 3-11 _____ 11-7 _____ To mother's room. Bonding noted, e.g., Calls by name; eye contact. MB Fussy, even p̄ feeding. M Barnes, RN
	1100	97²	40	118	++	P	40	FW	X2	M				

ASSESSMENT | **INTAKE/OUTPUT** | **ADDITIONAL DATA**

DATE: _____

Implementation

Discharge Summary

A discharge summary is a special nursing progress note written at the time a client is dismissed from the agency. It usually includes the following:

Current status of each client problem
Teaching and counseling that was done to prepare the client for dismissal
Current medications and treatments that are to be continued
Activities of daily living and self-care abilities
Support system, significant others
Mode of discharge (e.g., walking, wheelchair)
Person who accompanied the client
Where client is going (e.g., home, nursing home, another unit in the hospital)

Many institutions have a special discharge form that is used in conjunction with the nursing progress notes. This discharge record focuses on the information given to the patient at the time of dismissal. A copy is given to the patient, and the description of the client's condition and the problem status are recorded as a final entry on the progress notes.

Methods for Writing Nursing Progress Notes

As mentioned above, all client record systems provide a section for writing descriptive progress notes about the patient's status and progress. The four prevalent methods of writing progress notes are (1) chronological narrative, (2) SOAP format, (3) Focus charting©, and (4) charting by exception.

Chronological Narrative Charting

Narrative charting (e.g., Figure 7–5) is the traditional charting format. It is used primarily in source-oriented record systems. Nurses write notes in paragraph form for a given period of time (e.g., every two hours, or twice a shift). Events and client responses are recorded in chronological order. The disadvantage of this format is that it is not systematic; one entry may contain information about several problems or interventions. Because it is difficult to follow the progress of a specific problem without reading all of the recorded information, the narrative section is often combined with a flowsheet, as in Figure 7–4.

SOAP Charting

The SOAP method originated with the problem-oriented records system, but is now used in other systems as well. SOAP is an acronym for Subjective data, Objective data, Assessment, and Plan. SOAP charting is problem-oriented; that is, each SOAP note refers to a specific problem. Multiple problems require multiple SOAP notes. Most agencies require a SOAP note on each active problem every 24 hours, or more often if the problem status changes. An explanation of the SOAP elements follows.

S—**Subjective data** is information obtained from what the client says. It describes the client's perspectives, perceptions, and experience of the problem. When possible, quote the client's words; otherwise, summarize his statement. Include *subjective data* only when it is important and relevant to the problem.

244

DATE	TIME	NOTES	SIGNATURE
9-6-92	0800	Refused breakfast. States, "I feel too sick." abd. firm but not distended. No bowel sounds heard p̄ auscultating for 5 min. in @ quadrant. Using PCA (morphine) frequently for incision pain (see med. Record).	S. Fried, RN
	0900	200 cc. clear, yellow emesis	S. Fried, RN
	0930	100 cc. clear, yellow emesis. C/o severe nausea. Compazine 5 mg. given I M in LVG area. Closed door & advised to lie still to decrease sensation of nausea.	S. Fried, RN
	1030	States still nauseated, but less severe. No further emesis. T.E.D. hose removed for 15 min & reapplied. No edema or redness on legs. Dangled @ bedside for 5 min. Moves c̄ much reluctance. States, "Hurts too much."	S. Fried, RN

Shawnee Mission Medical Center
PATIENT PROGRESS RECORD

Figure 7–5. Patient Progress Record
Courtesy of Shawnee Mission Medical Center, Merriam, KS.

Implementation

O—Objective data consists of information that can be measured or observed by use of the senses (e.g., vital signs, bowel sounds, laboratory and X-ray results). The objective data section is also used to record interventions that have been carried out (e.g., "Taught correct procedure for drawing up insulin"). Note that this differs from the definition in Chapter 3, which states that *data* is information about the *client.* In the SOAP recording method, *objective data* refers to nursing interventions as well as client responses.

A—The Assessment is an interpretation or explanation of the subjective and objective data. During the *initial* assessment, the master problem list is created from interpretations and conclusions about the *S* and *O* data. At this time, the *Assessment* entry should be a statement of the problem. In all subsequent SOAP notes, the *A* should describe the client's condition and level of progress, not merely restate the diagnosis or problem. If a new problem develops later, it would be stated under the *A* at that time, but not in subsequent entries.

P—The Plan is the plan of care designed to resolve the stated problem. The person who enters the problem on the record writes the *initial* plan. For medical problems, the physician writes orders for diagnostic and treatment interventions; the nurse focuses on nursing interventions to monitor and support the medical treatment plan. Other disciplines, such as physical therapy, add their specific interventions to the plan. When writing subsequent SOAP notes for a problem, the plan is compared to plans in previous notes; then decisions are made about revising, continuing, or discontinuing previous interventions.

SOAPIE and SOAPIER are variations of the SOAP format. In these formats, the interventions (*I*) are written separately from the objective data (*O*), and an evaluation component (*E*) is added. The SOAPIER format adds a section for revision of the plan (*R*).

APIE is a similar format, developed by Groah and Reed (1983, p. 1184). In this format, the assessment (*A*) includes both subjective and objective data, as well as the nursing diagnosis; the plan (*P*) includes predicted outcomes with the nursing actions; and implementation (*I*) and evaluation (*E*) are the same as in the SOAPIE format. See Table 7–2 for a comparison of the SOAP, SOAPIER, and APIE formats. Compare these entries to Figures 7–5 and 7–6 on page 248, which contain the same information about nausea.

Focus Charting®

Like SOAP notes, Focus Charting uses key words to label and organize the progress notes, but the subject of the note is not necessarily a problem. According to Lampe (1985, p. 43), a focus can be any of the following:

A current client concern or behavior
A significant change in client status or behavior
A significant event in the client's therapy

A focus should be something that requires nursing care; therefore, it should not be a medical diagnosis. The focus can, however, describe needs and conditions that are *associated with* the medical diagnosis. For example, foci for a client with a medical diagnosis of fractured femur might include admission information, preoperative teaching, Pain, Risk for Constipation, and cast/traction assessment. The Focus method uses three columns: Date/Time, Focus, and Progress Notes. The progress notes column is organized in a DAR format.

Recording

Table 7–2. Comparison of the SOAP, SOAPIER, and APIE Formats

SOAP Format	SOAPIER Format	APIE Format
9/6/96 #5. Nausea 1030	9/6/96 #5. Nausea 1030	9/6/96 #5. Nausea 1030
S— Refused breakfast. "I feel too sick." c/o severe nausea during A.M. Stated less severe after IM Compazine.	S— Refused breakfast. "I feel too sick." c/o severe nausea during A.M.	A—Post-op nausea & vomiting. Refused breakfast. "I feel too sick." Abd. firm, not distended. No bowel sounds heard after auscultating 5 min. @ quadrant. Vomited × 2; total 300 mL clear, yellow emesis.
O—Abd. firm but not distended. No bowel sounds heard after auscultating for 5 min. @ quadrant. Vomited × 2: total 300 mL clear, yellow emesis. Closed door: advised to lie still to decrease sensations of nausea. Compazine 5 mg given IM in LVG area at 0930.	O—Abd. firm but not distended. No bowel sounds heard after auscultating for 5 min. @ quadrant. Vomited × 2: total 300 mL clear, yellow emesis.	P— Decrease nausea: Instruct to lie still. Compazine per order.
	A— Post-op nausea r/t decreased peristalsis; Compazine somewhat effective.	Prevent fluid deficit: Continue to assess N&V. Assess hydration q shift. Continue I&O. If nausea and vomiting continue, notify MD.
A—Post-op nausea r/t decreased peristalsis; Compazine somewhat effective. Possible ileus.	P— Instruct to lie still to decrease sensations of nausea. Medicate with Compazine. Continue I&O. Continue to assess for N&V. Assess hydration q shift.	I— Instructed to lie still. Compazine 5 mg given IM in LVG area at 0930.
P—Continue to observe for N&V. If nausea unrelieved by Compazine, notify MD. Continue I&O. Assess hydration q shift. Offer fluids 40 mL/hr if no further emesis.	I— Instructed to lie still to decrease sensations of nausea. Compazine 5 mg given IM in LVG area at 0930.	E— Lying still most of A.M. No emesis since Compazine given. States still nauseated, but less severe.
	E— States still nauseated but somewhat relieved after Compazine. Lying still most of A.M. No emesis after Compazine.	
	R— Offer fluids 40 mL/hr if no further emesis. If nausea unrelieved by Compazine, notify MD.	

D—The **data** includes the nurse's observations of client status and behaviors. This might include data from flowsheets (e.g., vital signs, intake, and output). It includes both subjective and objective data, but they are not labeled *S* and *O*. This section corresponds to the assessment step of the nursing process.

A—**Action** entries include interventions just performed as well as plans for further action. This step corresponds to the planning and implementation steps of the nursing process.

R—**Response** entries describe the client's responses to nursing and medical interventions. The data in this section consists of client measurements and behaviors, many of which will be recorded on flowsheets and checklists. This section corresponds to the evaluation step of the nursing process.

Focus notes can be used in source-, problem-, or computer-oriented record systems. Like the SOAP method, focus notes can be scanned to quickly find the desired subject; it is not necessary to read the entire set of notes, as in narrative

Date/Time	Focus	Progress Notes
9/6/96		
1430	Post-op nausea	D—Refused breakfast. Stated, "I feel too sick." c/o severe nausea throughout A.M. Vomited x 2, total of 300 cc clear, yellow emesis. Abd. firm but not distended. No bowel sounds auscultated after listening for 5 min. in @ quadrant.
		A—Closed door. Advised to lie still to decrease sensations of nausea. Compazine 5 mg given IM in LVG at 0930 per order. Continue to assess for N&V. If unrelieved by Compazine, notify MD. Continue I&O. Assess hydration x 1 per shift. Increase p.o. fluids to 40 cc/hr if no further emesis.
		R—Nausea somewhat relieved by Compazine. Stated "less severe." No emesis since Compazine administered. See flow sheet for I&O and VS.————R. Keeler, RN

Figure 7–6. Example of a Focus Charting® Note

charting. The focus method is useful for health-promotion and disease-prevention activities because charting can be organized around positive headings instead of problems. Figure 7–6 is an example of a Focus note containing the same information about nausea that appears in Figure 7–5 and Table 7–2.

Charting by Exception

Charting by exception (CBE) is a method of documenting nursing care developed at St. Luke's Hospital in Milwaukee to save time and eliminate repetitive charting of insignificant information. CBE is a system of record keeping that can be applied just to nursing documentation or to the entire patient record. CBE incorporates three key components for the documenting interventions (Burke and Murphy, 1988, p. 7):

1. *Unique flowsheets* that highlight significant findings and define assessment parameters and findings. Completed interventions are documented in the nursing progress notes or on one of the following four flowsheets: Nursing/Physician Order Flowsheet, the Graphic Record, the Patient Teaching Record, and the Patient Discharge Note. Guidelines on the back of the flowsheets specify what each assessment should include and the norms for each. A check mark beside the assessment indicates that it was made as specified and that the findings were within normal limits. For an exception, the nurse makes an asterisk instead of a check mark, and writes a narrative note describing the unusual finding. Following is an example of guidelines and norms from the Nursing/Physician Order Flowsheet:

GASTROINTESTINAL ASSESSMENT

Guidelines: GI assessment will include abdominal appearance, bowel sounds, palpation, diet tolerance, and stools.

Norms: The following will constitute a negative assessment: Abdomen soft, bowel sounds active (5–34/min). No pain with palpation. Tolerates prescribed diet without nausea and vomiting. Having BMs within own normal pattern and consistency (Burke and Murphy, 1988, p. 11).

If a client needs GI assessments, the nurse writes "GI Assessment" on the Order/Flowsheet. A check mark beside this order indicates that everything in the guidelines was done and that the findings were as described in the norms. If diet tolerance was not assessed, however, the nurse would place an asterisk beside "GI Assessment" and write in the progress notes, "*NPO—Diet tolerance not assessed."

2. *Documentation by reference to Standards of Nursing Practice.* An agency using CBE must develop its own specific, detailed Standards of Nursing Practice that identify the minimum criteria for patient care regardless of clinical area. Some units also have unit-specific standards unique to their type of patient. The following are examples of standards related to hygiene patterns:

The nurse shall ensure that the patient has oral care offered T.I.D.

The nurse shall ensure that the patient has a bath and backrub offered daily and a shampoo offered weekly (Burke and Murphy, 1988, p. 33).

Implementation

A check mark in the "Routine Standards" box on the Graphic Record indicates that all appropriate standards were implemented. No comment is written unless there are exceptions to the standards. This eliminates the need to document routine interventions such as repositioning, traction care, and care of the IV site. Exceptions to standards are clearly described in the progress notes.

3. *Bedside accessibility of documentation forms.* In the CBE approach, all flowsheets are kept at the bedside. Care is documented as it is implemented, eliminating the need to chart from memory or transcribe information from a worksheet to the permanent record.

In this system, only significant findings or exceptions to norms are written in the descriptive nursing progress notes. The nurse writes a progress note, in SOAP format, when she (1) activates a nursing diagnosis, (2) evaluates a goal, (3) resolves or discontinues a nursing diagnosis, (4) writes a discharge summary, or (5) makes a major revision of the care plan.

Guidelines for Charting

Legal requirements for record keeping vary from state to state and among agencies. Agency policies may describe which personnel are responsible for recording on certain forms, the frequency with which entries are to be made, which abbreviations are acceptable, and the preferred way to handle an error in recording. You should, of course, be familiar with legal and policy requirements. In addition, observe the following general guidelines.

When to Chart

Timing guidelines are critical for legal reasons as well as for their contribution to safe care.

1. *Date and time each entry.* Using the 24-hour (military) clock avoids confusion about whether a time is A.M. or P.M. For example, 9:30 A.M. would be written as 0930 in military time; 9:30 P.M. would be 2130.

2. For each entry, *indicate both the time the entry was made and the time the observation or intervention occurred,* if different. For example, in a chart entry timed 1445, you might write, "Drank 150 mL water at 1245, vomited 200 mL clear fluid at 1310."

3. When possible, *record the nursing action or client response immediately after it occurs.* The longer you wait, the less accurate your memory. Immediate recording is especially important for medications and treatments because it helps insure that the client will not be medicated or treated a second time by a different nurse. It is usually acceptable to record routine repetitive nursing actions at the end of the shift (e.g., hourly position changes, mouth care).

4. *Never leave the unit for an extended break unless all important information has been charted.* (Rationale is similar to that for Guideline 3.)

5. *Do not document interventions before carrying them out.* The client might refuse the treatment or you might encounter an emergency situation that prevents you from carrying out the intervention. Another staff member, seeing it charted, might conclude the action has been done and not wish to repeat it. The result would be that the client does not get the care he needs.

Comparison of Conventional and Military Time

Conventional	Military
12:01 A.M.	0001
12:15 A.M	0015
12:45 A.M	0045
1 A.M	0100
2 A.M	0200
3 A.M	0300
4 A.M	0400
5 A.M	0500
6 A.M	0600
7 A.M	0700
8 A.M	0800
9 A.M	0900
10 A.M	1000
11 A.M	1100
12 NOON	1200
12:01 P.M.	1201
12:15 P.M.	1215
12:45 P.M.	1245
1 P.M.	1300
2 P.M.	1400
3 P.M.	1500
4 P.M.	1600
5 P.M.	1700
6 P.M.	1800
7 P.M.	1900
8 P.M.	2000
9 P.M.	2100
10 P.M.	2200
11 P.M.	2300
12 MIDNIGHT	2400

What to Chart

1. *The nurse who makes the entry should sign it.* You should not sign someone else's notes. Remember that the person signing the entry is accountable for the entry.

2. In general, *you should not chart actions performed by someone else.* In some situations, it is permissible to chart an action you did not perform, but your note should identify the person who actually gave the care (e.g., "Assisted to car by nursing assistant. L. Woods, RN").

3. *Progress notes must be accurate and correct.* Never write an assessment you are unsure of. If you are not absolutely sure the patient's lungs are "clear to auscultation," ask someone else to check before you chart.

4. *Progress notes should be factual and specific.* Chart what you see, hear, smell or observe; not opinions and interpretations. To improve the precision of your charting, think, "Exactly what happened, and how, when and where did it happen?" For example, you would chart, "Talking constantly, pacing the floor; pulse 120," rather than "Patient is anxious." An exception is that in SOAP charting, the A *is* an interpretation of the S-O data. Any time you think an interpretation should be charted, be sure to include the supporting data.

5. *Progress notes should be clear and specific.* Do not use vague generalities, such as *good*, *normal*, or *sufficient*. It is better to say "a 2 × 2 cm area of blood" than "a small amount of blood."

6. *Do not use negative, prejudicial terms* (e.g., *uncooperative, noncompliant, unpleasant*). Instead, describe what the client did that was uncooperative (e.g., "Yelled, 'Go away!' and threw his tray on the floor").

7. *Chart entries should be appropriate and relevant.* You do not need to record everything you know about the client. Recording irrelevant data is a waste of time, and it is sometimes an invasion of privacy.

8. *Progress notes should be complete.* This is essential for communication among caregivers, as well as for legal purposes. For example, if there is no record of turning and skin care, nurses may be found negligent when the client develops a dermal ulcer. Box 7–4 is a guide suggested by Kozier et al. (1991) to help you select essential and complete information about clients.

9. To organize your narrative entry, *include **D—I—E***. Don't actually label the entry with these letters or words; use them as a memory device.

Data	What did you observe about the patient (*S-O*)?
Intervention	What actions did you take? What did you do?
Evaluation	What was the patient's response to the actions?
	What did he say or do? How did his condition change?

10. *Be brief.* Do not sacrifice completeness, but *omit unnecessary words*, such as *patient*. It is assumed the entry refers to the patient. Progress notes are usually written in incomplete sentences, but be sure to end each thought with a period. For example, write "300 mL clear emesis," rather than "The patient vomited 300 mL of clear fluid."

Implementation

How to Chart

1. *Use dark ink.* Most agencies specify black ink. Erasable ink is not acceptable.

2. *Write legibly, or print.* Narcan and Marcaine are different drugs, but they may look very much alike if handwriting is illegible or messy.

3. *Use correct grammar, spelling, and punctuation.*

4. *Use standard symbols, terminology, and abbreviations.* Many agencies have a list of abbreviations and terminology they accept. If not, use only those that are standard and used universally. Other professionals must be able to interpret the terms correctly, especially if the record is ever used as evidence in court. If you are in doubt about an abbreviation, write the term out fully.

5. *Sign each entry with your name and title* (e.g. "Kay Wittman, RN" or "K. Wittman, RN").

Box 7–4. Essential Charting Information

Essential charting information includes the following:

1. Any behavior changes, for example:
   Indications of strong emotions, such as anxiety or fear
   Marked changes in mood
   A change in level of consciousness, such as stupor
   Regression in relationships with family or friends

2. Any changes in physical function, such as:
   Loss of balance
   Loss of strength
   Difficulty hearing or seeing

3. Any physical sign or symptom that:
   Is severe, such as severe pain
   Tends to recur or persist
   Is not normal, such as elevated body temperature
   Gets worse, such as gradual weight loss
   Indicates a complication, such as inability to void following surgery
   Is not relieved by prescribed measures (such as continued failure to defecate or to sleep)
   Indicates faulty health habits, such as lice on the scalp
   Is a known danger signal, such as a lump in the breast

4. Any nursing interventions provided, such as:
   Medications administered
   Therapies
   Activities of daily living, if agency policy dictates
   Teaching clients self-care

5. Visits by a physician or other members of the health team

From Kozier, Erb, and Olivieri, *Fundamentals of Nursing*, 4th ed. (Redwood City, CA: Addison-Wesley Nursing, 1991), p. 313. Reprinted by permission.

6. *Chart entries on consecutive lines. Never skip a line or leave a line blank.* Draw a line through any blank spaces before or after your signature. For example, "Lungs clear to auscultation. Skin warm and dry._____ K. Wittman, RN."

7. *Correct errors by drawing a single line through the mistaken entry* and writing the word *error* above it. Initial the error, and then rewrite the entry correctly. These instructions may vary according to agency policy. Never try to erase or obliterate the entry: the incorrect entry should still be visible. Do not insert words above the line or between words.

8. *Be sure the client's name and identification number are on every page.*

ORAL REPORTS

In addition to written records, nurses use oral reports to communicate nursing interventions and client status. When the client's condition is changing rapidly, physicians and other caregivers must be constantly informed. Oral reports are also given when a client is transferred from one unit to another (e.g., from the emergency room to a medical floor), at change of shift, and when family members request reports of the client's condition. A report is given to communicate specific information about what has been observed, done, or considered. It should be concise, but still contain all pertinent information.

A **change-of-shift report** is given to the on-coming nurse by the nurse who has been responsible for the patient. The charge nurse may report to on-coming nurses for all clients on a team, or a primary nurse may report to the on-coming nurse for her own patients. Reports may be given in a meeting, on walking rounds, or on audiotape. Tape-recorded reports are less time-consuming, but do not allow for questions and clarification. A typical change-of-shift report includes the following:

1. *Basic identifying information for each client.* Name, room number, age, medical diagnosis or reason for admission, admission date, and physicians. This will vary depending on the setting (e.g., in a long-term care facility, you might omit the admission date).

2. *A description of the client's present condition.* Include only significant measurements. It is not necessary to report that the vital signs are normal, unless this is a change for the client (e.g., "After medication her temperature returned to 98.6°").

3. *Significant changes in the client's condition.* Report both deterioration and improvement in condition (e.g., "At 1400 her blood pressure was 150/94; baseline was under 130/80 until that time"). When reporting changes, organize your report as follows: State what you observed, its meaning (if appropriate), what action was taken, the client's response, and the continuing plan for the on-coming nurse.

   Example: "Her respirations are slow and shallow, and she has weak cough effort. I helped her turn and cough hourly. Her lungs are clear, but she still does not deep breathe well. You should continue to have her cough and deep breathe hourly unless you see improvement."

Implementation

4. *Progress in goal achievement for identified nursing diagnoses* (e.g., "Mrs. Martin has Risk for Impaired Skin Integrity. We are presently meeting our goal of intact skin").

5. *Results of diagnostic tests or other therapies performed in the last 24 hours* (e.g., "Blood cultures were negative").

6. *Significant emotional responses* (e.g., "She has been crying since she was told she won't be able to go home").

7. *Description of invasive lines, pumps, and other apparatus* (e.g., Foley catheter).

8. *Description of important activities* that occurred on your shift. This should not be a detailed catalog of the patient's day. Report only significant activities (e.g., there is no need to report that all clients showered and ambulated in the hall).

9. *Description of care the on-coming nurse needs to do.* This does not include routine care such as the daily linen change or routine vital signs, unless it is something you were unable to accomplish (e.g., "Her bed still needs to be changed"). Include laboratory and diagnostic tests and preps that the on-coming nurse should do or special observations that she should make (e.g., "She is scheduled for surgery in the morning, and should be NPO after midnight").

ETHICAL AND LEGAL ISSUES IN IMPLEMENTATION

As client advocates, nurses are obligated to protect clients' humanity; and it is during implementation of care that the choice exists for humanization or depersonalization of care. Issues of confidentiality and dignity arise frequently in the implementation step. In addition, Item 6 of the ANA code for Nurses (1985) indicates that delegation of care also has ethical implications (see Appendix A).

Respect for Dignity

Item 1 of the ANA Code of Ethics emphasizes *respect for human dignity*. Many of the procedures performed during implementation are invasive or require the client to be exposed or assume awkward positions. Nurses are obliged to respect the client's personhood by providing adequate draping and privacy for such interventions as enemas, catheterizations, and bed baths. These may seem like routine procedures to a busy nurse, but they can be very depersonalizing for the patient. The more skilled you become in technical procedures, the more you should be able to adopt and respect the patient's perspective on what is occurring.

The manner in which you address the patient can also preserve or diminish his dignity. It is easy to fall into the habit of addressing everyone as *dear* or *honey*. Some nurses do this in an effort to express caring; others do it because it is too hard to remember the patients' names. However, patients lose their individuality when they all have the same name—even if it is a "nice" name. This is a particularly disrespectful practice when the patient is older than the nurse. You should not call a patient by his first name unless you know that he prefers it, or you are on a reciprocal first-name basis with him.

Privacy and Confidentiality

Privacy and confidentiality are related to the issue of client dignity. Item 2 of the ANA Code treats these subjects as well: "The nurse safeguards the client's right to privacy by judiciously protecting information of a confidential nature". When you provide good nursing care, patients feel comfortable with you. They may trust you enough to disclose important and personal information (e.g., "This baby does not belong to my husband, but he doesn't know"). Do not chart such information unless it is important to the care plan, and do not share it with other staff members. Nurses are free to share only information that is pertinent to the client's health.

The law restricts access to the client's written record. Even if it did not, nurses would have a moral obligation to protect the confidentiality of the record. This means that insurance companies and other agencies have no right to the information in the record without the client's permission; nor does the client's family. Legally, the client must sign an authorization for review, copying, or release of information from the chart. When charts are used for educational or research purposes, the student or researcher is obligated to avoid using the client's name or identifying her in any way.

Widespread use of computer-based record systems increases the risk that the client's privacy will be accidentally or intentionally violated. To help ensure confidentiality, agencies issue passwords to those authorized to use the system. Be aware of the potential for abuse of computer data systems. Angry employees may break through system security to destroy, change, or distribute data, or computer hackers may break into the system simply for the challenge. You should not give unauthorized users your password or access to the computer.

CULTURAL AND SPIRITUAL CONSIDERATIONS

To provide meaningful nursing care, you must understand your own cultural values, beliefs, and behaviors. Box 7–5 offers suggestions for providing culturally competent nursing care.

When orienting clients to the nursing unit, you can provide information about hospital services and arrange for clients to participate in these as they are able. Many hospitals have full-time chaplains who assist with spiritual needs; and many nursing units have a list of clergy in the community who are on call when needed.

To intervene effectively for clients who have a nursing diagnosis of Spiritual Distress, you should have already examined and clarified your own spiritual beliefs and values. If you feel uncomfortable with spiritual interventions (e.g., praying with a client who requests it), you should verbalize your discomfort and offer to obtain someone else to help the client. It is important to respect the client's beliefs and be supportive; but it is equally important for nurses not to feel guilty about their own discomfort (Kozier, et al., 1994).

If there is a true conflict between the client's spiritual beliefs and medical therapy, you should encourage the client and physician to discuss the conflict and consider alternative therapies. The nurse always supports the client's right to make an informed decision.

Implementation

Box 7–5. Interacting with Clients of Differing Culture or Ethnicity

✓ Convey respect for the individual and respect for the individual's values, beliefs, and cultural and ethnic practices.

✓ Learn about the major ethnic or cultural groups with whom you are likely to have contact.

✓ Analyze your own communication (e.g, facial expression and body language) and how it may be interpreted.

✓ Recognize differences in ways clients communicate, and do not assume the meaning of a specific behavior (e.g, lack of eye contact) without considering the client's ethnic and cultural background.

✓ Understand your own biases, prejudices, and stereotypes.

✓ Relate clients' different cultural beliefs (e.g, the cause of swollen feet) to your own. In this way, you convey interest and respect for the clients' beliefs.

✓ Recognize that cultural symbols and practices can often bring a client comfort.

✓ Support the client's practices and incorporate them into nursing practice whenever possible, and not contraindicated for health reasons; for example, provide hot tea to a client who drinks hot tea and never drinks cold water.

✓ Don't impose a cultural practice on a client without knowing whether it is acceptable; for example, Vietnamese clients may prefer not to be touched on the head (Giger & Davidhizar 1991, p. 409).

✓ Remember that the color of a client's skin does not always determine the client's culture.

✓ Learn how a client views health, illness, grieving, and the health care system.

✓ Review your own attitudes and beliefs about health and objectively examine the logic of those attitudes and beliefs and their origins.

✓ Increase your knowledge about different beliefs and values and learn not to be threatened when they differ from your own.

✓ Remember that during illness clients may return to preferred cultural practices; for example, the client who has learned English as a second language may revert to the primary language.

SUMMARY

Implementation

✓ is action-focused.

✓ requires nurses to perform or delegate dependent, independent, and collaborative actions.

✓ may use one of six common systems for allocating tasks and authority: functional, team, primary nursing, differentiated practice, case management, or managed care.

✓ should preserve confidentiality and client dignity.

✓ relates to client readiness and the nurse's cognitive, technical, and interpersonal skills.

✓ is completed when the nursing actions have been carried out and recorded, along with the client's reactions to them. (The client record or chart is a permanent, legal document of the client's health care and status.)

✓ is documented in flowsheets and narrative notes and reported orally at change of shift and when a client is transferred.

✓ provides the opportunity for culturally and spiritually competent nursing care.

Practice in Critical Thinking: Analyzing Statements

Every day you hear or read many statements. Some statements seem to be correct when you first hear or read them; yet as you think further about them you find that you disagree. In these cases it is especially important to analyze why you agree or disagree.

Begin by considering the statement carefully to make sure you understand what the speaker or author is saying. Next, think about the subject and determine whether you agree with the statement. The following are examples of questions you could consider to help you. Has the author used key words in the same way you use them? Has the author made an assumption with which you do not agree? Has the author made a mistake, like faulty logic or incorrect mathematics? Finally, you should state clearly whether or not you agree, and give reasons for your judgment.

Step 1: Study the statement to make sure you understand what the author is saying.

Step 2: Determine whether or not you agree with the statement.

Step 3: State clearly whether or not you agree, and give reasons for your judgment.

Learning the Skill

Analyze the following statement about computer-based records. State clearly whether you agree or not, and state your reasons if you disagree. Try to go through the three steps mentally before writing.

> Computer-based records are a threat to patients' privacy because of the possibility they may be accessed by angry employees or hackers. A great deal of time and expense are involved in teaching nursing staff to use computers for charting and care planning. For these reasons, hospitals should not use computer-based records for charting and care planning.

Step 1. Study the statement to be sure you understand what the author is saying.

a. What is meant by computer-based records?

b. What is meant by patients' privacy?

Step 2. Determine whether or not you agree with the statement.

a. Has the author left anything out of the argument?

b. Has the author used any terms incorrectly?

c. Has the author used faulty logic?

Step 3. State clearly whether or not you agree, and give reasons for your judgment.

Applying the Skill

Analyze the following statement about "charting by exception." In your response, clearly state whether you agree or not, and state your reasons for disagreeing. Try to go through the three steps mentally before writing.

> Charting by exception should not be used because most people believe that if it isn't charted, it wasn't done.

* Adapted from *Critical Thinking Worksheets*, a supplement of *Addison-Wesley Chemistry*, by Wilbraham et al. (Menlo Park, CA: Addison-Wesley Publishing Company, 1990).

Case Study

Read the following case study. Several of the exercises will refer to it.

Nancy Atwell is a 32-year-old teacher who lives alone. She has been diagnosed as having rheumatoid arthritis for approximately 4 years. This change has made her knees painful and has limited the motion and weight-bearing ability of her knee joints. She has recently been diagnosed as having cervical cancer, and she now enters the hospital to have an abdominal hysterectomy.

On her previous admission for treatment of her arthritis, she was quiet, withdrawn, and extremely concerned for her privacy. Now she seems more outgoing and less overtly concerned about privacy. When questioned, Ms. Atwell states she has had no previous surgical experience, but denies feeling nervous about the operation. She says she is having "quite a bit" of abdominal cramping now.

Her preoperative orders follow:

1. S.S. enema at HS
2. NPO after midnight
3. pHisohex shower
4. Pre-op med: Demerol 50 mg and Vistaril 25 mg IM at 0600
5. Ibuprofen 500 mg p.o. every 3–4 hours prn for abdominal or joint pain

1. Define and give an example of each of the following types of nursing actions (you do not need to use the case study, but you may if you wish):

Type	Definition	Example
Dependent		
Independent		
Interdependent		

2. What activities may be a threat to Ms. Atwell's privacy and dignity?

3. A nursing diagnosis for Ms. Atwell is "Risk for Impaired Home Maintenance Management: Inability to manage own care on dismissal r/t single state (no one to help out), pain in knees, and post-op pain and weakness."

   a. What collaborative (interdependent) nursing action might be performed for this nursing diagnosis?

b. What independent nursing action might be performed?

4. Ms. Atwell's nurse is preparing to implement the order for a pHisohex shower. The nurse has the necessary supplies, but she does not know the rationale for giving a pHisohex shower. What should she do?

5. If you were Ms. Atwell's nurse, what would you do to prepare her before you implement the following new medical order: Nembutal 100 mg p.o. at H.S.?

6. What is an example of therapeutic communication that might be needed by Ms. Atwell? (One example is given for you.)

   Example: Talking to her to assess for feelings of grief related to her inability to bear children after the hysterectomy.

7. State the guideline for implementing nursing strategies that is demonstrated by the following situations (refer to Box 7–3 on page 235).

   a. It is important for Ms. Bates to be turned frequently, but it causes her a great deal of pain. It is 15 minutes past time to turn her, but she has a visitor—the first one she has had in several weeks. In order to meet Ms. Bates's emotional needs, the nurse decides to wait until the visitor leaves to do the turning.

   Guideline:

b. The physician has ordered Bromocriptine 2.5 mg p.o. The nurse does not know the side effects of this drug, so he looks it up in the Hospital Formulary.

Guideline:

c. The nurse pulls the curtain around the bed and drapes the client's legs and perineum before inserting an indwelling catheter.

Guideline:

d. The nurse asks a colleague to double-check her insulin dosage.

Guideline:

e. The nurse uses sterile technique to insert the urinary catheter.

Guideline:

f. The nurse takes the client's blood pressure before administering an antihypertensive medication.

Guideline:

8. Chart the following information in DAR format (focus charting): Mr. Jarrett says his head hurts. He has his eyes shut tightly; he says the light makes them hurt. The nurse places a cool cloth on his head and closes the door to his room. She gives him Tylenol #3, tabs. i, p.o., at 6 P.M., as ordered. When she reassesses Mr. Jarrett in one hour, he says it still hurts. She plans to disturb him as little as possible and keep the room dark. She wants the evening nurse to call Dr. King if Mr. Jarrett's headache is unrelieved after the second dose of medication.

9. Use Figure 7–7 to chart the following data about Ms. Atwell. Chart in the 1500–2300 column—you are the evening nurse. Much of the normal data can be recorded by making check marks. Everything else should be charted narratively under "Nursing Progress Notes." Notice that this is a two-page form, based on the Roy Adaptation model.

    Data

    Ms. Atwell seems outgoing and not overtly concerned about privacy. When questioned, she states she has had no previous surgical experience, but denies feeling nervous about the operation. She gets up to go to the bathroom and walks about in the room several times during the evening. She walks erect and with a steady gait.

    She eats all of her evening meal. At 9 P.M. (2100) you give her a soapsuds enema; she has a large, unformed stool. You tell her that she cannot have anything to eat or drink after midnight, explaining the rationale for this restriction. She says she understands this. You take this opportunity to do the rest of her preoperative teaching. She states, "I understand."

    Your assessment reveals that her oxygenation function is normal. She has +1 edema of her left ankle, which she says is normal for her. Her pedal pulses are strong and equal bilaterally; she has no numbness or tingling in her extremities. Her skin is warm and dry.

    She is alert and oriented. She says she is having "quite a bit" of abdominal cramping now. You give her the Ibuprofen at 1800, as ordered, and record it in the medication record (MAR). At 1900, she says, "I feel better now." You assess that she is cooperative (in the "self-concept, interdependence" mode).

10. Using the information in Exercise 9, chart in SOAP format all the data that are pertinent for the problem, #2, Risk for Noncompliance with Pre- and Post-op Instructions r/t lack of knowledge. Your plan for this problem will be to (1) remove the water pitcher at 2400 and (2) remind her when she wakes up not to drink anything.

	DATE	2300-0700	0700-1500	1500-2300
	SIGNATURE			

EXERCISE/REST	Type of activity
	How far? How long?
	Repositioned
	ROM
	Aides (walker, cane, crutches, etc.)
	Sleep
		___Bedrest
		___Reposition
		    q 2 hrs
		___BRP/BSC
		___Chair/WC
		___Walk
		___Sleeping
		___Check q hr
		___Request SR down
		___Tx ___hrs
		Patient Response
			___Bedrest
			___Reposition
			    q 2 hrs
			___BRP/BSC
			___Walk
			___Up ad lib
			___Tx ___hrs
			Patient Response
				___Bedrest
				___Reposition
				    q 2 hrs
				___BRP/BSC
				___Walk
				___Up ad lib
				___Tx ___ hrs
				Patient Response

NUTRITION/ FLUID/ELEC	N/V Feeding assistance Tube feedings	___No Problems identified ___Not assessed/sleeping ___NPO	___No Problems identified ___Feed ___Assist Feed ___NPO	___No Problems Identified ___Feed ___Assist Feed ___NPO
ELIMINATION	Stool: freq/char Urine: freq/char Bowel sounds flatus, distention	___No Problems Identified ___Urine ___Abd. status ___Stool ___Incontinent	___No Problems Identified ___Urine ___Abd. status ___Stool ___Incontinent	___No Problems Identified ___Urine ___Abd. status ___Stool ___Incontinent

OXYGENATION	Breathing pattern
	Breath sounds
	Chest tubes
	Sputum
	O$_2$
	Tissue perfusion
		___Eupneic
		___Lungs clear to
		    auscultation
		___O$_2$
		___IS c assist
		___Cough/sputum
			___Eupneic
			___Lungs clear to
			    auscultation
			___O$_2$
			___IS c assist
			___Cough/sputum
				___Eupneic
				___Lungs clear to
				    auscultation
				___O$_2$
				___IS c assist
				___Cough/sputum

CIRCULATION	Pulse quality/presence
	Heart sounds
	Edema
		___No problems identified
		___Pedal pulses
		___Cap Refill
		___Numbness/tingling
		___Edema
		___TED Hose
		___R/L toes/fingers
		    pink/pale & warm/cool
			___No problems identified
			___Pedal pulses
			___Cap refill
			___Numbness/tingling
			___Edema
			___TED Hose
			___R/L toes/fingers
			    pink/pale & warm/cool
				___No problems identified
				___Pedal pulses
				___Cap refill
				___Numbness/tingling
				___Edema
				___TED Hose
				___R/L toes/fingers
				    pink/pale & warm/cool

TEMP REGUL/ SKIN INTEGRITY	Skin assessment
	Wound/incision
	Rash
	Heparin Lock Site
		___Hep Lock
		___Dressing/incision
		    Normal
		___Warm/dry
		___Cast dry/intact
		___Brace/splint
		___Checked q 2 hr
		    for fit/position
			___Hep Lock
			___Dressing/incision
			    normal
			___Warm/dry
			___Cast dry/intact
			___Brace/splint
			___Checked q 2 hr
			    for fit/position
				___Hep Lock
				___Dressing/incision
				    Normal
				___Warm/dry
				___Cast/dry intact
				___Brace/splint
				___Checked q 2 hr
				    for fit/position

PATIENT DAILY ASSESSMENT SUMMARY FLOW SHEET
2 NORTH (PILOT)

Figure 7–7. Patient Daily Assessment Summary Flowsheet. Courtesy of Shawnee Mission Medical Center, Merriam, KS.

→

		DATE	2300-0700	0700-1500	1500-2300
		SIGNATURE			

SENSORY/ NEURO		Visual/hearing aid
		Communication aid
		Perceptual ability
		Pain
		Neuro assessment
		Level of conscious.
			__Alert/oriented
			__No c/o pain
			__C/o pain
			  (Location)
			
			__See MAR
			__Dorsi/Plantar flex
			__Indicates pain relief
				___Alert/oriented
				___No c/o pain
				___C/o pain
				  (Location)
				
				___See MAR
				___Dorsi/Plantar flex
				___Indicates pain relief
					___Alert/oriented
					___No c/o pain
					___C/o pain
					  (Location)
					
					___See MAR
					___Dorsi/Plantar flex
					___Indicates pain relief

ENDOCRINE		Uterine/prostate
		  status
		Menstrual/lactation
		Pregnancy
		Endocrine status
			___NA
			
			___No s/s hypo/hyper
			  glycemia
			
			___See Diabetic Record
				___NA
				
				___No s/s hypo/hyper
				  glycemia
				
				___See Diabetic Record
					___NA
					
					___No s/s hypo/hyper
					  glycemia
					
					___See Diabetic Record

SELF CONCEPT/ INTERDEPENDENCE		Emotional status
		Coping mechanisms
		Role of S.O.
			___Cooperative
			___Freq call lite use/
			  demands
			__Safety assessment
			  min/mod/intense
			  Posey/wrist
			  restraints
			___Pt/family emotional
			  support (Mod/intense
				___Cooperative
				___Freq. call lite use/
				  demands
				__Safety assessment
				  min/mod/intense
				  Posey/wrist
				  restraints
				__Pt/family emotional
				  support (mod/intense
					___Cooperative
					___Freq call lite use/
					  demands
					__Safety assessment
					  min/mod/intense
					  Posey/wrist
					  restraints
					___Pt/family emotional
					  support (Mod/intense)

ROLE FUNCTION		Knowledge deficit
		Learning abilities
		Discharge planning
		Adaptive difficulty
		  to new roles
			___Nursing cares/
			  procedures explained
			
			___Special teaching:
			
			___Pt. indicates
			  understanding
				___Nursing cares/
				  procedures explained
				
				___Special teaching:
				
				___Pt. indicates
				  understanding
					___Nursing cares/
					  procedures explained
					
					___Special teaching:
					
					__Pt. indicates
					  understanding

NURSING PROGRESS NOTES

TIME	

Figure 7–7. (concluded)

266

REFERENCES

American Nurses Association. (1993). The American Nurses Association position statement on registered nurse utilization of unlicensed assistive personnel. *American Nurse,* February: 6–8.

American Nurses Association. (1985). *Code for Nurses.* Kansas City, MO: ANA.

American Nurses Association. (1991). *Standards of Clinical Nursing Practice.* Kansas City, MO: ANA.

Barter, M., and Furmidge, M. (1994). Unlicensed assistive personnel: Issues relating to delegation and supervision. *Journal of Nursing Administration, 24*(4):36–40.

Burke, L., and Murphy, J. (1988). *Charting by Exception: A Cost-Effective, Quality Approach.* New York: John Wiley and Sons.

Bulechek, G., and McCloskey, J. (1985). *Nursing Interventions: Treatments for Nursing Diagnoses.* Philadelphia: W.B. Saunders.

Christensen, P., and Bender, L. (1994). Models of nursing care in a changing environment: Current challenges and future directions. *Orthopaedic Nursing, 13*(2):64–70.

Conger, M. (1994). The nursing assessment decision grid: Tool for delegation decision. *The Journal of Continuing Education in Nursing, 25*(1):21–27.

Feutz, S. (1989). *Nursing and the Law.* 3rd ed. Eau Claire, WI: Professional Education Systems.

Gordon, M. (1994). *Nursing Diagnosis: Process and Application.* 3rd ed. St. Louis: Mosby.

Groah, L., and Reed, E. (1983). Your responsibility in documenting care. *Association of Operating Room Nurses Journal, 37*(May):1174, 1176–77, 1180–85.

Guzzetta, C. (1987). Nursing diagnoses in nursing education: Effect on the profession. Part 1. *Heart and Lung. 16*(November):629–635.

Jellinek, M., Herzog, D., and Stoddard, F. (1994). Primary nursing: Psychological implications. *Nursing Management, 25*(5):40–42.

Kozier, B., Erb, G., Blais, K. and Wilkinson, J. (1995). *Fundamentals of Nursing.* 5th ed. Redwood City, CA: Addison-Wesley.

Kozier, B., Erb, G., and Olivieri, R. (1991). *Fundamentals of Nursing.* 4th ed. Redwood City, CA: Addison-Wesley.

Lampe, S. (1985). Focus charting: Streamlining documentation. *Nursing Management, 16*(7):43–46.

Lengacher, et al. (1993). Redesigning nursing practice: The partners in patient care model. *Journal of Nursing Administration, 23*(12):31–37.

Malkin, K. (1993). Primary nursing: Job satisfaction and staff retention. *Journal of Nursing Management, 1*(3):119–124.

Modrcin, M., Rapp, C., and Chamberlain, R. (1985). *Case Management and Psychiatrically Disabled Individuals: Curriculum and Training Program.* Lawrence, KS: University of Kansas School of Social Welfare.

Olson, L. (1994). Commentary on voice-activated nursing documentation: On the cutting edge. *AONE's Leadership-Prospectives, 2*(1):14.

Skinner, P. (1995). The role of the family in the strengths model of psychiatric community case management. *The Kansas Nurse, 70*(1):3–4.

Trofino, J. (1993). Voice-activated nursing documentation: On the cutting edge. *Nursing Management, 24*(7):40–42.

Wiggins, M., Farias, J., and Miller, J. (1990). The role of the patient care technician at the New England Deaconess Hospital. In G. Mayer, M. Madden, and E. Lawrenz, Eds., *Patient Care Delivery Models.* Gaithersburg, MD: Aspen Publishers.

CHAPTER 8

EVALUATION

OBJECTIVES

On completing this chapter, you should be able to do the following:
- Define evaluation as it relates to (1) the nursing process and (2) quality assurance.
- State the importance and purpose of evaluation in (1) the nursing process and (2) quality assurance.
- Explain how nurses use critical thinking when evaluating.
- Describe the process of evaluating client progress toward outcome achievement.
- Given predicted outcomes and client data, write two-part evaluative statements.
- Describe a process for modifying the nursing care plan.
- Explain the relevance of culture and spirituality to evaluation in the nursing process.
- Describe a process for nursing quality assurance.
- Differentiate between criteria and standards.
- Explain how quality-assurance evaluation supports the moral principles of beneficence and nonmaleficence.

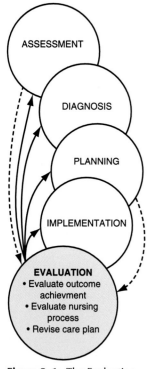

Figure 8–1. The Evaluation Step in the Nursing Process

INTRODUCTION

In the course of their work, nurses make frequent and varied evaluations. Because the client is the nurse's primary concern, the most important evaluations involve the following:

1. The client's progress toward health goals
2. The value of the nursing care plan in helping the client to achieve desired outcomes
3. The overall quality of care given to defined groups of clients

This chapter first examines the universal characteristics of evaluation and then discusses evaluation as a step of the nursing process (see Figure 8–1). Finally, it explains the process of quality assurance.

UNIVERSAL CHARACTERISTICS OF EVALUATION

Before examining evaluation as it is used in the nursing process, it may be helpful to analyze a more universal definition of the term. In general, **formal evaluation** is a deliberate, systematic process in which a judgment is made about the *quality,* value, or worth of something by comparing it to *previously identified criteria or standards*. Almost anything can be the subject of evaluation (e.g., a painting, a highway system, a teaching method, or a person's character). Furthermore, various aspects or properties of a thing can be evaluated. If you are evaluating a painting, for instance, you can assess the artist's use of color or the extent to which the painting elicits emotion. If you were evaluating teaching methods, you might measure the teacher's ability to hold student interest, promote student learning, or minimize student stress. The important thing to remember is that you must decide *in advance* what properties you are going consider and how you will measure those properties.

Universal Characteristics of Evaluation

Standards and Criteria

Although *standards* and *criteria* are sometimes used interchangeably, most texts differentiate between these terms. A **standard** is established by authority, custom, or consensus as a model of what should be done. In nursing, standards describe quality nursing care and are used for comparison when evaluating job performance. Nursing standards should be based on scientific and ethical knowledge and research, as well as on currently accepted nursing practice. Some standards, like those written for routines of care on a nursing unit, are specific enough to serve as criteria. Others are broad and abstract, as in the ANA's *Standards of Clinical Nursing Practice* (1991). The following example compares standards from each of these sources. Note the difference in specificity.

Distinctive Characteristics of Evaluation:
- ✓ Determination of quality or value
- ✓ Use of predetermined criteria or standards

> **Example:**
>
> *Broad:*
> (*ANA Standard I, Criterion 4*)
> The data collection process is systematic and ongoing.
>
> *Specific:*
> (*Standard for a Nursing Unit*)
> Temperature will be taken q4h. (Assess q2h if membranes ruptured.) Temp. will be assessed qh if > 99.6.

When standards or criteria are broad, more specific criteria must be developed to guide the collection of data for evaluation. **Criteria** are measurable or observable qualities that describe specific skills, knowledge, behaviors, attitudes, and so on. Two more specific criteria that could be used to evaluate Criterion 4 of ANA Standard I follow:

1. Vital signs are taken and recorded on the flowsheet every hour.
2. Flowsheets are kept on a clipboard at the foot of the bed while in use and transferred to the chart daily by 0700.

Because they are concrete and specific, criteria serve as guides for collecting evaluation data, as well as for making judgments about such data. The patient outcomes you learned to write in Chapter 6 are examples of criteria. The preceding standard for the nursing unit could also be used as a criterion for evaluating because it describes specific, observable behaviors.

Criteria should be both valid and reliable. A criterion is **valid** if it actually measures what it is intended to measure. For example, the white-blood-cell count is often used to "measure" the presence of infection. However, it would not be valid if used alone, because the white count is not elevated in all infections; in addition, the white count is sometimes elevated when there is no infection. More valid indicators might be a blood culture or a bacterial count of a body fluid.

A **reliable** criterion yields the same results every time it is used, no matter who uses it (e.g., determining a patient's age by asking his friends is less reliable than asking the patient or checking his birth certificate). Box 8–1 presents a comparison of standards and criteria.

Types of Evaluation

Evaluation is often classified into three types: (1) structure, (2) process, and (3) outcome. Each type of evaluation requires different criteria and methods, and each has a different focus. In a health care agency, the structure in which care is given, the caregiving processes, and the outcomes produced are interrelated.

Structure evaluation focuses on the setting in which care is given. It answers the question, What effect does the setting have on the quality of care? Structure evaluation examines the organization of the system for delivering care, looking at such factors as administrative and financial procedures, communication and staff-development processes, staffing patterns, qualifications of personnel, physical facilities, and availability of supplies and equipment.

Process evaluation focuses on the activities of the caregiver. It is concerned with actual performance in relation to the client's needs, and answers questions like the following:

In what manner is the care given?
Is care relevant to the client's needs?
Is care appropriate, complete, and timely?
What is the level of the caregiver's skills? The quality of the caregiver's performance?

Your nursing instructor probably uses a process-oriented tool to evaluate your clinical performance.

	Standards	**Criteria**
Box 8–1. Comparison of Standards and Criteria		
Similarities	Describe what is acceptable or desired	Describe what is acceptable or desired
	Serve as basis for comparison	Serve as basis for comparison
Differences	Describe nursing care	Describe expected nurse or client behaviors
	May be broad or specific	Are specific, observable, measurable
Example	ANA standards	Patient outcomes on a care plan

Outcome evaluation focuses on the client's health status and satisfaction with the results of care. Outcomes are evaluated by comparing clients' changes or responses to their health goals. Outcome evaluation answers the following questions:

To what degree were the client's health goals/outcomes achieved?
To what degree, and in what way, did the interventions contribute to outcome achievement?

Determining the relationship between nursing interventions and achievement of patient outcomes is one example of outcome evaluation.

Aspect of Care	Focus	Criterion Examples
Structure	Setting	Exit signs are clearly visible.
		A resuscitation cart will be housed on each unit. There is a family waiting room on each floor.
Process	Caregiver activities	Initial interview is completed within 8 hours after admission of client.
		Client responses to medications are charted.
		Patients will receive oral hygiene on each shift.
		Nurse introduces self to client before giving care.
Outcome	Patient responses	B/P < 140/90 at all times.
		Walks to bathroom unsupported by third day.
		Abdomen will be soft and nontender by day 5.

EVALUATION IN NURSING PROCESS

In the context of the nursing process, **evaluation** is a planned, ongoing, deliberate activity in which the client, family, nurse, and other health care professionals determine (1) the client's progress toward outcome achievement and (2) the effectiveness of the nursing care plan. Recall the two universal characteristics of evaluation:

Determination of quality or value
Use of preselected criteria or standards

The nurse and client determine the *quality* of the client's health by using as *predetermined criteria* the predicted responses identified in the planning step. They determine the *value* of the nursing care plan by using as *standards* the excellent application of each step of the nursing process.

271

Evaluation

Universal Definition	Nursing Process Definition
Determination of quality or value	**1.** of the client's health. **2.** of the nursing care plan.
Use of predetermined criteria or standards	Criteria/standards are: **1.** the outcomes identified in the planning step. **2.** Use of the nursing process according to guidelines such as those in the "Guidelines for Writing Nursing Orders" in Chapter 6.

Evaluation is an ongoing process that begins with the initial baseline assessment and continues during each contact with the client. Frequency of evaluation depends on frequency of contact, which is determined by the client's status or the condition being evaluated. When a patient has just returned from surgery, the nurse may evaluate for signs of change in status every 15 minutes. The following day, the nurse may evaluate the client only every 4 hours. As the client's condition improves and she approaches dismissal, evaluation gradually becomes less frequent.

Critical Thinking in Evaluation

Critical thinking is an integral part of the evaluation step. You will use it to apply knowledge, identify relevant facts, analyze data, and test hypotheses. When developing the criteria for evaluation, you will apply knowledge of physiology, psychology, and other fields to the specific client situation in order to know what outcomes can reasonably be expected. When collecting evaluation data, you will use critical thinking to determine the significant data for the goal being evaluated. Critical thinking continues as you analyze the data to judge the congruence between predicted and actual outcomes. In a sense, you hypothesized during the planning step that a particular nursing intervention would produce a desired client outcome; in the evaluation step you test that hypothesis.

Relationship to Other Steps

Evaluation is a planned, ongoing, deliberate activity in which the nurse, client, significant others, and other health care professionals determine
1. the extent of client outcome achievement, and
2. the effectiveness of the nursing care plan.

Effective evaluation depends on the effectiveness of the steps that precede it. Assessment data must be accurate and complete so that the outcomes written in the planning step will be appropriate for the client. The predicted outcomes (planning) must be stated in concrete, behavioral terms if they are to be useful for evaluating actual client outcomes. Finally, without the implementation step, there would be nothing to evaluate.

Evaluation overlaps with assessment. During evaluation, the nurse collects data (assessment), but for the purpose of evaluating (evaluation) rather than diagnosing. The *act* of data collection is the same; the differences are in (1) when it is collected and (2) how it is used. In the assessment step the nurse uses data to make nursing diagnoses; in the evaluation step, it is used to assess the effect of nursing care on the diagnoses.

	Assessment Data	*Evaluation Data*
When Collected	In assessment step Before care is given	In evaluation step After care is given
Purpose/Use	Diagnosis of client status	Evaluation of change in client status

Evaluation in Nursing Process

Although it is the fifth and final step in the nursing process, evaluation does not end the process; the information it provides is used to begin another cycle. After implementing the care plan, the nurse compares client responses to predicted outcomes and then uses this information in reviewing the care plan and each step of the nursing process.

Evaluation of Client Progress

In the context of the nursing process, outcome evaluation focuses primarily on the client's progress toward achieving health goals. The nurse compares the **actual outcomes** (client responses) to the **predicted outcomes** identified during the planning step and makes a judgment about whether or not they have been achieved. Evaluation data is collected by observing the client's behavior and responses, examining care plans and client records, and talking to the client, family, friends, and other health team members.

Evaluation of client outcomes may be ongoing or intermittent. **Ongoing evaluation** is done while, or immediately after, implementing an intervention to enable you to make on-the-spot modification. **Intermittent evaluation,** performed at specified times, shows the amount of progress toward outcome achievement and enables you to correct any inadequacies in the client's care and modify the care plan as needed. Evaluation continues until the client's health goals are achieved or until he is discharged from the agency.

Terminal evaluation indicates the client's condition at the time of discharge. It includes understanding of follow-up care and status of outcome achievement, especially with regard to self-care abilities. Most agencies have a special Discharge Record for the terminal evaluation, as well as for instructions regarding medications, treatments, and follow-up care. As you work with the client throughout her stay, you should prepare her for eventual discharge by gradually promoting more self-care and talking about the time when she will be leaving.

Responsibility for Evaluation

Professional standards of practice (see Box 8–2) identify evaluation as a mutual nurse-client activity. Family and other team members provide data and participate, but the nurse is responsible for initiating and recording the evaluation.

By performing organized, systematic evaluation of client outcomes, nurses demonstrate caring and responsibility. Examining outcomes shows that nurses care not only about planning and delivering care, but also about its effect on those whose lives they touch. Without evaluation, nurses would not know whether the care they give actually meets the client's needs.

Evaluation enables the nurse to improve care. It promotes efficiency by eliminating unsuccessful interventions and allowing the nurse to focus on actions that are more effective. Only by evaluating the client's progress in relation to the plan of care can the nurse know whether to continue, change, or terminate the plan.

Evaluation

Finally, by linking nursing interventions to improvements in client status, evaluation can demonstrate to employers and consumers that nurses play an important role in achieving client health.

Procedure for Evaluating Client Progress

For each of the client's nursing diagnoses you will (1) review the stated goals or outcomes, (2) collect data about the client's responses to nursing interventions, (3) compare actual outcomes to predicted outcomes and draw a conclusion about whether they have been achieved, (4) record the evaluative statement, and (5) relate the nursing orders to the client outcomes. The following discussion provides a step-by-step guide for evaluating client progress.

Review Stated Outcomes   The outcomes identified in the planning stage describe how the client is expected to look, feel, or be, or what he will be able to do if the nursing interventions are effective. A nursing diagnosis may have only one outcome, but usually there are several. You may find it helpful to make a working list of the predicted outcomes before collecting evaluation data. Table 8–1 illustrates this and the following step in the evaluation process.

Collect Evaluation Data   Collect data about the client's responses to the nursing interventions. Use the nursing diagnosis and its list of outcomes from the care plan to guide your ongoing focus assessment. In the example in Table 8–1, in order to get the data under "Actual Outcomes" during interactions with Sam Rizzo, the nurse focused on his facial expression and muscle tension and listened for statements reflecting his level of anxiety and his knowledge of routines and treatments.

The professional nurse responsible for the care plan is also responsible for evaluating the client's response to care. The client is the best source of information about subjective symptoms such as pain, nausea, or anxiety. Family input is often helpful as well, especially in ambulatory or home health settings where you are not present to observe client responses. To help make their data useful, you need to provide detailed guidelines (e.g., when to make observations, what to look for, how to get the data, how to describe what they experience or observe).

Box 8–2. ANA Standard VI: Evaluation

The nurse evaluates the client's progress toward attainment of outcomes.
Measurement Criteria:
1. Evaluation is systematic and ongoing.
2. The client's responses to interventions are documented.
3. The effectiveness of interventions is evaluated in relation to outcomes.
4. Ongoing assessment data are used to revise diagnoses, outcomes, and the plan of care, as needed.
5. Revisions in diagnoses, outcomes, and the plan of care are documented.
6. The client, significant others, and health care providers are involved in the evaluation process, when appropriate.

Source: American Nurses Association, *Standards of Clinical Nursing Practice,* 1991, p. 11. Used with permission.

The nature of the outcome determines the type of information you will collect. Outcomes can be classified as cognitive, psychomotor, or affective, or as pertaining to body appearance and functioning. For cognitive outcomes, you might ask the client to repeat information or apply new knowledge (e.g., choose low-fat foods from a menu). For psychomotor outcomes, you could ask the client to demonstrate a skill, such as drawing up insulin. For affective outcomes, you might talk to the client and observe her behavior for cues to changes in values, attitudes, or beliefs. You can obtain data about body appearance and functioning by interviewing, observing, and examining the client, as well as from secondary sources such as laboratory results. Some examples of data-collection methods for the different types of outcomes appear in Table 8–2.

***Evaluation in
Nursing Process***

Compare Actual and Predicted Outcomes, and Draw a Conclusion
Comparing data to preestablished criteria is a necessary component of evaluation: without this step, evaluation has not occurred. If the nursing process has been effective up to this point, it is relatively simple to determine if a goal has been met. Is the client's response (actual outcome) what you wanted it to be (predicted outcome)? Is it at least the best you can expect given the time and circumstances? Include the client in decisions about the level of outcome achievement. Go over the predicted outcomes with the client, and ask him if he believes they have been achieved. Three possible conclusions about outcome achievement are possible:

1. Outcome achieved   The desired client response occurred, and
The actual outcome is congruent with the predicted outcome.

Table 8–1. Evaluation Example: Sam Rizzo

Nursing Diagnosis: Moderate Anxiety r/t unfamiliar environment and dyspnea

Compare Predicted Outcomes . . .	to Actual Outcomes (Data) . . .	Conclusion
Broad goal: Will experience reduced anxiety, as evidenced by outcomes:		
1. verbalization of feeling less anxious	When dyspneic, states "What should I do? Can you help me?"	Outcome not achieved.
2. relaxed facial muscles	Face relaxed except during episodes of dyspnea.	Outcome partially achieved.
3. absence of skeletal muscle tension	No skeletal muscle tension except during episodes of dyspnea.	Outcome partially achieved.
4. verbalization of understanding of hospital routines and treatments	States, "I feel better since you explained about the fire drill. I thought there was a real fire."	Outcome achieved.
	States, "I understand about the hospital routines and the breathing treatments. Those things really aren't causing any anxiety."	

Evaluation

2. Outcome partially achieved — Some, but not all, desired behaviors were observed, or The predicted outcome is achieved only part of the time.

3. Outcome not achieved — The desired client response did not occur by the target time, or The actual outcome does not match the predicted outcome.

Table 8–1 shows how actual outcomes would be compared to predicted outcomes in order to draw conclusions about Sam Rizzo's goal achievement.

Write the Evaluative Statement An evaluative statement consists of two parts: (1) the judgment about whether the outcome was achieved ("Conclusion" in Table 8–1) and (2) data to support the judgment ("Actual Outcomes" in Table 8–1). Following are the evaluative statements that would be written for Sam Rizzo, using the data and conclusions in Table 8–1.

Predicted Outcome	*Evaluative Statement*
1. Verbalization of feeling less anxious	2/14. Outcome not achieved. When dyspneic, states, "What should I do? Can you help me?" No statements of feeling less anxious.
2. Relaxed facial muscles	2/14. Outcome partially achieved. Face relaxed except during episodes of dyspnea.
3. Absence of skeletal muscle tension	2/14. Outcome partially achieved. No skeletal muscle tension except during episodes of dyspnea.
4. Verbalization of understanding of hospital routines and treatments	2/14. Outcome achieved. States, "I feel better since you explained about the fire drill. I thought there was a real fire." Also states, "I understand about the hospital routines and the breathing treatments. Those things really aren't causing any anxiety."

Table 8–2. Evaluation Data-Collection Methods

Type of Outcome	Outcome Statement	Example of Data Collection Activity
Cognitive	By the end of the week, names foods to avoid on a low-fat diet.	Using a chart of the Food Guide Pyramid, ask the client to tell you which foods to avoid.
Psychomotor	Within 24 hours after delivery, positions baby correctly at breast.	Observe the mother breastfeeding the infant.
Affective	After orientation to routines and procedures, states he is feeling less anxiety.	Listen for spontaneous statements about anxiety, or ask, "How are you feeling?"
Body function and appearance	Heart rate < 100 at all times.	Auscultate apical heart rate.

Some care plans have a special column for the evaluative statement; in other systems you may record the evaluative statement in the progress notes. In still other systems you may record the evaluation data but not the conclusion about outcome achievement.

Relate Nursing Interventions to Outcomes It is important to establish whether or not the patient outcomes were actually caused by the nursing actions. You cannot automatically assume that a nursing intervention was the reason a goal was or was not met. A number of variables can have an impact on outcome achievement, for example:

Actions and treatments performed by other health care professionals
Influence of family members and significant others
Client's attitudes, desire, and motivation
Client's failure to give accurate or sufficient information during data collection
Client's prior experiences and knowledge

Nurses cannot control all the variables that might influence the outcome of care; therefore, in determining the effect of a nursing action, you should try to identify other factors that might have promoted or interfered with its effectiveness.

The preceding steps should tell you whether or not the care plan has been effective in achieving outcomes and resolving or preventing the client's problems. The final step—whether or not the outcomes were achieved—is to review the nursing care plan and each of the nursing process steps in its development. This step should always follow the step comparing interventions to outcomes. However, because it uses a different type of evaluative process than just explained, this final step is considered separately in the next section.

Evaluation of the Nursing Care Plan

Changes in the client's condition and the status of her goal achievement determine whether, but not how, the care plan should be revised. After finishing the outcome evaluation, examine the nursing care plan to see if it needs modification. You will probably modify the care plan if (1) the client's condition changes or (2) if the health goals were not met.

Some agencies use a pink or yellow highlighter to mark through discontinued sections of the care plan. Others have a status column in which to write the date of any revisions. These methods do not obliterate the original plans; thus they can be photocopied or used for reference as needed. Computerized care plans are easily changed on-screen, and a copy of the revised plan can be printed out.

The nursing care plan is evaluated primarily by process evaluation while the client is still receiving care, so that modifications can benefit the client. Data is obtained from client examination, interviews and records, or from staff conferences. In evaluating a care plan, you need to (1) draw conclusions about the status of client problems, and (2) review each step of the nursing process, evaluating the quality of the diagnoses, goals, and nursing orders, and also review the manner in which each step was performed.

Evaluation in Nursing Process

Evaluation

Process for Evaluating Client Outcomes

1. Review the predicted outcomes on the client's care plan.
2. After implementing the nursing order, collect data relevant to the predicted outcomes.
3. Compare actual outcomes (data) to predicted outcomes, and draw one of the following conclusions: outcome achieved, partially achieved, or not achieved.
4. Record the two-part evaluative statement: Outcome status + supporting data.
5. Relate nursing actions to outcome achievement.
6. Review and modify care plan as needed, depending on outcome achievement and changes in client's condition.

Draw Conclusions about Problem Status

Decisions about care plan modifications depend in part on whether client outcomes were achieved, not achieved, or partially achieved. The fact that outcomes have been achieved usually indicates that nursing interventions are no longer needed for a particular problem. However, you will sometimes need to continue or modify a care plan, even though outcomes were achieved. You will draw one of the following conclusions about the client's problem **when evaluation indicates that an outcome has been achieved.**

1. *Problem Resolved.* When the problem stated in the actual or potential nursing diagnosis has been resolved, nursing care is no longer needed for that problem. You can conclude that the problem has been resolved if all the outcomes for that problem have been achieved. If this is the case, document that outcomes were achieved, and discontinue the nursing diagnosis. In Mr. Rizzo's case (Table 8–1), the Anxiety problem can be considered resolved when Outcomes 1, 2, and 3 have been met.

2. *Potential Problem Prevented; Risk Factors Remain.* When the potential problem stated in the nursing diagnosis has not occurred, but the risk factors are still present, nursing care is still required for continued outcome achievement. You will probably continue with the same nursing diagnosis, outcomes, and nursing orders. For example, suppose that Tamara Jordan's nursing diagnosis is Risk for Puerperal Infection r/t membranes having ruptured several days before delivery of her baby. The desired outcome is that she will not develop puerperal infection. When the home health nurse evaluates her progress on day 3 postpartum, Tamara's temperature is normal and she has no other signs of infection—all outcomes for this problem are being met. However, this problem could still develop, so the nurse keeps it in the care plan and continues to assess for it.

3. *Possible Problem Ruled Out.* In this case you should discontinue the problem, outcomes, and nursing orders.

4. *Actual Problem Still Exists.* Even though the outcome was achieved, the problem may still exist, particularly if the outcome was only one of several written for the problem. The Anxiety diagnosis in Table 8–1 illustrates this point. One of Mr. Rizzo's outcomes was met: he verbalized understanding of hospital routines and treatments. However, the others were either not met or only partially met, so his diagnosis of Anxiety still exists. The nursing orders related to explaining routines and treatments can probably be discontinued, but the other nursing interventions for Anxiety should be continued or modified to make them more effective.

5. *All Problems Resolved; No New Problems.* When all outcomes have been achieved and no new problems have developed, the client is discharged from nursing care. In an acute-care setting this is not likely to occur before dismissal from the institution.

It is important to identify variables that have contributed to outcome achievement, so that you can reinforce positive behaviors and use them in promoting continued and future goal achievement. For example, if your evaluation shows that a child eats better for his mother, you could arrange his mealtimes so that his mother feeds him when she is there.

You may have some, but not enough, evidence that the outcome has been achieved; or perhaps it is being achieved at one time and not another. One of Mr. Rizzo's outcomes, for instance, is absence of muscle tension. He does achieve this outcome at times, but not when he is dyspneic. You will conclude one of the following when evaluation indicates that an **outcome has been partially achieved.**

1. *The problem has been reduced; care plan needs revisions.* As in Mr. Rizzo's case, you may conclude that the problem has been reduced but that nursing interventions are still needed. Since the outcome is not being fully achieved, the care plan may need to be modified.

2. *The problem has been reduced; continue with the same plan, but allow more time.* After examining the care plan, you may wish to continue with the same plan but give the client more time to achieve the outcome. To decide, you must assess why it has not been fully achieved.

Even when outcomes have not been achieved, you cannot automatically conclude that the care plan needs revision. Recall that client, family, and other variables also influence the success of the plan; therefore, you must reexamine the entire care plan and each step of the nursing process. You may conclude one of the following **when an outcome has not been achieved:**

1. The problem still exists. Continue with the same plan.
2. The problem still exists. Revise the plan.

Critically Review All Steps of the Nursing Process

As you can see, whether or not outcomes have been achieved, there are a number of decisions to make about continuing, modifying, or terminating nursing care for each problem. Before making specific modifications, you must first determine why the plan was not effective. This requires that you review the entire care plan and the nursing process steps involved in its development. This section provides a checklist of questions and actions for use in your review of each step of the nursing process.

Assessment Step   Examine the initial and ongoing assessment data in the client's chart (e.g., data base, progress notes). Errors or omissions in data influence subsequent steps of the nursing process and may require changes in every section of the care plan.

Example: Wasumita Singh answers the nurses in brief phrases; she does not initiate conversation. Her nurses initially believed her communication problem was caused by her difficulty with English. When evaluating her progress, the nurse concludes that her Impaired Verbal Communication problem still exists. However, on reviewing Ms. Singh's chart, she finds new data: a psychiatric consultation note indicating that Ms. Singh is deeply depressed. The nurse realizes now that Ms. Singh's communication problem is more than simply a language barrier.

You may find that new data have become available since the client's initial assessment, or perhaps the client's condition has changed. For example, Ms. Ray's care plan states that she can ambulate "with help of one." However, she has become progressively weaker and now cannot bear weight at all; thus the nursing order is no longer appropriate.

Evaluation

The following checklist will help you to review the assessment step. Ask yourself each of the questions. If you answer no, proceed to the next question. If you answer yes to a question, take the suggested actions, and then move to the next question.

EVALUATION CHECKLIST—ASSESSMENT STEP

Questions to Ask	*Actions to Take*
1. Were the assessment data incomplete or inaccurate?	☐ Yes. Reassess the client. Record the new data. Change care plan as indicated.
2. Are there data that still need to be validated?	☐ Yes. Validate with client (by interview and physical examination), significant others, or other professionals. Record validation (or failure to validate). Change care plan as indicated.
3. Have new data become available that require changes in the plan (e.g., a different problem etiology, new goals/outcomes, new nursing orders)?	☐ Yes. Record the data in the progress notes. Change care plan as indicated.
4. Has the client's condition changed?	☐ Yes. Record data about client's present status. Change care plan as indicated.

Move to a review of the diagnosis step.

Diagnosis Step If your examination of the assessment step results in a revision of the data base, you may need to revise or add new nursing diagnoses. Even if data were complete and accurate, you must still analyze the diagnostic process and each of the diagnostic statements. The nursing diagnosis could be incorrect because of errors in the diagnostic process, or the diagnostic statement may have been poorly written. Perhaps the nurse who wrote the statement had a clear idea of the client's problem, but was unable to communicate the idea when writing the diagnostic statement. Other nurses might therefore have focused their interventions inappropriately.

Use the following list of questions to help you review the diagnosis step. Take the suggested actions as needed.

EVALUATION CHECKLIST—DIAGNOSIS STEP

Questions to Ask	*Actions to Take*
1. Is the diagnosis irrelevant or unrelated to the data base?	☐ Yes. Revise the diagnosis.
2. Is the diagnosis inadequately supported by the data?	☐ Yes. Collect more data. Support or revise diagnosis.
3. Has the problem status changed (actual, possible, potential)?	☐ Yes. Relabel the problem.

EVALUATION CHECKLIST—DIAGNOSIS STEP (concluded)

Questions to Ask	*Actions to Take*
4. Is the diagnosis stated unclearly?	☐ Yes. Revise the diagnostic statement.
5. Does the etiology incorrectly reflect the factors contributing to the problem?	☐ Yes. Revise the etiology.
6. Is the problem one that cannot be treated primarily by independent actions?	☐ Yes. Label as collaborative and consult appropriate health care professional.
7. Is the diagnosis broad and general (rather than individualized for *this* patient)?	☐ Yes. Revise diagnosis. Revise outcomes and nursing orders as suggested by the new nursing diagnosis.
8. Has the nursing diagnosis been resolved?	☐ Yes. Delete diagnosis and related outcomes and nursing orders.

Proceed to a review of client goals.

Planning Step   If you have made additions to the data or changed the nursing diagnosis, you will need to revise the outcomes and nursing orders. However, if the data and the diagnostic statement are satisfactory as initially written, the reason for lack of outcome achievement may lie in the outcomes themselves. Perhaps they were unrealistic, or perhaps the best nursing strategies were not chosen. The following questions will help you decide whether your outcomes should be revised.

EVALUATION CHECKLIST—PATIENT OUTCOMES

Questions to Ask	*Actions to Take*
1. Have nursing diagnoses been added or revised?	☐ Yes. Write new outcomes.
2. Is the outcome unrealistic in terms of patient abilities and agency resources?	☐ Yes. Revise outcome.
3. Was insufficient time allowed for outcome achievement?	☐ Yes. Revise time frame.
4. Are there aspects of the client's problem that the outcomes do not address?	☐ Yes. Write additional outcomes.
5. Do the predicted outcomes, as written, fail to demonstrate resolution of the problem specified in the nursing diagnosis?	☐ Yes. Revise outcomes.
6. Have client priorities changed? Has the focus of care changed?	☐ Yes. Revise outcomes.
7. Were they the nurse's goals instead of the client's?	☐ Yes. Get client input. Write outcomes valued by the client.

Proceed to review of nursing orders.

EVALUATION CHECKLIST—NURSING ORDERS

Questions to Ask

Actions to Take

1. Have nursing diagnoses or outcomes been added or revised in previous review steps?

   ☐ Yes. Write new nursing orders.

2. Do the nursing orders seem unrelated to the stated client outcomes?

   ☐ Yes. Revise or develop new nursing orders.

3. Is the rationale insufficient to justify the use of the nursing order?

   ☐ Yes. Revise or develop new nursing orders.

4. Are the nursing orders unclear or vague, so that other staff may have had questions about how to implement them?

   ☐ Yes. Revise nursing orders. Add details to make more specific and/or individualized to the client.

5. Do the nursing orders lack instructions for timing of the strategies?

   ☐ Yes. Revise nursing orders. Add times.

6. Was the order clearly ineffective?

   ☐ Yes. Delete it.

7. Are the orders unrealistic in terms of staff and other resources?

   ☐ Yes. Revise orders or obtain resources.

8. Have new resources become available that might enable you to change the goals or nursing orders?

   ☐ Yes. Write new goals or nursing orders reflecting the new capabilities.

9. Do the nursing orders fail to address all aspects of the client's health goals?

   ☐ Yes. Add new nursing orders.

Proceed to review of implementation step.

Implementation Step If all sections of the nursing care plan appear to be satisfactory, perhaps the lack of outcome achievement is due to the manner in which the plan was implemented. To find out what went wrong in the implementation step, consult the progress notes, the client, significant others, and other caregivers. Use the following checklist as a guide.

EVALUATION CHECKLIST—IMPLEMENTATION

Questions to Ask

Actions to Take

1. Did the nurse fail to get client input at each step in developing and implementing the plan?

   ☐ Yes. Obtain client input, revise plan and implementation as needed.

2. Were the nursing interventions unacceptable to the client?

   ☐ Yes. Consult client; change nursing orders or implementation approach.

3. Did the nurse fail to prepare the client for implementation of the nursing order (e.g., fail to explain what client should expect or do)?

   ☐ Yes. Continue plan. Prepare client before implementing. Reevaluate.

EVALUATION CHECKLIST—IMPLEMENTATION (concluded)

Questions to Ask	Actions to Take
4. Did the nurse lack the knowledge or skill to perform techniques and procedures correctly?	☐ Yes. Continue same plan. Have someone else implement or help the nurse to acquire the knowledge or skills. If neither of these is possible, delete nursing order.
5. Did client and/or family fail to comply with the therapeutic regimen? Were strategies performed incorrectly?	☐ Yes. Reassess motivation, knowledge, and resources. Add outcomes and nursing orders aimed at teaching, motivating, and supporting client in carrying out the regimen. Set time for reevaluation.
6. Did other personnel fail to carry out nursing orders? Why?	☐ Yes. Implement the nursing order or ensure that others will do so. Set time for reevaluation.
7. Was the plan of care implemented in a manner that failed to communicate caring?	☐ Yes. This is a problem that must be addressed by staff development and personal development.

After making the necessary modifications to the care plan, implement the new plan, and begin the nursing process cycle again.

Cultural and Spiritual Considerations

When planned outcomes have not been achieved, review the client's cultural values, beliefs, and practices to determine what effect they may have had. You must consider these factors in addition to other physiologic, psychologic, social, and developmental factors when you review the nursing process and revise the treatment plan. Complete evaluation includes evaluating your own competence in providing culturally competent care to determine whether you need to improve your ability to work with clients from culturally diverse backgrounds.

When evaluating whether clients have accomplished spiritual goals, you will need skill in observation, helping relationships, and communication. You will need to observe the client when alone and when interacting with others and listen to what the client says and does not say. The following are characteristics that indicate spiritual well-being and achievement of spiritual goals: a sense of inner peace, compassion for others, reverence for life, gratitude, appreciation of unity and diversity, humor, wisdom, generosity, ability to transcend the self, and the capacity for unconditional love (Carson, 1989).

Evaluation Errors

Probably the most common evaluation error is failure to perform systematic evaluation of patient outcomes. Many nurses are more action-oriented than analytic and reflective, so it is easy in the press of a busy day to make a plan and act; you may have to make determined efforts to find time to observe and record the client's responses to the actions. Remember that quality care is not guaranteed simply because you have implemented the nursing orders. Only when you evaluate client outcomes can you be assured that the care has met the client's needs.

Evaluation

Usually the nurse does, in fact, observe the client's response, but she may not document it or consciously use it in an evaluation process that would enable her to modify interventions. You must be sure to document the evaluative statements in the client's record so that other nurses will be able to judge the effectiveness of your interventions. Otherwise, they might continue with approaches that you have already discovered to be ineffective.

Another error may occur when a nurse uses irrelevant data to judge the level of goal achievement. You should consider only data that is clearly related to the predicted outcome. Box 8–3 provides examples of both relevant and irrelevant data related to Mr. Rizzo's Anxiety problem from Table 8–1 (on page 275).

Errors are also possible in judging the congruence between actual and predicted client outcomes; actual outcomes may be measured inaccurately, or data may be incomplete. In the example of Table 8–1, if the nurse observed Sam Rizzo only during periods when he was not dyspneic, she might erroneously conclude that his anxiety was relieved.

QUALITY ASSURANCE

In addition to evaluating outcome achievement for individual clients, nurses are also involved in evaluating and modifying the overall quality of care given to groups of clients. Table 8–3 compares quality assurance and nursing process evaluation.

A **quality-assurance program** is an ongoing, systematic process designed to evaluate and promote excellence in health care given to groups of clients. Quality assurance frequently refers to evaluation of the level of care provided in an agency, but it may be as limited in scope as an evaluation of the performance of one nurse or as broad as the evaluation of the overall quality of care in an entire country.

Quality assurance evaluation is done both because it benefits professions and because consumers and government agencies mandate it. As health costs rise, increasingly sophisticated consumers demand accountability from professionals. The public wants to know that it receives maximum quality for the high price it pays.

Box 8–3. Relevant and Irrelevant Data: Sam Rizzo	
Relevant data	When dyspneic, states "What should I do? Can you help me?"
	Face relaxed; no skeletal muscle tension except during episodes of dyspnea.
	States, "I feel better since you explained about the fire drill. I thought there was a real fire."
	States, "I understand about the hospital routines and the breathing treatments. Those things really aren't causing any anxiety."
Irrelevant data	Temperature 98.6°.
	Watching television except when wife is here.

Background

Quality Assurance

Quality assurance is not a new concept. Florence Nightingale (1858) developed standards for patient care, which she supported with evidence gathered from hospital wards. Evaluation of health care has changed in the past twenty-five years in response to consumer pressures and government concerns about cost containment and quality control. Since the United States government mandated professional review of health care services in 1972, it has been increasingly required by other private and government agencies. The 1972 Joint Commission for Accreditation of Hospitals standards were an impetus for institutions, as well as the nursing profession, to place more emphasis on evaluating the quality of nursing care. Since that time, regulatory agencies such as the Joint Commission for Accreditation of Healthcare Organizations and state boards of nursing have required documentation that nursing care is being given according to nursing standards. Nursing quality assurance is now a major part of the overall evaluation of care in an institution. Nurses are involved in developing standards to describe quality nursing care in their setting and in conducting quality-assurance evaluations.

In 1982 a system of peer review organizations (PROs), managed on a state-wide basis, replaced the earlier professional standards review organizations (PSROs) (Werner, 1985). Hospitals receiving federal funds must now conduct utilization reviews through PROs. The PROs use **peer review**, which means that the members of the profession delivering the care develop and implement the process for evaluating that care. This has been a further impetus for nurses to become involved in developing standards that describe good nursing care.

Nursing Quality Assurance

Quality assurance enables nursing to demonstrate accountability to society for the quality of its services. Consumers, administrators, and bureaucrats do not always clearly perceive the relationship between quality nursing care and improved patient outcomes; professional survival requires that nurses demonstrate this link.

Table 8–3. Comparison of Quality Assurance and Nursing Process Evaluation

	Nursing Quality Assurance	The Nursing Process
Scope of evaluation	Groups of clients	Individual clients
Subject of evaluation	Overall quality of care	1. Progress toward achieving client outcomes
		2. Review of nursing care plan
Type of evaluation	Structure, process, outcome	1. Outcome evaluation of patient progress
		2. Process evaluation of nursing care plan
Responsibility for evaluation	Chief nurse in the institution	Nurse caring for client

285

Evaluation

In an effort to control health-care costs, Medicare began in 1983 to use a prospective payment system (PPS), in which hospitals are reimbursed on the basis of the client's diagnosis rather than on the number of days the client stays in the hospital. This method provides strong incentive for early discharge and has raised both professional and consumer concerns about quality. Since the advent of the PPS, there has been a great deal of pressure on home-health and extended-care agencies to accommodate those discharged from acute-care settings. Clients frequently complain of being discharged from hospitals before they feel ready to leave, of bed shortages in nursing care facilities, and of abuses in home health care. Unfortunately, while resources for treating clients in hospitals are becoming more limited, sufficient alternative treatment settings are not yet available. Providing adequate care is difficult under these circumstances, and nurses are challenged to provide a satisfactory level of care. Monitoring and promoting quality of care is an important nursing function.

Types of Quality-Assurance Evaluations

Quality assurance requires evaluation of three essential components of care: structure, process, and outcome, which were defined in the first part of this chapter; this section explains how they relate to nursing quality assurance. Nurses were traditionally evaluated by supervisors on characteristics such as dependability, communication, and clinical skills. However, such process evaluation does not consider whether the nursing care was effective in improving the client's health. On the other hand, outcome evaluation by itself does not take into account that variables other than the nursing care may affect the client's health. Quality assurance requires consideration of the interaction of these three components.

Quality assurance usually involves a **nursing audit**, in which client records are reviewed for data about nursing competence. A committee establishes standards of care (e.g., for safety measures, documentation, preoperative teaching), and a number of charts are randomly selected and reviewed to compare nursing interventions against these standards.

Structure Evaluation

Structural standards describe desirable environmental and organizational characteristics that indirectly influence care. Pertinent data includes information about policies, procedures, fiscal resources, facilities, equipment, and the number and qualifications of personnel. The data is obtained by direct observation of the physical facilities and examination of written records such as policies and financial records. Criteria that might be written for structure evaluation include (1) "Call light is within reach," (2) "Narcotics are kept in double-locked cabinet," (3) "Policies for medication errors are written and easily accessible." Although adequate staff and resources do not insure quality care, they are certainly important factors.

Process Evaluation

In nursing quality assurance, process evaluation concentrates on the activities of the nurse. Process standards focus on the manner in which the nurse uses the nursing process. They describe what the nurse should do for the client or what constitutes proper performance of a procedure. The ANA *Standards of Clinical Nursing Practice* (1991) are an example of process standards. Some examples of specific, observable criteria for evaluating process standards follow:

Checks client's identification band before giving medication.

Performs and records chest assessment, including auscultation, once per shift.

Explains procedures (e.g., catheterization) prior to implementation.

Quality Assurance

Data for *concurrent process evaluation* is obtained by observing nursing performance, by interviewing the client, and by auditing the client's records while he is still in the institution. Process questions that might be asked concurrently are (1) Does the nurse administer medications safely? and (2) Is privacy provided during treatments and procedures?

A positive relationship should exist between the quality of the nurse's practice and the outcomes for the patient. This is an important premise of the nursing profession and an important focus for nursing research. Of course, the patient's health may become worse instead of better no matter how expertly the nurse performs, but overall, good nursing care should improve patient outcomes.

Process evaluation after the client is discharged involves an audit of client records to obtain evidence of the nurse's application of the nursing process. This emphasizes the need for careful documentation of nursing care and client responses (see Chapter 7). *Retrospective process evaluation* may also use post-discharge questionnaires or telephone interviews as sources of data. Examples of process questions that might be answered retrospectively follow:

Were medications given on time?

How soon after admission was the client's nursing history complete?

Is the nursing care plan complete?

Do the nursing progress notes provide evidence that the care plan was implemented?

Outcome Evaluation

Outcome evaluation focuses on demonstrable changes in the client's health status that occur as a result of nursing care. Evaluation criteria are written in terms of client responses or health states—just as they are for evaluation of an individual client's progress (e.g., "Verbalizes feelings about cesarean birth"; "Skin over bony prominences is intact and free from redness"). Additionally, the criterion states what percent of clients are expected to have this outcome when nursing care is satisfactory.

> **Example:** Skin over bony prominences is intact and free from redness. *Expected compliance: 100%*

Taken alone, this means that you would expect that with good care, no clients in the institution will develop redness over a bony prominence. If used alone, however, outcome evaluation fails to consider the effect of variables other than nursing care; some clients' nutritional and mobility status may be so compromised that no amount of care can prevent redness over bony prominences. A process evaluation for such a client might show that a good care plan was written and that the client received hourly turning and skin care—indicating that the nursing care was adequate even though the outcome was poor. A structure evaluation might also show that the nursing unit was chronically understaffed, which would validate a process evaluation that reveals that the client often went for more than 2 hours without being repositioned—providing the reason for the poor processes and poor outcome.

Evaluation

Client responses are the data used for outcome evaluation. Data is obtained from nursing audits, as well as client interviews and questionnaires. Judgments made after the client is discharged can be used to determine whether the nursing care plan was effective. Of course, the information comes too late to improve outcomes for that particular client, but it can contribute to improved care for future clients.

It is not always easy to demonstrate the relationship between nursing care and client outcomes. Medical, or disease-related, outcomes are easy to observe. For instance, a temperature of 98.6° and a white-blood-cell count of 8,000 provide good evidence that there is no infection, and it is easy to attribute these results to the effects of the antibiotic that was given. The nursing perspective is more holistic, so it is sometimes difficult even to define the outcomes desired. Emotional, social, or spiritual responses, for instance, are hard to write in measurable terms. It is also difficult to measure the degree to which the outcome was caused by the nursing care, since many variables contribute to improvement (or deterioration) in the client's health (e.g., the nature of the client's illness, medical interventions, quality of nursing care, availability of resources, client motivation, and family participation).

A Procedure for Quality-Assurance Evaluation

The quality-assurance process is similar to the nursing process; it involves data collection, comparison of data to criteria, identification of problems, generation and implementation of solutions, and reevaluation. It is different in that it focuses on nurses and institutions rather than patients, does not rely as heavily on outcome evaluation, and is concerned with groups of clients rather than individuals. The following steps are included in the quality-assurance models of most organizations:

1. *Decide the topic to be evaluated.* The topic might be the care for a group of clients with a particular medical diagnosis, care for all clients in a hospital, or record keeping on a nursing unit.

2. *Identify standards of care.* Determine whether structure, process, or outcome standards are appropriate. Recall that standards are broad guidelines and are not measurable or useful in data collection. Therefore, this step is sometimes omitted, and only the criteria are actually written.

3. *Establish criteria* for measuring the standards of care. Process and outcome criteria are specific, observable characteristics that describe the desired behaviors of the nurse or client.

4. *Determine expected compliance or performance levels.* A performance level is the percent of times you would expect the criterion to be met. This may vary from 0% to 100%, depending on how the criterion is stated. For example, you might expect that 95% of the time, an admission data base would be completed within 4 hours after the client was admitted.

5. *Collect data related to the criteria.* Data may be obtained from client interviews, chart audits, direct observation of nursing activities, questionnaires, or special evaluation tools, depending on the criterion you are evaluating.

6. *Analyze the data.* Identify discrepancies between the data and the criteria. Determine reasons for the discrepancies, using information about structures, processes, and outcomes. Identify problems. In the example in Item 4, if fewer than 95% of the admission data bases were completed in the specified time, it would be important to find out why this is happening.

7. *Generate solutions for correcting discrepancies and solving problems.* For instance, more in-service education may be needed for nurses, or perhaps the staffing pattern should be changed, or a new data-collection form used.

8. *Implement the solutions.* The purpose of evaluation is to maintain the quality of care being delivered. Once problems have been identified, action must be taken to see that they do not recur.

9. *Reevaluate* to determine if the solutions were effective.

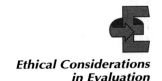

Ethical Considerations in Evaluation

ETHICAL CONSIDERATIONS IN EVALUATION

The moral principle of **beneficence** holds that we ought to do good things for other people, that is, benefit them. A nurse who holds the hand of a dying patient honors this principle. The principle of **nonmaleficence** holds that we should not harm others. For example, a nurse upholds this principle when she withholds morphine from a client whose respirations are already depressed. You can think of these principles as being on a continuum, with the duty to do no harm taking precedence over the other duties:

Nonmaleficence ⟶ Beneficence
↓ ↓
Do no harm → Try to prevent harm → Remove harmful things → Do good

Some simple examples to help you understand this continuum follow:

Nonmaleficence	Do no harm	Do not push a stranger into the lake.
	Try to prevent harm	If a stranger starts to fall into the lake, try to grab him and keep him from falling in.
	Remove harmful things	If you see that a person is about to stumble over a rock, which will cause him to fall in the lake, warn him or remove the rock.
Beneficence	Do good	If you happen on the scene after a stranger has fallen into the lake, jump in and rescue him.

It is easy to see how the first situation is a stronger duty than the last one.

Evaluation

> ## Critical Thinking: Developing Evaluation Criteria
>
> In the past three months, several medication errors have been made on your nursing unit. The unit has instituted some policies and procedures to enhance the safety of this task. Develop criteria to use to evaluate whether this practice problem has been solved. Include criteria to measure structure, process, and outcomes. To begin, answer these questions:
> ✓ What is the purpose of the evaluation?
> ✓ What is being evaluated; what is the function of the thing being evaluated?
> ✓ What different points of view might exist?
> Now write your criteria.

Nurses are morally obligated under the principles of beneficence and nonmaleficence to seek to benefit patients and not harm them. Quality assurance and evaluation of client progress fulfill this obligation by enabling nurses to improve the quality of care they deliver. Quality assurance not only contributes to improved nursing care, it can produce changes in the total health care system and improve communication and collaboration between health care disciplines.

The ANA code of ethics (1985) in Appendix A includes at least four items that imply that evaluating care is a nursing responsibility:

Item 4.   The nurse assumes responsibility and accountability for individual nursing judgments and actions.

Item 8.   The nurse participates in the profession's efforts to establish, implement, and improve standards of nursing.

Item 9.   The nurse participates in the profession's efforts to establish and maintain conditions of employment conducive to high-quality nursing care.

Item 11.   The nurse collaborates with members of the health professions and other citizens in promoting community and national efforts to meet the health needs of the public.

SUMMARY

Evaluation
- ✓ is a deliberate, systematic process in which the quality, value, or worth of something is determined by comparing it to previously identified criteria or standards.
- ✓ in nursing, is a planned, ongoing, deliberate activity in which the nurse, client, significant others, and other health care professionals determine the client's progress toward goal achievement and the effectiveness of the nursing care plan.
- ✓ considers *structure* (focusing on the setting in which care is given), *process* (focusing on nursing activities), and *outcomes* (focusing on the changes in client health status that result from nursing care).
- ✓ does not end the nursing process, because the information it provides is used to begin another cycle.
- ✓ involves five steps: (1) *review* of the stated client goals or predicted outcomes, (2) *collection* of data about the client's responses to nursing interventions, (3) *comparison* of actual client outcomes to the predicted outcomes and drawing a conclusion about whether the goals have been met, (4) *recording* of evaluative statements, and (5) *relating* the nursing orders to the client outcomes.
- ✓ requires the nurse to consider all variables, including cultural and spiritual, that may have influenced goal achievement and to modify the care plan as needed.

Quality-assurance evaluation
- ✓ is an ongoing, systematic process designed to evaluate and promote excellence in health care.
- ✓ is usually concerned with the care given to groups of clients.
- ✓ frequently refers to evaluation of the level of care provided in an agency, but it may be as limited in scope as an evaluation of the performance of one nurse or as broad as the evaluation of the overall quality of care in an entire country.
- ✓ commonly uses the methods of retrospective chart audit and peer review.
- ✓ effects the moral principles of beneficence and nonmaleficence.

The word *synthesis* means putting things together to form something new. Chemists synthesize new compounds for use as medicines by thoughtfully com-

Nurses synthesize when they use concepts and ideas from nursing theories and related knowledge to bring patient data together into meaningful relationships.

bining various kinds of reactants and determining what the products are. We can also put ideas together to develop new ideas. Concepts, data, ideas, and methods from one source are linked with those from other sources. We call this process *synthesizing ideas*. It is an important skill because it allows us to come up with new ideas to deal with the different situations we encounter in everyday life.

First, cues are clustered by identifying relationships between them. Knowledge of physiological and psychological norms is combined with knowledge of nursing theories and other concepts to explain the clustered data. Further synthesis is done as the information is formed into a meaningful whole: the nursing diagnosis.

Applying the Skill

Max Dupree is 75 years old. He has a medical diagnosis of peripheral arterial disease, characterized by decreased circulation in both his lower legs. Mr. Dupree has atherosclerosis and arteriosclerosis, which have caused his arteries and arterioles to become stiff and resistant, as well as smaller in radius. He is a heavy smoker. Even if you are not familiar with the nursing care of a patient with peripheral arterial disease, you should be able to synthesize a *potential (risk)* nursing diagnosis (problem + etiology) for Mr. Dupree, based on the following facts.

All body cells need oxygen and nutrients and are sensitive to any reduction in their supply.

Oxygen and nutrients are carried to the tissues in the arterial blood.

Vessel resistance (including vessel size) is one of the most important factors in determining arterial blood flow.

The physiological effects of decreased peripheral circulation depend on the degree to which *reduced blood flow* exceeds *tissue demands* for oxygen and nutrients. If tissue needs are high, then even a small reduction in flow can create symptoms.

Metabolic rate is a measure of the rate at which energy is being expended. An increased metabolic rate causes an increase in oxygen use.

Physical exercise greatly increases the metabolic rate.

Metabolic activity in muscles that lack oxygen results in hypoxia and a buildup of metabolites, producing muscle spasms.

(*Note:* Do not write a diagnosis of Altered Peripheral Tissue Perfusion, since independent nursing interventions for that diagnosis are limited in this case. Additionally, if you use this diagnosis, the etiology will either consist of pathophysiology or a medical diagnosis, neither of which can be addressed by nursing orders.)

As you work your way through the following questions, you will practice the skill of synthesizing a new idea by combining the seven original ideas you were given.

1. First, use synthesis to determine a potential (risk) problem for Mr. Dupree.

   a. What is the connection between the radius of the arteries/arterioles and the amount of blood flow to the tissues?

   b. What is the connection between decreased blood flow and the amount of oxygen that reaches the tissues?

   c. Knowing Mr. Dupree's diagnosis, and using the facts in (*a*) and (*b*), what can you say about the probable state of oxygenation of the muscle tissues in Mr. Dupree's lower legs?

   d. What is the connection between hypoxia, muscle spasms, and pain?

   e. How does the balance (imbalance) between reduced blood flow and tissue demands affect the severity of symptoms or the likelihood that the patient will have symptoms?

   f. Taking (*d*) and (*e*) into account, you could say that Mr. Dupree will probably have Pain **if**

   g. Therefore, you could diagnose the problem: Risk for Pain in Lower Legs. Given that Mr. Dupree has a constant state of reduced blood flow to his legs, he will probably have pain whenever his legs experience an increased need for oxygen.

2. Now use synthesis to determine an etiology for Mr. Dupree's potential problem of Pain.

   a. What determines the likelihood that a symptom will be produced by a reduction in peripheral blood flow?

   b. What is the connection between metabolic rate and oxygen use?

c. What is the connection between exercise and metabolic rate?

d. Combine the ideas in (*a*) and (*b*). What is the connection between exercise and the demands of the skeletal muscle tissues for oxygen (especially in Mr. Dupree's legs)?

e. Combine the ideas in (*a*) and (*d*). Under what circumstances is Mr. Dupree most likely to experience the problem (symptom) of Pain?

f. Therefore, for Mr. Dupree, the etiology of Risk for Pain in Lower Legs is exercise. Your diagnosis is: Risk for Pain in Lower Legs r/t exercise. You do not have enough information to determine how much exercise it will take to produce pain, nor how severe the pain would be.

Reviewing What You Have Learned

In your own words, explain what synthesizing an idea means.

Adapted from *Critical Thinking Worksheets*, a Supplement of *Addison-Wesley Chemistry*, by Wilbraham et al. (Menlo Park, CA: Addison-Wesley Publishing Company, 1990).

Applying Nursing Process

1. Place a check mark (✔) beside the criteria that are specific, measurable, or observable.

   a. ___ The nurse gives safe care.

   b. ___ Medications are recorded at the time they are given.

   c. ___ Every patient will have an arm band with name and hospital number.

   d. ___ Temperature will be less than 100.1° during entire stay.

   e. ___ Each unit will have an adequate number of wheelchairs.

   f. ___ Data collection is systematic.

2. Match the data source to the letter of the type of evaluation for which it would be used.

   a. Structure

   b. Process

   c. Outcome

   1. ___ Charts

   2. ___ Procedure manuals

   3. ___ Verbal data from the client

   4. ___ Observation of the client (e.g., VS)

   5. ___ Observation of nursing activities

   6. ___ Staff orientation plans

   7. ___ Most performance-evaluation forms

   8. ___ System for measuring client acuity

3. Match the criterion (or question) to the letter of the type of evaluation for which it would be used.

   a. Structure

   b. Process

   c. Outcome

   1. ___ Client will state he is free from pain.

   2. ___ The nurse washes her hands before drawing up the medication.

   3. ___ How many wheelchairs are kept on the unit?

   4. ___ Client's B/P will be < 130/90.

   5. ___ All direct caregivers are registered nurses.

   6. ___ Bed is in low position with wheels locked.

   7. ___ Are all monitors in working order?

4. Your client has a nursing diagnosis of Altered Oral Mucous Membrane r/t prolonged NPO and mouth breathing. Some of the nursing orders follow:

1. Instruct client to rinse mouth as needed with a solution of 25% acetic acid and water.
2. Reinforce importance of oral hygiene after meals and as needed.
3. Remind client to breathe through nose as much as possible.
4. Lubricate lips with mineral oil.

    a. Write at least two outcome criteria you could use to determine whether this problem has been resolved.

    b. State how you would obtain the data needed to determine if each criterion has been met (e.g., interview the patient, etc.)

Case Study

Refer to the following case study for Exercises 5 and 6.

Ms. Nancy Atwell is a 32-year-old unmarried teacher who has been diagnosed as having rheumatoid arthritis for approximately 4 years. This change has made her knees painful and has limited the motion and weight-bearing ability of the knee joints themselves. She has recently been diagnosed as having uterine cancer, and now enters the hospital to have a hysterectomy. On her previous admission for treatment of her arthritis, she had been quiet, withdrawn, and extremely concerned for her privacy. Now she seems more outgoing and less overtly concerned about privacy. When questioned, Ms. Atwell states that she has had no previous surgical experience, but denies feeling nervous about the operation. Her preoperative orders follow:

1. S.S. enema at HS
2. Nembutal 100 mg p.o. at HS
3. NPO after midnight
4. pHisohex shower in A.M.
5. Pre-op med: Demerol 50 mg and Vistaril 25 mg IM at 0600.

5. The nurse identified for Ms. Atwell a diagnosis of "Risk for Anxiety r/t lack of knowledge of effects and procedure of hysterectomy." Her goal is to find out whether Ms. Atwell is anxious and if she is, to relieve her anxiety. (The first answer is provided for you.)

   a. Give an example of a verbal cue that would indicate achievement of this objective.

      Ms. Atwell states, "I'm confident everything will go all right. I certainly don't have any experience with this kind of thing, but I know you will tell me what I need to know. I feel pretty relaxed, actually."

   b. Give an example of a nonverbal cue that would indicate achievement of this objective.

   c. Give an example of a verbal cue that would indicate the objective has not been achieved.

   d. Give an example of a nonverbal cue that would indicate the objective has not been achieved.

6. The following nursing diagnoses and outcomes appear on Ms. Atwell's care plan. Using the new data charted by the nurse after implementing care for each diagnosis, write an evaluative statement for each diagnosis.

Nursing Diagnosis	Outcomes	New Data (Progress Notes)
Risk for Anxiety r/t lack of knowledge of effects and procedure of hysterectomy	Will state not anxious about effects of surgery Will show no physical signs of anxiety.	Pre-op teaching done. States understanding of surgical procedure. Says she expects to have some post-op pain, but is sure she can manage with meds. No facial tension, hands folded loosely in lap while talking.
Evaluative statement for care plan:		

Nursing Diagnosis	Outcomes	New Data (Progress Notes)
Risk for Grief r/t loss of childbearing ability 2° hysterectomy	Will express her feelings about sterility/desire for children, prior to discharge.	During pre-op teaching, ct. was told she would not have periods after her hysterectomy and would not be able to become pregnant. She stated "Periods are a nuisance anyway," but did not comment further.

Evaluative statement for care plan:

Nursing Diagnosis	Outcomes	New Data (Progress Notes)
Risk for Noncompliance with NPO order r/t lack of understanding of importance	Will state reasons for remaining NPO for O.R. after pre-op teaching. Will remain NPO after midnight.	9 P.M.—Pre-op teaching done. States relationship of NPO to anesthesia, aspiration, etc. this evening. 11:50 P.M.—Water pitcher removed; NPO sign up. 2:30 A.M.—Ct. up to bathroom, drinking water from cupped hands. Stated she forgot about drinking restriction and would not drink any more.

Evaluative statement for care plan:

7. For the three nursing diagnoses in Exercise 6, draw a line through parts of the care plan that could be discontinued after evaluation.

8. The nursing diagnosis is "Risk for Impaired Skin Integrity: Dermal Ulcer r/t inability to move about in bed and poor nutritional status." The desired outcome is, "Skin integrity will be maintained." The nurse notes that the client's skin is intact, with no redness over bony prominences, and concludes that the goal has been met. Circle the letter of the correct action. The nurse should

a. decide the problem no longer exists, document that the outcome was achieved, and discontinue the nursing care for that outcome.

b. decide that the problem still exists even though the outcome was achieved, and continue the same nursing interventions.

REFERENCES

American Nurses Association. (1991). *Standards of Clinical Nursing Practice*. Kansas City, MO: ANA.

American Nurses Association. (1985). *Code for Nurses with Interpretative Statements*. Kansas City, MO: ANA.

Buchanan, L. (1994). Therapeutic nursing intervention knowledge development and outcome measures for advanced practice. *Nursing and Health Care, 15*(4):190–195.

Carson, V. B. (1989). *Spiritual Dimensions of Nursing Practice*. Philadelphia: W. B. Saunders.

Harvey, G., (1991). An evaluation of approaches to assessing the quality of nursing care using (predetermined) quality assurance tools. *Journal of Advanced Nursing, 16*(3):277–286.

Joint Commission on the Accreditation of Hospitals. (1973). *Joint Commission on the Accreditation of Hospitals: Procedure for Retrospective Patient Care Audit in Hospitals, Nursing Edition*. Chicago.

Nightingale, F. (1858) *Notes on Matters Affecting the Health, Efficiency, and Hospital Administration of the British Army*. London: Harrison and Sons.

O'Brien, B. and McHugh, M. (1994). Quality circles: One organization's experience. *Journal of Nursing Care Quality, 8*(4):20–24.

Patterson, O. (1994). Critical pathways . . . care paths cut length of stay, reduce charges. *OR Manager, 10*(7):12.

Werner, J. (1985). PSROs and hospital accreditation. In McCloskey, J., and Grace, H., eds., *Current Issues in Nursing*. 2nd ed. Boston, MA: Blackwell Scientific Publications.

CHAPTER 9

CREATING A PATIENT-CARE PLAN

OBJECTIVES

On completing this chapter, you should be able to do the following:
- Describe the content of a comprehensive patient-care plan.
- Compare and contrast standardized and individually written care plans.
- Explain how model care plans, standards of care, protocols, and policies are used in creating a patient-care plan.
- Compare and contrast individualized nursing care plans with multidisciplinary care plans or critical pathways.
- List guidelines for writing patient-care plans.
- Explain how a well-written care plan supports two conventional ethical principles of nursing.
- Develop a complete plan of care for a client using either inductive or deductive diagnostic reasoning and a nursing framework.
- Describe the steps necessary in using the nursing process to develop a comprehensive patient-care plan.

INTRODUCTION

Chapters 3 through 8 presented the five steps of the nursing process and illustrated how each step is applied, using nursing models as frameworks for collecting, organizing, and analyzing data. The nursing process steps are summarized for you in Figure 9–1.

This chapter describes and provides examples of each section of a comprehensive care plan. It next presents a step-by-step Care-Planning Guide, which summarizes how the entire nursing process is used to develop a care plan for a client. Finally, the Luisa Sanchez case (begun in Chapter 3) is used to demonstrate how to create a comprehensive care plan by combining standard (preprinted) and individually written care plans.

Benefits of a Written Plan

The most obvious benefit of a written care plan is that it *provides continuity of care*. It is important—sometimes essential—that all caregivers use the same approach with a patient.

Example: Jed Goldstein is being treated on an adolescent mental health unit. The staff has been trying to modify his manipulative behavior. Val Benitez, RN, has been floated to the mental health unit from the intensive care unit. She

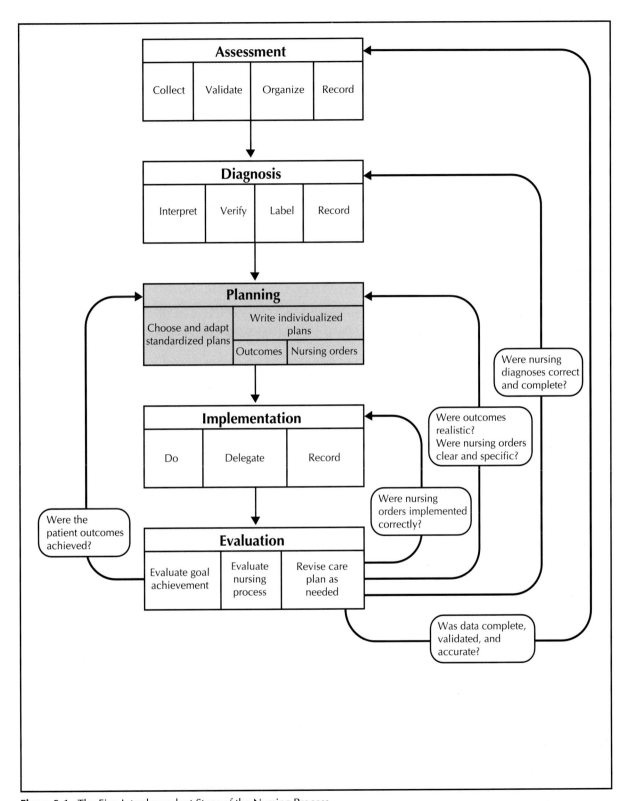

Figure 9-1. The Five Interdependent Steps of the Nursing Process

Creating a Patient-Care Plan

does not know Jed, but she reads an order on the nursing plan: "Do not respond to negative talk about staff on other shifts." Later, Jed begins to complain about the night nurse. Val's usual response with ICU patients is to remain neutral but encourage them to express their feelings. Instead, she remembers the nursing order and changes the subject. Val is not an experienced psychiatric nurse; without the care plan, her nurturing instincts and past experience might have prompted her to respond differently. This would not have been therapeutic for Jed, and would have undermined the work of the nurses on the other shifts.

A written care plan *promotes efficient functioning of the nursing team* by assuring that time is not wasted on ineffective approaches (as in the Jed Goldstein example, above) and that efforts are not duplicated. By specifically outlining nursing interventions and expected client responses, written plans provide a convenient reference for organizing the nursing progress notes. They also help to assure adequate discharge planning (see Chapter 6), provide documentation for third-party reimbursement, and serve as a guide for making staff assignments.

Systems for Storing Care Plans

Care plans must be easily accessible to all members of the health care team, and stored so that the nurse does not have to wait while someone else is using the records. They may be kept at the bedside or all the care plans for a unit may be stored together in a central location, either on special forms or in a computer to be printed out as needed.

A **Kardex** (see Figure 9–4 on page 306) is a holder for care plans written on specially designed 6 × 11-inch cards. Each Kardex holds several care plans. Some institutions keep the care plans for a group of patients in an 8½ × 11-inch notebook in a central location. This is similar to the Kardex system. In agencies that use problem-oriented medical records (POMR), the nursing care plan is documented in a special format and kept in the patient's chart. In this system, the patient's problems, goals, and nursing orders are recorded in the progress notes.

Computerized Care Plans

Computers are being used to create both standardized and individualized care plans (see Figure 9–9 on page 326 for an example of a computer-generated care plan). The nurse can access the patient's stored care plan from a centrally located terminal at the nurses' station or from terminals in patient rooms.

With this system, the nurse chooses the appropriate nursing diagnoses from a menu suggested by the computer. The computer then lists possible outcomes and interventions for those diagnoses. The nurse chooses those appropriate for the patient and types in any additional outcomes or interventions not listed in the menu. The nurse can read the plan on the computer screen or print out an updated working copy each day. Computerized care plans are easy to review and update, and since they do not rely on human memory, they are likely to be thorough and accurate. Charting is also more thorough and accurate. While the nurse is charting, the computer reads the specific interventions on the care plan and prompts the nurse to document the patient's responses to each intervention.

One disadvantage is that some nurses are not yet computer-literate. It takes time and effort to learn to use each new system, but it pays off in more efficient use of the nurse's time. For this reason, more and more agencies are using computerized record systems. In this era of information explosion, computer literacy is becoming another essential nursing skill.

Format for Nursing Care Plans

Care plan forms differ from agency to agency. However, the format usually consists of at least three columns: nursing diagnoses, patient outcomes, and nursing orders. Some agencies add a column for assessment data (the *A.M.B.* part of the nursing diagnosis), and some add a column for evaluating patient responses to the nursing interventions. Planning usually progresses horizontally across the page: Nursing Diagnosis → Patient Outcomes → Nursing Orders → Evaluation. Figure 9–2 shows a typical format. In this format, you could write the assessment data in the same column as the nursing diagnosis if you use the *A.M.B.* format. A few agencies add a column for a **rationale**, which consists of principles or scientific reasons for selecting a specific nursing action. It may also explain why the action is expected to achieve the outcome. Professional functioning requires an understanding of the rationale underlying the nursing orders, even when the rationale is not written on the care plan.

Date	Nursing Diagnosis	Predicted Outcomes	Nursing Orders	Rationale	Evaluation
7/15/96	Decisional Conflict r/t value conflicts regarding termination of treatment A.M.B. tearfulness. Statements of inability to decide.	1. By 7/16 will discuss feelings about the situation with nurse and significant other. 2. etc.	1. Spend at least 15 minutes sitting with client during each visit. 2. Listen without making judgements. 3. etc.	1. Demonstrates support and caring. 2. Demonstrates acceptance of client's value and worth unconditionally. 3. etc.	7/16 Goal #1 Goal met. Discussed feelings of guilt with wife.

Figure 9–2. Sample Format for Nursing Care Plan

Creating a Patient-Care Plan

If care plans are to be useful in the clinical setting, they must be concise and easy to use. Still, the format chosen should include adequate space to write individualized nursing orders, even when preprinted plans are used.

Student Care Plans

Care plans in practice settings are designed primarily for nurses to use in delivering care. Student care plans are designed, in addition, to provide a learning experience. Student care plans are commonly assigned for these purposes:

1. To help the student learn and apply the nursing process.

2. To provide a guide for giving nursing care to meet the client's needs while in the clinical setting.

3. To help the student learn about the client's pathophysiology or psychopathology and the associated nursing care.

Therefore, you will probably be required to handwrite your student care plans without incorporating any preprinted plans. You may be expected to develop a list of all your patient's actual and risk (potential) nursing diagnoses and collaborative problems, not just the unusual ones, and to develop detailed nursing interventions for them. Your instructors may also ask you to provide an in-depth rationale for your nursing interventions, and perhaps to cite literature to support your rationale.

THE PATIENT-CARE PLAN

There are two kinds of care plans: comprehensive nursing care plans and multidisciplinary (collaborative) care plans. Both types may contain sections that are: (1) standardized, preplanned, and preprinted and/or (2) individualized to fit the unique needs of an individual patient. This section explains how standardized and individualized approaches are used to create both nursing and multidisciplinary care plans.

Comprehensive Nursing Care Plans

A **comprehensive care plan** is made up of several different documents that (1) address the patient's nursing diagnoses and collaborative problems; (2) describe any routine care needed to meet basic needs (e.g., bathing elimination); and (3) specify nursing responsibilities in carrying out the medical plan of care (e.g., preparing the patient for a laboratory test, keeping the patient NPO before surgery). A complete plan of care integrates dependent, interdependent, and independent nursing functions into a meaningful whole, providing a central source of patient information.

The **nursing diagnosis care plan** is the section of the comprehensive care plan that prescribes the independent nursing actions for the patient's nursing diagnoses and collaborative problems. Some nurses also use the term *care plan* to mean the outcomes and nursing orders written for a *single* nursing diagnosis, as in, "Ms. Sifuentes needs a *care plan* for Impaired Skin Integrity related to total immobility," and "What is your *plan of care* for Mr. Debicki's Anxiety?" A comprehensive care plan usually contains several of these single-problem care plans.

Content of the Comprehensive Care Plan

A comprehensive patient-care plan covers all aspects of the patient's care. Any nurse, even one who does not know the patient, should be able to find in the care plan the instructions needed to provide competent care. Regardless of whether it is preplanned (standardized) or written from scratch, every comprehensive care plan should include (1) a brief patient profile, (2) instructions for meeting basic care needs, (3) nursing responsibilities for the medical plan, and (4) the care plan for the patient's identified nursing diagnoses and collaborative problems (the nursing diagnosis care plan). Many care plans also include special sections for discharge and teaching plans. Figure 9–3 illustrates the various components of a comprehensive care plan.

Client Profile The client profile includes the client's name, age, admitting diagnosis, support people, and other pertinent personal or demographic data. This should be a brief summary, available at a glance, to give a quick overview of the client. On the computer care plan (see Figure 9–9), the profile data appears at the top of each page. The Kardex (Figure 9–4) shows Luisa Sanchez's profile data, taken from Figure 3–3 in Chapter 3. This profile data is grouped in a section at the bottom of the Kardex. Notice that even if the nurse is not acquainted with Mrs. Sanchez, she can quickly find out how to reach Mr. Sanchez in case of an emergency. She can also see the date and type of surgery, as well as the physician to call if she needs medical orders.

The Patient-Care Plan

Figure 9–3. Components of a Comprehensive Care Plan

SHAWNEE MISSION MEDICAL CENTER

Date ord.	Radiology	Date Sch	DONE	Date ord.	Laboratory	Date Sch	DONE	Date ord.	Special Procedures	Date Sch	DONE
4/16/96	Chest Xray PA + lateral	4/16	✓	4/16	Blood Culture	4/16	✓	4/16	C+S Sputum		✓
				4/16	Urine specific gravity	4/16	✓	4/16	24-hr urine		
				4/16	Blood gases	4/16	✓				
				4/16	serum Electrolytes	4/16	✓				
				4/16	CBC with diff.	4/16	✓				

Daily Tests

Ancillary Consults

Daily Weight

Diet: Clear liquid, then as tol.

Food Allergies: none

Hold:

Feeding/Fluids

- ☒ Self
- ☐ Assist
- ☐ Feeder
- ☒ Force 3,000 ml/day
- ☐ Restrict c̄ IV

	meal	Ext	IV
7-3			
3-11			
11-7			

☒ I&O

☒ IV O₅LR, 100/hr

☐ Other_____

Safety Measures

- ☐ Siderails
- ☐ Restraints
- ☐ Other_____

Activities

- ☐ Bedrest
- ☒ BRP
- ☐ Dangle
- ☒ Chair
- ☐ Commode
- ☐ Up ad Lib
- ☐ Turn
- ☐ Ambulate

Transportation

per _____

Hygiene

- ☐ Bedbath
- ☒ Assist
- ☐ Self Bath
- ☒ Shower
- ☐ Tub
- ☐ Vanity
- ☐ Oral Care

Bowel/Bladder

- ☐ Foley IN _____ OUT _____
- ☐ Cath care Bid
- ☐ Incontinent
- ☐ Colostomy
- ☐ Ileostomy
- ☐ Urostomy

Communication

Fowlers or semi-fowlers position

V.S. q̄4h

Physical Therapy	Date	Treatments

Cardio-Pulmonary
4/16 Postural drainage 0900 daily
4/16 Incentive spirometer q̄ 3 hrs
4/16 O₂ per cannula at 5L
4/16 Nebulizer q̄4h

Drug Allergies: Penicillin

Isolation: _____ In _____ Out _____

Emergency Instructions: Out of Town until 4/17.
Relatives: Michael Sanchez
Phone: 641-1212

Clergy: None
Religion: Catholic

Religious Rites: Last Rites only

Code Blue: Yes

Diagnosis: Pneumonia

Surgery & Dates:

Consults & Dates:

Room	Name	Adm Date	Age	Physician
416	Luisa Sanchez	4-16-96	28	R. Katz

Figure 9–4. Kardex Care Plan: Client Profile, Basic Needs, Medical Plan. Courtesy of Shawnee Mission Medical Center, Merriam, KS.

Instructions for Meeting Basic Needs   Regardless of the client's nursing diagnoses, the nurse must know what routine assistance is needed for hygiene, nutrition, elimination, and other basic needs. Most comprehensive care plans have a separate section for these instructions, often on a Kardex or basic care flowsheet, where they can be found quickly and conveniently. From Figure 9–4, the nurse can quickly determine that Mrs. Sanchez can feed herself, can have clear liquids and then solid foods as she can tolerate them, can get out of bed to go to the bathroom, has an IV, and should have 3,000 mL of fluids per day. Because instructions for meeting basic needs change rapidly as the client's condition changes, this section of the care plan is usually marked with pencil so it can be easily altered.

In addition to the routine care marked on the form, you may need to write individualized nursing diagnoses for clients who have special basic needs requirements, for example, those with Bathing/Hygiene Self-Care Deficit, Urinary Incontinence, or Altered Nutrition. These would be written in the nursing care plan section (Figure 9–2).

Aspects of the Medical Plan to Be Implemented by the Nurse   A comprehensive care plan includes nursing activities necessary for carrying out medical orders, for example, dressing changes and IV therapy. It also includes a section for scheduling prescribed diagnostic tests and treatments to be carried out by other departments (e.g., physical therapy). In Figure 9–9 this type of information is listed under "Active Doctor's Orders" and "Active Ancillary Orders." In Figure 9–4 it appears mainly in the top section of the form.

It is better to have a separate section for these activities, but you may also see them included as a part of the nursing care plan for a nursing diagnosis or collaborative problem; for example, in the section for "Laboratory" in Figure 9–4, a physician-ordered "Blood Culture." However, if you were creating a student care plan, you might not have a Kardex form to work with. So, for Mrs. Sanchez, you might write a collaborative problem: Potential Complication of Pneumonia: Sepsis. The medical order for a blood culture would then be incorporated into the nursing interventions for that problem.

Example:

Medical order (in bold print) included in student care plan.

Problem	*Nursing Orders*
Potential Complication of Pneumonia: Sepsis	1. **Blood cultures today, per order.** Explain reason for blood cultures
	2. Temperature q4hr. Hourly if >101°

Nursing Diagnoses and Collaborative Problems   The **nursing diagnosis care plan**, a part of the comprehensive patient-care plan, includes a list of all the client's actual and potential health problems, as well as the outcomes and nursing orders for those problems. This part of the care plan reflects the independent component of nursing practice, and is the part that best demonstrates the nurse's clinical expertise. For predictable, routine problems, the outcomes and nursing orders are often available in preplanned, printed standards of care, standardized care plans, protocols, and agency policies and procedures. A special plan of care is handwritten for unusual problems or ones that need special attention. For example, a standardized care plan for "all clients with a medical

Creating a Patient-Care Plan

diagnosis of pneumonia" would probably include a nursing diagnosis of Fluid Volume Deficit and direct the nurse to assess the client's hydration status. On a respiratory unit, this is a common nursing diagnosis; therefore, Luisa Sanchez's nurse was able to obtain a standardized plan for Fluid Volume Deficit (see Figure 9–6 on page 311). However, the nursing diagnosis, Risk for Altered Family Processes would not be common to all clients on this unit; it is specific to Mrs. Sanchez. Therefore, the plan for that diagnosis was handwritten by the nurse.

Regardless of whether nursing orders are handwritten or chosen from a preprinted plan, the nursing care plan must be individualized to fit the unique needs of each patient. The problem list you develop for the patient (Chapters 4 and 5) will help to individualize care because each patient will have a different set of problems and etiologies.

Multidisciplinary (Collaborative) Care Plans

Like the traditional nursing care plan, a multidisciplinary care plan specifies patient outcomes and nursing orders to address client problems. However, it includes medical and other treatments as well, and may be structured around a medical diagnosis instead of, or in addition to, nursing diagnoses. Typically, it is a standardized plan, developed and revised in multidisciplinary team conferences. As discussed in Chapter 7, a critical pathway is a standardized form of the multidisciplinary plan that outlines the care required for patients with common, predictable conditions. It is a structured document, organized with a column for each day of hospitalization. There are as many columns on the plan as the preset number of days allowed for the client's diagnostic related group (DRG).

The communication that occurs in multidisciplinary care planning tends to enhance collaborative practice. In addition, critical pathways can result in cost savings, and increased patient satisfaction (Gage, 1994). However, such plans are time-consuming to develop, and there is concern that individualization of care may be lost in this system. The focus of these plans is sometimes more medical than holistic, and the need to achieve outcomes within rigidly specified time frames creates the possibility of focusing on efficiency more than quality of care. (See Chapter 4 for using nursing diagnoses to individualize critical pathways.)

Standardized Approaches to Care Planning

Obviously it would take a great deal of time to handwrite every bit of nursing care needed for all clients that a nurse cares for. Nurses know to perform certain routine interventions for all patients, and it would be inefficient to write these for every patient. Standardized, preprinted instructions are frequently used for "generic" care given to all patients on a unit or for the "usual" interventions for patients with certain medical conditions or nursing diagnoses. One example of a standardized care plan is the critical pathway, discussed in the preceding section.

Standards of Care

According to Carpenito (1993, p. 77) **standards of care** are "detailed guidelines that represent the predicted care indicated in specific situations" such as the following:

A medical diagnosis (e.g., preeclampsia, abdominal hysterectomy)
A defined situation (e.g., postpartum, relinquishing infant)
A treatment or diagnostic test (e.g., artificial ventilation, colonoscopy)

A selected nursing diagnosis label (e.g., Anticipatory Grieving)
A collaborative problem (e.g., Potential Complication of
Thrombophlebitis: Pulmonary Embolus

The Patient-Care Plan

Standards of care are preplanned, preprinted directions for care, developed by nurses for groups of clients rather than individuals. The standards identify the nursing diagnoses and collaborative problems that occur in a defined situation. They describe achievable rather than ideal nursing care for those problems, taking into account the particular circumstances and client population of the institution. Standards define the interventions for which nurses are held accountable. They do not contain medical orders.

Standards of care are not necessarily placed in the client's care plan or medical record, but are reference documents, stored as permanent hospital records. They are either filed on the unit or in the computer for easy reference. If they are not actually kept as a part of the client's care plan, then the problem list (see Table 9–1 on page 323) should indicate which standards of care apply to the patient.

Depending on the institution, standards of care may or may not be organized according to problems or nursing diagnoses. Figure 9–5 is an example of standards of care that list only the nursing interventions, without identifying the problems to which they apply.

For some clients, all necessary nursing care may be contained in the standards of care; others will need additional interventions. These can be added as printed model care plans or developed by the nurse and handwritten on a blank care plan form.

Model (Standardized) Care Plans

Do not confuse **standardized care plans** with *standards of care.* To avoid confusion, some nurses prefer to call them **model care plans.** Although they have some similarities, there are important differences between standards of care and model care plans:

1. Model care plans are kept with the client's active care plan (in the Kardex or computer). When no longer active, they become a part of her permanent medical record. This is not usually true of standards of care.

2. Model care plans provide more detailed instructions than standards of care. They contain deviations (either additions or deletions) from the standards for the agency.

3. Unlike standards of care, model care plans take the usual nursing process format:

   Problem → Outcomes → Nursing orders → Evaluation.

4. Model care plans allow you to add addendum care plans. They usually include checklists, blank lines, or empty spaces to allow you to individualize goals and nursing orders. This is not usually true for standards of care.

Model care plans are similar to standards of care in that they are preplanned, preprinted guides for nursing interventions for specific nursing diagnoses or for all the nursing diagnoses associated with a particular situation or medical condition. They are developed by nurses, and while they are not standards of care, following them ensures that acceptable standards of care are provided. Refer to Figure 9–6 on page 311 for a model care plan for a single problem, Fluid Volume Deficit.

STANDARDS OF CARE: Patient with Thrombophlebitis

Goal: **1.** To monitor for early signs and symptoms of compromised respiratory status.

        2. To report any abnormal signs and/or symptoms promptly to the medical staff.

        3. To initiate appropriate nursing actions when signs and/or symptoms of compromised respiratory status occur.

        4. To institute protocol for emergency intervention should the client develop cardiopulmonary dysfunction.

SUPPORTIVE DATA: The purpose of these standards of care is to prevent, monitor, report, and record the client's response to a diagnosis of thrombophlebitis. Thrombophlebitis places the client at risk for pulmonary embolism. The hemodynamic consequences of embolic obstruction to pulmonary blood flow involve increased pulmonary vascular resistance, increased right ventricular workload, decreased cardiac output, and development of shock and pulmonary arrest.

CLINICAL MANIFESTATIONS: Nursing assessments performed q3–4h should monitor for the following signs/symptoms:

- Dyspnea (generally consistently present)
- Sudden substernal pain
- Rapid/weak pulse
- Syncope
- Anxiety
- Fever
- Cough/hemoptysis
- Accelerated respiratory rate
- Pleuritic type chest pain
- Cyanosis

PREVENTIVE NURSING MEASURES:

- Encourage increased fluid intake to prevent dehydration.
- Maintain anticoagulant intravenous therapy as prescribed (See Protocol for Anticoagulant Administration).
- Maintain prescribed bedrest.
- Prevent venous stasis from improperly fitting elastic stockings; Check q3–4h.
- Encourage dorsiflexion exercises of the lower extremities while on bedrest.

INDIVIDUALIZED PLANS/ADDITIONAL NURSING/MEDICAL ORDERS

   Do not massage lower extremities.

   Intake and output q8h.

Initiated by: *S. Ibarra, RN*   Date: *4-9-96*

Figure 9–5. Example of Non-Problem-Oriented Standards of Care.

Standardized Care Plan for Nursing Diagnosis of FLUID VOLUME DEFICIT		
Etiology	**Expected Outcomes**	**Nursing Order** (Identify Frequency)
✓Decreased oral intake	✓Urinary output > 30 mL/hr	✓Monitor intake and output q _1_ h
✓Nausea	✓Urine specific gravity 1.005–1.025	✓Weigh daily
__Depression		✓Monitor serum electrolyte levels X 1 or *until normal*
✓Fatigue, weakness	✓Serum Na⁺ normal	✓Check skin turgor and mucous membranes q _8_ h
__Difficulty swallowing	✓Mucous membranes moist	
__Other:_____		✓Monitor temperature q _4_ h
✓Excess fluid loss	✓Skin turgor good	✓Administer prescribed IV therapy (Monitor according to protocol for "Intravenous Therapy") 1000 mL D₅ LR at 100 mL/hr
✓Fever or increased metabolic rate	✓No weight loss	
✓Diaphoresis	✓8-hour intake =	✓Offer oral liquids q _1_ h
✓Vomiting	_400 mL oral_	Type _clear, cold_
__Diarrhea	Other:	✓Instruct client regarding amount, type, and schedule of fluid intake.
__Burns		✓Assess understanding of type of fluid loss; teach accordingly
__Other_____		✓Mouth care prn with _mouthwash_
		✓Institute measures to reduce fever (eg, lower room temperature, remove bed covers, offer cold liquids.)
Defining Characteristics		Other Nursing Orders:_____
✓Insufficient intake		_Monitor urine specific gravity_
✓Negative balance of intake and output		_q shift_
✓Dry mucous membranes		_____
✓Poor skin turgor		_____
__Concentrated urine		_____
__Hypernatremia		_____
✓Rapid, weak pulse		_____
__Falling B/P		_____
__Weight loss		

Plan Initiated by: _M. Medina RN_   **Date** _4-15-95_

Plan/outcomes evaluated_____ **Date**_____

Plan/outcomes evaluated_____ **Date**_____

Client: _Luisa Sanchez_

Figure 9–6. A standardized care plan for nursing diagnosis of **Fluid Volume Deficit**.

Creating a Patient-Care Plan

Many commercial books of model care plans are available. They can be used as guides when developing your care plans, but remember that they do not address the client's individualized needs, and they can cause you to focus on predictable problems and miss cues to important special problems the client is experiencing. If you use a model care plan as a student, do the following:

1. Consult your instructor to be sure you are using a reliable source.

2. First perform a nursing assessment and make your own list of all the client's actual and potential problems. You can then consult the model care plan to be sure your list is complete.

3. Using client input, establish specific, individualized goals before consulting the model care plan. Consulting the model first may inhibit your creativity.

4. Write as many of your own nursing orders as you can. Refer to the model to be sure you have not omitted any important interventions.

5. Be sure the nursing interventions in the model are appropriate for your client and possible to implement in your institution. Delete any that do not apply.

6. Individualize the outcomes and nursing orders to fit your client.

> **Example:**
>
> | *Standardized Nursing Order* | *Individualized Nursing Order* |
> |---|---|
> | Force fluids as ordered or as tolerated by patient. | Force fluids to 2400 mL per 24 hours: |
> | | 7–3: Offer 200 mL water or apple juice hourly. |
> | | 3–11: Offer 200 mL water or apple juice hourly while awake. |
> | | 11–7: Offer water or juice when awakening patient for VS or meds. |
> | | Pt. prefers ice in his water or juice. |

Protocols

Protocols are preplanned and preprinted. Like standards of care and model care plans, they can cover the common actions required for a particular medical diagnosis, defined situation, treatment, or diagnostic test. For example, there may be a protocol for admitting a patient to the intensive care unit, or a protocol covering the administration of magnesium sulfate to a preeclampsia patient. Protocols are different, though, because they may include both medical orders and nursing orders. When a protocol is used, it can be added to the nursing care plan and become a part of the patient's permanent record. An alternative is to keep all protocols in the hospital's file of permanent records and write "See protocol" on the care plan, as in Table 9–1 on page 323.

Policies and Procedures

When a situation occurs frequently, an institution is likely to develop a **policy** to govern how it is to be handled. A hospital may have a policy that specifies the number of visitors a patient may have; a policy may also be similar to a protocol and specify, for example, what is to be done in the case of cardiac arrest. As with protocols and standing orders, the nurse must recognize the situation and then use judgment in implementing the policy. Hospital policies must be interpreted to meet patient needs.

   Example: While on a business trip, Fred Gonzalez was in an automobile accident. He has been hospitalized in serious condition for several days. It is 8:55 P.M., and Mr. Gonzalez's wife has just arrived on the unit for her first visit. Even though hospital policy requires that visitors leave at 9 P.M., the nurse decides that implementing the policy would not meet Mr. Gonzalez's needs.

If a policy covers a situation pertinent to the patient-care plan, it is usually simply noted on the care plan (e.g., "Make Social Service referral per Unit Policy"). Hospital policies and procedures are institution records, not patient records, so they are not actually placed in the care plan.

Special Teaching Plans

In response to health care trends such as shorter hospital stays and emphasis on wellness, teaching has become an essential part of the nursing role. At the same time, nurses are caring for more and sicker patients and find they have less time for teaching. Careful planning is therefore essential. To assure that teaching is emphasized, many institutional care plans include a special section for teaching needs. Teaching needs may also be addressed in standards of care, in model care plans, or by individually written nursing diagnoses. It is usually better to include teaching interventions as a part of the nursing orders for every nursing diagnosis, rather than write a single Knowledge Deficit problem to cover all the patient's various learning needs (see the *Nursing Diagnosis Guide* at the end of this text).

   When a patient has complex learning needs (e.g., a newly diagnosed diabetic, a new mother without a support system), a Knowledge Deficit problem *may* be appropriate. For such patients you may wish to develop a special teaching plan to ensure efficient use of your time and maximize the patient's learning. Figure 9–7 is an example of a section of an individualized teaching plan.

Addendum Discharge Plans

All clients need some degree of discharge planning, but a separate, formal discharge plan may not always be needed. Often, you can include discharge assessments and teaching in the nursing orders for other nursing diagnoses. For example, one nursing order for Mrs. Sanchez is to teach her to continue taking her antibiotics after discharge until they are all gone, even if she begins to feel better. Such routine discharge planning is called **standard discharge planning** and is the responsibility of the nurse caring for the client and family (Carpenito, 1991, p. 26). Many institutions have a standardized, preprinted discharge plan, like the one in Figure 9–8 (on page 315).

   A separate discharge plan is required for clients with special needs; for example, those who are to be placed in a nursing home or other continuing-care agency, those with newly diagnosed long-term diseases such as diabetes, those with complex self-care needs, those who lack financial or social support, and so forth. Such **addendum discharge plans** require collaborative action and usually involve a discharge-planning coordinator or case manager other than the staff nurse (Carpenito, 1991, pp. 26–27).

Nursing Diagnosis: Risk for Altered Health Maintenance r/t lack of knowledge of insulin therapy				
Met	Learning Objective	Content	Teaching Strategy	Learning Strategy
	1st Session Client will describe the basic patho-physiology of diabetes mellitus (cognitive).	Location and function of pancreas How cells use glucose Function of insulin Effects of insulin deficiency (elevated blood sugar, mobiliza-tion of fats and protiens, ketones, etc.)	Explain. Transparency of the pancreas.	Read pamphlet, "Your Pancreas."
	2nd Session Ct. will demonstrate ability to draw up correct amount of insulin (psychomotor).	Syringe markings Sterile technique Preparation	Point out on enlarged drawing; then actual syringe. Demonstrate and discuss. Demonstrate and discuss: How to mix insulin. Read label carefully, be sure syringe and label concentrations match. Clean top of bottle with alcohol. Withdraw correct amount.	Practice with syringe and vial of sterile water.

Figure 9–7. Sample Teaching Plan (Partial): Diabetes Mellitus

HEALTH MIDWEST

Discharge Summary Record

1. Discharge Date: _____ **2. Discharge Time:** _____ _____

Section I: DISCHARGE MODE

3. TO: [Home] [SNU] [Rehab] [ECF] [Mental Health] [Other:] _____ 4. MODE: [Ambulatory] [WC] [Cart]

If discharged to SNU, Rehab, ECF or other facility stop here and complete interagency transfer form.

5. TRANSPORTATION: [Car] [Ambulance] [WC Van] [Other:]   6. Personal items (valuables, home meds, assist devices per NDB) returned [N/A] [YES]

Section II: CARE AT HOME

7. MEDICINE	DOSE	TIME						REASON / SPECIAL INSTRUCTIONS	TIME NEXT DOSE	PRE-SCRIPTION GIVEN	USE HOME SUPPLY
		AM	NOON	AFTERNOON	EVENING	BEDTIME	NIGHT				

☐ Addendum   ***** Medication Instructions Completed by: _____

INSTRUCTIONS

8. ☐ Call your doctor for the following _____

9. ☐ Appointment(s) with Dr. _____ Within _____ Phone _____
   Appointment made for _____ at _____

10. ☐ Appointment(s) with Dr. _____ Within _____ Phone _____
    Appointment made for _____ at _____

11. ☐ Appointment(s) with Dr. _____ Within _____ Phone _____
    Appointment made for _____ at _____

12. ☐ Outpatient appointment arranged (location/phone) _____

13. ☐ Diet (specify) _____

14. ☐ Food and your Medicine (specify food/drug interaction) _____

15. ☐ Exercise/Activity (specify) _____

16. ☐ Skin/Wound Care (Instructions) _____

17. ☐ Treatment/Therapy/Catheter/Lines/Tubes (specify) _____

18. ☐ Equipment, supplies (specify) _____
    Providing Company (name/phone) _____

19. ☐ Instructional Material (list what is given) _____

20. ☐ Home Health visits arranged (name/phone) _____

21. I have reviewed and understand the above instructions and I have also received a copy to take home for future reference.

                                                                    RN
_____ _____ _____
PATIENT or AGENT   DISCHARGE NURSE   REVIEWED BY

HM 10-36-605   Distribution: White - Medical Record   Yellow - Patient Copy   Pink - Physician Copy

Figure 9–8. Discharge Plan. Courtesy of Research Medical Center, Kansas City, MO.

Creating a Patient-Care Plan

CARE-PLANNING GUIDE

Now that you are familiar with the various documents that make up a comprehensive care plan, you should be able to follow the steps of the nursing process and make a care plan for an actual patient. The guide in Box 9–1 compresses all the steps of the nursing process into a concise but detailed reference to use in planning care. The care plan developed for Luisa Sanchez in this chapter follows this guide.

Each chapter in this book included a detailed guide for carrying out a particular step of the nursing process. For example, Box 4–6 (in Chapter 4) is a list of steps to follow in the diagnostic process. If you need to review any of the steps in the following care-planning guide, refer to the appropriate chapter in this book, where the step is expanded for you. In addition to proceeding step-by-step through the care-planning guide, you should refer to Box 9–2 on page 318 when writing care plans.

CREATING A COMPREHENSIVE CARE PLAN

Read the following case study, which describes the course of Luisa Sanchez's hospitalization. Then follow the steps of the care-planning guide (Box 9–1) and the guidelines in Box 9–2 to develop a comprehensive plan for Ms. Sanchez.

Case Study: Luisa Sanchez

Framework: Functional Health Patterns, Gordon
Medical Diagnosis: Pneumonia

Luisa Sanchez, a 28-year-old married attorney, was admitted to the hospital with an elevated temperature, a productive cough, and rapid, labored respirations. During the nursing interview, she told Mary Medina, RN, that she has had a "chest cold" for two weeks and has been short of breath on exertion. She stated, "Yesterday I started having a fever and pain in my lungs." Mrs. Sanchez's complete assessment data appears in Figure 3–3 in Chapter 3, so it is repeated here only in part. Admission medical orders included:

CBC with differential	PA and lateral chest X ray
Arterial blood gases	Blood culture (repeat ×2 if temp over 101°)
Urine specific gravity	24-hour urine
Sputum C & S	Serum electrolytes
Postural drainage daily	Incentive spirometer q3h
Pulse oximeter	Nebulizer q4h
IV of D_5 LR, 100 mL / hr	Vancomycin 0.5 Gm IV q6h
Tylenol 650 mg q4h po	O_2 per cannula, 5L
for temp > 101°	

Assessment

Step 1: Collect Data

To begin collecting Mrs. Sanchez's data, you could use a data collection form such as Figure 3–3 in Chapter 3, organized by body systems and specific nursing concerns, rather than one based on a single nursing model. Next you would

Box 9–1. Care-Planning Guide

1. **Collect data.**
   a. Interview, physical exam.
   b. Validate data.
   c. Organize according to framework.
2. **Analyze and synthesize data.**
   a. Group related cues according to framework.
   b. Form new cue clusters as needed.
   c. Identify deviations from normal.
3. **List all problems (working list).**
   a. Human responses that need to be changed.
   b. Medical, nursing, collaborative.
   c. Actual, risk, possible
4. **Make formal list of labeled problems.**
   a. Label nursing diagnoses (Problem + Etiology)
      (1) Problem: Compare pt. data to defining characteristics, definitions, and risk factors.
      (2) Etiology: Related factors (risk, causal, contributing factors).
   b. Label Collaborative Problems (Potential complications of . . .).
5. **Determine which problems can be addressed by**
   a. standards of care.
   b. model care plans.
   c. protocols.
   d. policies/procedures (e.g., note on formal problem list: Risk for Pulmonary Embolus—See Standards of Care).
6. **Individualize model care plans, protocols, and so forth, as needed.**
7. **Transcribe medical, collaborative, ADLs, and basic care needs to Kardex.**
8. **Develop individualized care plan for remaining nursing diagnoses and collaborative problems.**
   a. Develop individualized outcomes.
      (1) State desired client responses.
      (2) Opposite of problem response.
      (3) Measurable/realistic.
   b. Choose nursing orders.
      (1) Address etiology: reduce/remove related factors.
      (2) Address problem: relieve symptoms.
      (3) Address outcomes: how to bring about desired behaviors.
      (4) Health promotion, prevention, treatment, observation.
      (5) Physical care, teaching, counseling, environment management, referrals, emotional support, activities of daily living.
      (6) For complex orders, refer to policies and protocols (See "Unit Procedure for IV Therapy").
   c. Include any special, complex teaching or discharge plans.
9. **Implement care plan (do or delegate; record in chart).**
10. **Evaluate results of care.**
    a. Compare patient progress to original goals.
    b. Revise care plan as needed.
       (1) Collect more data, if needed.
       (2) Revise, discontinue, or continue problem.
       (3) Change outcomes if unachievable.
       (4) Revise, discontinue, or keep nursing orders.

Box 9–2. Guidelines for Writing Comprehensive Care Plans

1. **Include each of these components:**
   a. Client profile
   b. Basic needs
   c. Aspects of medical plan
   d. Nursing diagnoses and collaborative problems
   e. Special or complex teaching or discharge needs

2. **Date and sign the initial plan and any revisions.** The date is important for evaluation; the signature demonstrates nursing accountability.

3. **List or number the nursing diagnoses in order of priority.** Priorities can be changed as the client's needs change.

4. **List the nursing orders for each problem in order of priority** or in the order in which they should be done. For instance, you would assess the client's level of knowledge before you teach him to log-roll.

5. **Write the plan in clear, concise terms.** Use standard medical abbreviations and symbols. Use key words rather than complete sentences. Leave out unnecessary words, like *client* and *the* (e.g., write "Turn & reposition q2h" rather than "Turn and reposition the client every two hours").

6. **Write legibly, in ink.** When the plan cannot be erased, accountability is emphasized and more importance is placed on what is being written. If a nursing diagnosis is resolved, write "Discontinued" and a date beside it, highlight it, or date a special "Inactive" column. Outcomes and nursing orders can be discontinued similarly.

7. **For detailed treatments and procedures, refer to other sources** (e.g., standards of care) instead of writing all the steps on the care plan. You might write, "See unit procedure book for diabetic teaching," or you might attach a standard nursing care plan for a problem (e.g., "See standard care plan for Ineffective Breastfeeding"). This saves time, and focuses the written part of the care plan on the unique needs of the client.

8. **Be sure the plan is holistic.** It should consider the client's physiological, psychological, sociocultural, and spiritual needs.

9. **Be sure the plan is individualized** and addresses the client's unique needs. Include the client's choices about how and when care is given. For example, "Prefers evening shower."

10. **Include the collaborative and coordination aspects of the client's care.** You may write nursing orders to consult a social worker or physical therapist, or you may simply coordinate tests and treatments. The medical plan should be incorporated into the nursing care plan so that the two plans do not conflict.

11. **Include discharge plans** (e.g., arrangements for follow-up by a social worker or community health nurse).

organize the data according to a nursing model (Gordon's Functional Health Patterns) in order to have a worksheet to use during data analysis. Box 4–2 on page 105 summarizes the admission data collected in each of the patterns.

Diagnosis

Step 2: Analyze and Synthesize Data

Next underline all the cues that seem significant or outside the norm (see Box 4–2, page 105). For example, in the Role-Relationship pattern, the nurse underlined "husband out of town" and "child with neighbor." Next, think about how the abnormal (significant) cues in one group might be related to cues in another group—inductively forming new cue clusters (refer to Table 4–5 on page 107). For instance, in the Coping/Stress-Tolerance pattern, Luisa shows signs of Anxiety (e.g., tense facial muscles, trembling). You might wonder if the data in the Role-Relationship pattern might be related to that anxiety. It would be logical to think: "Perhaps part of Mrs. Sanchez's anxiety might be caused by worry about her child being without a parent or by her need for emotional support from her husband, who is away." Because those cues seem related, they are inductively grouped, together with other related cues, into a new cue cluster (Cluster 9 in Table 4–5). Cluster 9 represents a problem that is essentially psychological and fits best in the Self-Perception/Self-Concept pattern.

Notice in Box 4–2 (page 105), that the cues "urinary frequency and amount decreased ×2 days" and "diaphoretic" cannot be interpreted accurately using only the cues in that pattern. To interpret their meaning, you need to think how those abnormal cues relate to the cues in the Nutritional-Metabolic pattern. Notice, too, that even in the new, inductively formed groupings, a single piece of data may appear in more than one cluster. For example, in Table 4–5 (on page 107), "Can't breathe lying down" appears in Clusters 4 and 6. In Cluster 4, it is one of the causes of Sleep Pattern Disturbance; in Cluster 6, it indirectly causes Self Care Deficit by causing Mrs. Sanchez to lose sleep and become too tired and weak to perform self-care activities. Examine Box 4–2 and Table 4–5 to see if you can follow the reasoning for each of the cue clusters. If you need to review Functional Health Patterns, refer to Table 3–6 on page 67 and the form in Appendix B.

Step 3: Make a Working Problem List

Recall that a nursing diagnosis is a judgment about the client's responses to health problems or life processes. In this step you made a judgment about the most likely explanation for each cue cluster; then decide whether it represents an actual, potential (risk), or possible problem. Also decide whether the problem is medical, collaborative, or a nursing diagnosis. Tentative conclusions for Luisa Sanchez are listed in Table 4–5 on page 107.

For Cluster 1, there are no abnormal cues in the Health Perception/Health Management pattern; the pattern represents patient strengths: a healthy lifestyle and understanding of and compliance with treatment regimens (e.g., taking her Synthroid as directed).

Cluster 2 represents a problem of inadequate nutrition. A likely explanation is that Mrs. Sanchez's poor appetite is a result of her disease process. Her appetite will probably return on successful medical treatment of the pneumonia. In the meantime, Mrs. Sanchez will need nursing care to assess for and encourage adequate nutrition.

Creating a Patient-Care Plan

Cluster 3 represents a nursing diagnosis, Fluid Volume Deficit. It is probably caused by excess fluid loss secondary to fever and diaphoresis, and inadequate fluid intake because of nausea and poor appetite. Mrs. Sanchez's poor skin turgor, decreased urinary frequency, dry mucous membranes, and hot skin are defining characteristics that help to identify the problem.

Cluster 4 cues indicate a Sleep-Rest pattern nursing diagnosis. Apparently, when she lies down to sleep, she is unable to breathe. In addition, her cough and pain keep her awake. Undoubtedly her fever, diaphoresis, and chills (in Clusters 3 and 7) also keep her awake. As a result, she feels weak and is short of breath on exertion.

Cluster 5 represents a medical problem, hypothyroidism, for which Mrs. Sanchez is already receiving medication. Therefore, the problem requires no nursing intervention and would not be included in the care plan. The medication order would appear in the medication record and would be given to Mrs. Sanchez routinely while she was in the hospital.

Cluster 6 contains cues for a nursing diagnosis of either Activity Intolerance or Self Care Deficit, which are being caused by cues and problems in other clusters. For example, the Sleep-Rest problem in Cluster 4, and the oxygenation problem in Cluster 11 are both contributing to the overall pattern of weakness in Cluster 6.

The problem in *Cluster 7* is that Mrs. Sanchez is uncomfortable because she is having chills. The chills are being caused by fever secondary to the pneumonia, and will stop when her illness is treated. The fever will be treated medically (by the order for Tylenol); however, there are nursing interventions that can be instituted to increase Mrs. Sanchez's comfort.

Cluster 8 contains risk factors for a potential nursing diagnosis, Risk for Altered Family Processes; however, there is not enough data to indicate an actual problem. In any event, the problem will resolve itself the next day, as soon as Mr. Sanchez returns home. You might decide to include it in the care plan, to be sure that the necessary follow-up assessments are made.

Cluster 9 represents a nursing diagnosis of Anxiety. Mrs. Sanchez expressed anxiety but she had no other signs of anxiety, such as trembling and tense facial muscles. She said she was worried about leaving her child with a neighbor, and about getting behind at work. In addition, her anxiety is obviously caused by periodic difficulty breathing. This is a nursing diagnosis with more than one etiology.

Cluster 10 indicates a nursing diagnosis of Chest pain, which is caused by the pneumonia-induced cough. Until the antibiotic therapy can treat the pneumonia, nursing measures will be needed to promote comfort.

Cluster 11 contains the defining characteristics for the nursing diagnosis, Ineffective Airway Clearance (productive cough, shallow respirations, decreased chest expansion, and inspiratory crackles). The other cues (e.g., pale mucous membranes) are signs of pneumonia, the medical problem creating the Ineffective Airway Clearance. You can infer that problems in other patterns are contributing to the oxygenation problem as well: Fluid Volume Deficit creates thick, tenacious mucus, and Pain and weakness contribute to shallow respirations and decreased chest expansion.

In addition to the problems identified from the cue clusters, you should identify collaborative problems that exist for Mrs. Sanchez because of her disease process and her IV and medical therapies. Recall that collaborative problems are potential problems for which nursing care focuses on assessment and prevention. The following is a working problem list for Luisa Sanchez, before being put into standard NANDA terminology:

Cue Cluster	Probable Explanation
1	No problem. Strength: Healthy lifestyle; understanding of and compliance with treatment regimens.
2	Actual nursing diagnosis. Altered Nutrition: Less than Body Requirements. Probably caused by nausea and poor appetite; and also by increased metabolism secondary to fever and pneumonia.
3	Actual nursing diagnosis. Fluid Volume Deficit, caused by excess fluid loss (diaphoresis) secondary to fever; and inadequate intake secondary to nausea and loss of appetite.
4	Actual nursing diagnosis. Difficulty sleeping; probably NANDA label of Sleep Pattern Disturbance, caused by cough, pain, orthopnea, fever, and diaphoresis.
5	No problem as long as patient takes Synthroid. Be sure it is on medical administration record.
6	Actual nursing diagnosis. Probably Self Care Deficit (perhaps Activity Intolerance). Lack of oxygen and sleep loss are causing weakness and fatigue. As a result, she is unable to perform self-care activities.
7	Actual nursing diagnosis. Chills are causing discomfort.
8	Potential nursing diagnosis. There could be a problem with child care if Mr. Sanchez's return is delayed. Probably Altered Family Processes because both parents are unavailable to care for child; but probably self-limiting (tomorrow).
9	Actual nursing diagnosis. Anxiety. Caused by difficulty breathing, worry about child, and of "getting behind" at work.
10	Actual nursing diagnosis. Chest pain from cough. Medical treatments will help alleviate.
11	Actual nursing diagnosis. Airway clearance problem. Unable to cough up thick sputum, which has been created by infection, fever, weakness, pain, and fluid deficit.

Creating a Patient-Care Plan

Collaborative Problems

Potential Complication of pneumonia: Septic shock

Potential Complication of pneumonia: Respiratory insufficiency

Potential Complications of IV therapy: Infiltration, phlebitis

Potential Complications of antibiotic therapy: Allergic reaction, GI upset

Step 4: Make a Formal List of Labeled Problems

To make the formal list of nursing diagnoses and collaborative problems, refer to the list of NANDA diagnostic labels (see inside back cover for the list of diagnostic labels organized by Functional Health Patterns). Compare the data in the cue clusters to the defining characteristics in the *Nursing Diagnosis Guide* to be sure you have chosen the correct NANDA label for each nursing diagnosis. After verifying the diagnoses with Mrs. Sanchez, you would write them on the care plan in order of priority (see Table 9–1). Note that in addition to listing all the problems identified for Mrs. Sanchez on the day of her admission, Table 9–1 indicates changes that a nurse might make to the list after implementing the care plan and evaluating the outcomes.

Planning

Step 5: Determine Which Problems Can Be Addressed by Standards of Care, Standardized Care Plans, Protocols, Policies, and Procedures.

After developing the formal problem list, decide how each of the problems is to be addressed (i.e., with preplanned interventions or individualized plans). For each problem, ask the following series of questions.

1. *Are there* **standards of care** *for clients with this medical diagnosis or situation?* Mrs. Sanchez was admitted to 2-South, a medical unit that has written standards of care for patients having pneumonia. These standards describe all the care necessary for Problems 1, 5, 6, and 10 (Ineffective Airway Clearance, Self Care Deficit, Chest Pain, and Potential Complications of Pneumonia). Most patients with pneumonia experience these problems, so it is possible to plan in advance the care these patients are expected to need. Because no special plan is necessary, you would simply list the problems and write beside them, "See Unit Standards of Care for Pneumonia," as shown in Table 9–1.

2. *Is there a* **model nursing care plan** *for the client's medical diagnosis or condition?* In Mrs. Sanchez's case, because there were standards of care for pneumonia patients, and because her needs did not exceed the standards, you would not look for a model care plan for this medical diagnosis.

3. *For the* **collaborative problems** *not completely covered by the standards of care, do any of the following exist to direct your interventions?*

   Physician's orders (you may need to call to obtain these)
   Standing orders
   Protocols
   Policies and procedures

Mrs. Sanchez has two collaborative problems not addressed by standards of care: Problems 11 and 12. For Problem 11, the physician's orders specify the type of IV fluid and prescribe the rate of flow. You would note this information on an IV flowsheet or a Kardex form (Figure 9–4 on page 306). The 2-South procedure manual contains a section on IV therapy, which specifies how often IV tubing is to be changed, what focus assessments to make, and so forth. This resource is noted on the formal problem list beside Problem 11 (in Table 9–1).

Because Vancomycin is not routinely given to all pneumonia patients, it would not be included in the unit's Standards of Care for Pneumonia. However, because it is often given to patients who are allergic to penicillin, it would not be unusual to give it. Furthermore, the nurses must be aware of

Creating a Comprehensive Care Plan

Table 9–1. Formal Prioritized Problem List for Luisa Sanchez

Prioritized Problems	Type of Plan Used
1. Ineffective Airway Clearance related to viscous secretions and shallow chest expansion secondary to pain, fluid volume deficit, and fatigue.	See "Unit Standards of Care for Pneumonia"
2. ~~Fluid volume Deficit related to intake insufficient to replace fluid loss secondary to fever, diaphoresis, and nausea~~ *Resolved 4/17/96 JW*	See Standardized Care Plan for Fluid Volume Deficit
3. Anxiety related to difficulty breathing and concerns over work and parenting roles	Individualized nursing diagnosis care plan
4. Sleep Pattern Disturbance related to cough, pain, orthopnea, fever, and diaphoresis	Individualized nursing diagnosis care plan
5. Self-Care Deficit (Level 2) related to Activity Intolerance secondary to Ineffective Airway Clearance and Sleep Pattern Disturbance	See "Unit Standards of Care for Pneumonia"
6. Chest Pain related to cough secondary to pneumonia	See "Unit Standards of Care for Pneumonia"
Risk for 4/17/96 JW 7. Altered Comfort: Chills related to fever and diaphoresis	Individualized nursing diagnosis care plan
8. ~~Risk for Altered Family Processes related to mother's illness and temporary unavailability of father to provide child care~~ *Resolved 4/17/96 JW*	Individualized nursing diagnosis care plan
9. Altered Nutrition: Less than Body requirements related to decreased appetite and nausea and increased metabolism secondary to disease process	See Standardized Care Plan for Altered Nutrition: Less than Body Requirements
10. Potential Complications of Pneumonia: Septic shock and respiratory insufficiency	See "Unit Standards of Care for Pneumonia"
11. Potential Complications of IV Therapy: Infiltration, phlebitis	See Unit Procedures: "IV Insertion and Maintenance"
12. Potential Complications of Vancomycin Therapy: Ototoxicity, Hepatotoxicity, Allergic reaction, GI upset	See "Protocol for Administration of Intravenous Vancomycin"

**Creating a
Patient-Care
Plan**

assessments and interventions that apply to Vancomycin that are over and above those routinely performed when administering penicillin. Therefore, 2-South developed a preprinted multidisciplinary protocol that specifies how the drug is to be administered: for example, that the drug is to be given no faster than 100 mL/hour and that it is never given IM. It also specifies the important nursing observations to make: for example, monitor for tinnitus, oliguria, hypotensive reaction, rash, chills, and itching. You would simply note on the formal problem list the reference to the protocol (See Table 9–1). In some institutions, a copy of the protocol is kept with the patient's care plan, and the physician may sign the order for the dosage and administration rate.

If there are collaborative problems that are not covered by any of the above documents, they must be written on the care plan, and individualized nursing orders must be developed for them. This is not needed for Mrs. Sanchez.

4. *For the **nursing diagnoses** not covered by the standards of care, determine the following:*

a. *Which nursing diagnoses really need individualized nursing care plans?* Remember that an individualized plan is needed only if the care is not completely covered by standards of care, protocols, or other routine nursing care. For Luisa Sanchez, Problems 2 through 4 and 7 through 9 need care beyond that specified in the standards of care and unit procedures. You would not expect all pneumonia patients to have these problems (Fluid Volume Deficit, Anxiety, Sleep Pattern Disturbance, Risk for Altered Family Processes, and Altered Nutrition). Therefore, they would not be found on the standardized care plan or on unit standards of care for pneumonia.

b. *Is there a preprinted model care plan for the nursing diagnosis?* Recall that model care plans may exist for a medical diagnosis or for a single nursing diagnosis. For Problem 2, Fluid Volume Deficit, 2-South has a standardized (model) nursing diagnosis care plan (see Figure 9–6 on page 311). You would indicate that resource on the formal problem list (Table 9–1).

For beginning student care plans, you may not use the procedure in Step 5 (Planning step); but you will certainly use it when you develop working care plans as a professional nurse. While you are learning to write care plans, your instructors may ask you to make a complete list of the client's nursing diagnoses and collaborative problems, and to write your own outcomes and nursing orders for each problem—even the ones that are routine. You will usually not have the option of using standards of care, standing orders, protocols, and model care plans.

Step 6: Individualize Standardized Documents as Needed
Besides the handwritten care plans for the three nursing diagnoses, you would use the following documents to direct Mrs. Sanchez's care:

"Unit Standards of Care for Pneumonia"
"Standardized Care Plan for Fluid Volume Deficit"
"Standardized Care Plan for Altered Nutrition: Less than Body Requirements"
"Unit Procedures: IV Insertion and Maintenance"
"Protocol for Administration of Intravenous Vancomycin"

Assume that the "Unit Standards of Care for Pneumonia," the "Unit Procedures for IV Insertion and Maintenance," and the "Protocol for Administration of Intravenous Vancomycin" are all in the 2-South files and require no alterations for Mrs. Sanchez. Because they are a part of the permanent agency records and reflect the care given to all patients with those conditions and therapies, you would not add copies of them to Mrs. Sanchez's comprehensive care plan. However, the standardized care plans for Fluid Volume Deficit and Altered Nutrition are meant to be individualized to a specific patient. Therefore, you would make the appropriate check marks, sign (as shown in Figure 9–6 on page 311), and place a copy with Mrs. Sanchez's complete care plan.

Step 7: Transcribe Medical, Collaborative, ADLs, and Basic Care Needs to Special Sections of the Kardex

Because 2-South uses computerized care plans, you would type the medical orders into the computer. Each day you can obtain a list of orders in effect for that day (see Figure 9–9, "Active Doctor's Orders"). Instructions for Mrs. Sanchez's diet, activity, hygiene needs, intravenous therapy, and so on, are also found on the care plan; some appear under "Active Ancillary Orders." (Note: page 1 of Mrs. Sanchez's computerized care plan, her Problem List, is not shown.)

Step 8: Develop Individualized Care Plan for Remaining Nursing Diagnoses and Collaborative Problems

Examining the formal problem list (Table 9–1 on page 323), you can see that you would need to develop outcomes and nursing orders for Problems 3 (Anxiety), 4 (Sleep Pattern Disturbance), 7 (Altered Comfort: Chills), and 8 (Risk for Altered Family Processes). You would type these into the computer or, in some systems you would be able to choose appropriate outcomes and nursing orders from a list provided by the computer. See Figure 9–9 on page 326 for an example of what a computerized plan for two of Mrs. Sanchez's nursing diagnoses might look like.

Implementation

Step 9: Implement the Care Plan (Do or Delegate)

On the day of admission, care was instituted immediately for Mrs. Sanchez's two highest-priority problems, Ineffective Airway Clearance and Fluid Volume Deficit. Medical orders for oxygen and intravenous antibiotics were begun, diagnostic tests were performed, and routine nursing care was given according to the Unit Standards of Care for Pneumonia, as well as other documents listed in Table 9–1. Problems 3 and 4 (Anxiety and Sleep Pattern Disturbance) were addressed by nursing orders on the nursing diagnosis care plan, and constant monitoring was done for the collaborative problems (10, 11, and 12). As a part of the Implementation step, all of this care would have been charted and passed on to other caregivers in oral reports.

Evaluation

Step 10: Evaluate Results of Care, Revise Plan as Needed

During evaluation, you will compare patient progress to the predicted outcomes and revise the care plan if necessary. Using a computerized plan, such as Figure 9–9, you would simply key in the changes and print out a new plan. On this form, there is a column for problem "Status" and a "Start/Stop" column in which one can enter the date that a problem is discontinued. Of course not all agencies have computerized care plans. Table 9–1 on page 323 indicates how changes might

STORMONT VAIL REGIONAL MED CTR   04/16/96   17:15
TOPEKA, KS 66604

Patient: SANCHEZ, LUISA
Location: 221A   Sex: F   Age: 28   Birthdate: 1/25/72   Wt.: 125 lbs
Account #: 8-37838-1 MRN: 299333 Vst#: 00279 3   Admitted date: 04/16/96
Discharge Date: / /   Admitting Diagnosis: PNEUMONIA
Surgical Procedure: NONE
Drug Allergies: PENICILLIN   Admitting Dr.: KATZ, R
Food Allergies: NONE   Consult Dr. 1:
Other Allergies: NONE   Consult Dr. 2:
Religion: CATHOLIC   Consult Dr. 3:
Marital Status: MARRIED   Pri Care Phy: KATZ, R
Diabetic? N   Pregnant? N   Smoker? N   Infectious? Y   Fasting? N
Hygiene? Help bath 4/15/96

ACTIVE DOCTOR'S ORDERS

	Start	Stop	Entered by
ACTIVITY			
BRP, CHAIR	04/16/96		MLM
INTAKE & OUTPUT	04/16/96		MLM
ROUTINE			
IV THERAPY/FLUIDS			
PERIPHERAL – D$_5$LR @ 100CC/HR	04/16/96		MLM
PULSE OXIMETER	04/16/96		MLM
MEDICATIONS			
VANCOMYCIN 0.5 GM IV q6HR	04/16/96		MLM
TYLENOL 650 MG Q4HR PO FOR TEMP>101°	04/16/96		MLM
OXYGEN PER CANNULA, 5L	04/16/96		MLM

ACTIVE ANCILLIARY ORDERS

LABORATORY	Ord#	Freq	Priority	Ord Dt	Status	Entered by
CBC WITH DIFF	1	X1	ROUT	04/16/96	ORDERED	MLM
ABG'S	2	X1	STAT	04/16/96	ORDERED	MLM
BLOOD CULTURE	10	X2IF	STAT	04/16/96	ORDERED	MLM
		TEMP>101				
SERUM ELECTROLYTES	12	X1	ROUT	04/16/96	ORDERED	MLM
URINE SPEC GRAVITY	3	X1	ROUT	04/16/96	ORDERED	MLM
24-HOUR URINE	11	X1	ROUT	04/16/96	ORDERED	MLM
SPUTUM C&S	4	X1	ROUT	04/16/96	ORDERED	MLM
DIAGNOSTIC RADIOLOGY						
PA & LATERAL CHEST XRAY	9	X1	STAT	04/16/96	ORDERED	MLM
RESPIRATORY THERAPY						
POSTURAL DRAINAGE	5	DAILY	ROUT	04/16/96	ORDERED	MLM
INCENTIVE SPIROMETER	13	q3HR	ROUT	04/16/96	ORDERED	MLM
NEBULIZER	14	Q4HR	ROUT	04/16/96	ORDERED	MLM

Figure 9–9. Initial Care Plan for Luisa Sanchez. Adapted courtesty of Stormont Vail Regional Medical Center, Topeka, KS.

STORMONT VAIL REGIONAL MED CTR   04/16/96   17:15
TOPEKA, KS 66604

Patient: SANCHEZ, LUISA
Location: 221A   Sex: F   Age: 28   Birthdate: 1/25/72   Wt.: 125 lbs
Account #: 8-37838-1 MRN: 299333 Vst#: 00279 3   Admitted date: 04/16/96

NURSING CARE PLAN

Prob.
No.   Start   Stop   Status
3. Nursing Diagnosis: ANXIETY (MODERATE)   04/16/96   IN PROGRESS
   Related to: DIFFICULTY BREATHING AND CONCERNS
                       OVER WORK AND PARENTING ROLES

   Outcomes: • LISTENS TO AND FOLLOWS INSTRUCTIONS   04/16/96   IN PROGRESS
                      FOR CORRECT BREATHING AND COUGHING
                      TECHNIQUE, EVEN DURING DYSPNEIC PERIODS.
                    • VERBALIZES UNDERSTANDING OF   04/16/96   IN PROGRESS
                      CONDITION, TESTS, AND TREATMENTS
                      (BY 04/16/95, 2200).
                    • DECREASED REPORTS OF FEAR AND   04/16/96   IN PROGRESS
                      ANXIETY; (NONE WITHIN 12 HOURS).
                    • VOICE STEADY, NOT SHAKY.   04/16/96   IN PROGRESS
                    • RESP. RATE 12-22/MIN.   04/16/96   IN PROGRESS
                    • FREELY EXPRESSES CONCERNS ABOUT   04/16/96   IN PROGRESS
                      WORK AND PARENTING ROLES, BUT
                      PLACES THEM IN PERSPECTIVE IN
                      VIEW OF HER ILLNESS.

   Nursing Orders: • STAY WITH CLIENT WHEN SHE IS   04/16/96   IN PROGRESS
                      DYSPNEIC. REASSURE HER YOU WILL STAY.
                    • REMAIN CALM; APPEAR CONFIDENT.   04/16/96   IN PROGRESS
                    • ENCOURAGE SLOW, DEEP BREATHING   04/16/96   IN PROGRESS
                      WHEN CLIENT IS DYSPNEIC.   04/16/96   IN PROGRESS
                    • GIVE BRIEF EXPLANATIONS OF
                      TREATMENTS AND PROCEDURES.
                    • WHEN ACUTE EPISODE OVER, GIVE
                      DETAILED INFORMATION ABOUT NATURE
                      OF CONDITION, TESTS, AND TREATMENTS.
                    • AS TOLERATED, ENCOURAGE TO EXPRESS   04/16/96   IN PROGRESS
                      AND EXPAND ON HER CONCERNS ABOUT
                      HER CHILD AND HER WORK. EXPLORE
                      ALTERNATIVES.
                    • NOTE WHETHER HUSBAND RETURNS AS   04/16/96   IN PROGRESS
                      EXPECTED. IF NOT, INSTITUTE CARE
                      PLAN FOR ACTUAL ALTERED FAMILY
                      PROCESSES.

Figure 9–9. (continued)

```
┌──────────────────────────────────────────────────────────────────────────────┐
│              DAILY CARE ACTIVITY SHEET                        PAGE 4           │
│                                                                                │
│ STORMONT VAIL REGIONAL MED CTR                      04/16/96      17:15        │
│ TOPEKA, KS 66604                                                               │
│                                                                                │
│ Patient: SANCHEZ, LUISA                                                        │
│ Location: 221A    Sex: F    Age: 28    Birthdate: 1/25/72    Wt.: 125 lbs      │
│ Account #: 8-37838-1 MRN: 299333 Vst#: 00279 3      Admitted date: 04/16/96    │
│                                                                                │
│                        NURSING CARE PLAN                                       │
│ Prob.                                                                          │
│ No.                                                      Start  Stop  Status   │
│ 4. Nursing Diagnosis: SLEEP PATTERN DISTURBANCE        04/16/96     IN PROGRESS│
│    Related to:        COUGH, PAIN, ORTHOPNEA, FEVER,   04/16/96     IN PROGRESS│
│                       DIAPHORESIS                                              │
│                                                                                │
│    Outcomes:        • OBSERVED SLEEPING AT NIGHT ROUNDS.  04/16/96  IN PROGRESS│
│                     • REPORTS FEELING RESTED IN A.M.      04/16/96  IN PROGRESS│
│                     • DOES NOT EXPERIENCE ORTHOPNEA       04/16/96  IN PROGRESS│
│                       (BY DAY 2).                                              │
│                                                                                │
│    Nursing Orders:  • PROVIDE COMFORT MEASURES, SUCH AS   04/16/96  IN PROGRESS│
│                       BACK RUB, QUIET ENVIRONMENT, DIM                         │
│                       LIGHTS, DRY LINEN WHEN DIAPHORETIC,                       │
│                       AND MOUTH CARE.                                          │
│                     • MONITOR AND INSTITUTE COLLABORATIVE 04/16/96  IN PROGRESS│
│                       MEASURES TO CONTROL                                      │
│                       PAIN, FEVER, AND DYSPNEA.                                │
│                     • USE FLASHLIGHT WHEN MAKING NIGHT    04/16/96  IN PROGRESS│
│                       ROUNDS.                                                  │
│                     • USE SEMI-FOWLER'S POSITION IF       04/16/96  IN PROGRESS│
│                       CLIENT CANNOT FALL ASLEEP IN FOWLER'S.                   │
│                     • INQUIRE DAILY IF CLIENT FEELS RESTED 04/16/96 IN PROGRESS│
└──────────────────────────────────────────────────────────────────────────────┘
```

Figure 9–9. (concluded)

be made on a handwritten problem list; Table 9–2 shows how changes to Mrs. Sanchez's care plan would look if it were not computerized. For brevity, only Problem 3 is shown in Table 9–2. The following scenario illustrates how the evaluation step might have been done for Mrs. Sanchez on the next morning after her admission.

The intravenous fluids quickly restored Mrs. Sanchez's fluid balance, and by the next morning, she showed no signs of Fluid Volume Deficit (Problem 2). As you would expect, her Ineffective Airway Clearance, along with Problems 4, 5, 6, and 9, did not improve as rapidly. These problems would resolve more slowly, as the antibiotics gradually controlled the pneumonia and her oxygenation improved. Therefore, Problems 1, 4, 5, 6, and 9 are unchanged in Table 9–1, the problem list.

Improvement was noted in Problem 7. Because the oral Tylenol was effective in lowering Mrs. Sanchez's temperature, she was no longer experiencing chills. Her husband returned as expected, removing the risk factor for Altered Family Processes (Problem 8). Table 9–1 shows how these problems were redefined to reflect Mrs. Sanchez's changing condition.

Table 9–2. Revised Care Plan for Luisa Sanchez (Anxiety Only)

Nursing Diagnosis	Expected Outcomes	Evaluation Statements	Nursing Orders	Rationale
Anxiety r/t difficulty breathing and concerns about work and parenting roles (4/16/96. MM)	Demonstrates decreased anxiety, as evidenced by:		(a) When client is dyspneic, stay with her; reassure her you will stay.	(a) Presence of a competent caregiver reduces fear of being unable to breathe. Control of anxiety will help client to maintain effective breathing pattern.
	1. Listens and follows instructions for correct breathing and coughing technique, even during periods of dyspnea.	1. Outcome met. Performed coughing techniques as instructed during periods of dyspnea.	(b) Remain calm, appear confident.	(b) Reassures client the nurse can help her.
	2. Verbalizes understanding of condition, diagnostic tests, and treatments (by end of day 1).	2. Outcome met. See nurses' notes for 3–11 shift. Stated "I know I need to try to breathe deeply even when it hurts." Demonstrated correct use of incentive spirometer and stated understanding of the need to use it. Understands IV is for hydration and antibiotics. (Evaluated 4/17/96. JW)	(c) Encourage slow, deep breathing to feel in control and decrease anxiety.	(c) Focusing on breathing may help client.
			(d) When dyspneic, give brief explanations of treatments and procedures.	(d) Anxiety and pain interfere with learning. Knowing what to expect reduces anxiety.
			(e) ~~When acute episode is over, give detailed information about nature of condition, treatments, and tests.~~ *Reassess whether client needs any information about condition, etc. (4/17/96 JW)*	(e) *Detailed information has been given. Because client shows understanding, there is no need to repeat information.*
	3. Reports of fear and anxiety decrease; none within 12 hrs.	3. Outcome met. States, "I know I can get enough air, but it still hurts to breathe."	(f) As client can tolerate, encourage her to express and expand on her concerns about her child and her work. Explore alternatives as needed.	(f) Awareness of source of anxiety enables client to gain control over it.
	4. Voice steady, not shaky.	4. Outcome met. Speaks in steady voice.		
	5. Respiratory rate of 12–22 per min.	5. Outcome not met. Rate 26–36 per minute.		
	6. Freely expresses concerns about work and parenting—places them in perspective in view of her illness.	6. Outcome partially met. Discussed only briefly on 3–11 shift. Not done on 11–7 shift because of client's need to rest. (Evaluated 4/17/96 JW)	(g) ~~Note whether husband returns as scheduled. If he does not, institute care plan for actual Altered Family Processes.~~ *(4/17/96 Mr. Sanchez returned JW)*	(g) Husband's continued absence would constitute defining characteristic for this nursing diagnosis. It is important that this assessment be made right away so child care can be arranged if needed.

329

The evening and night nurses were able to effectively implement the nursing orders for Problem 3 (Anxiety). Resulting changes in the care plan for Anxiety are shown in Table 9–2. However, Anxiety remains on the problem list (Table 9–1) because not all the outcomes were achieved.

Critical Pathway for Luisa Sanchez

Because pneumonia is a common illness, some agencies would use a critical pathway, such as Figure 9–10, for Luisa Sanchez instead of an individualized, comprehensive care plan. The expected length of stay for pneumonia is 5 or 6 days, so the complete critical pathway would have six columns, one for each day. However, to save space, Figure 9–10 includes only days 1, 3, and 4.

When a critical pathway is used, the nurse must nevertheless assess the client for problems that the standardized pathway does not address—the same as when using any type of standardized or prewritten plan. For Problems 3 (Anxiety), 4 (Sleep Pattern Disturbance), and 8 (Risk for Altered Family Processes), you would need to write an individualized plan of care. Additionally, because Vancomycin is not a "typical" therapy for pneumonia, you would also need to write a plan for collaborative Problem 12.

WELLNESS IN THE ACUTE-CARE SETTING

Even in an acute-care setting, nurses do not focus entirely on problems and illness needs. You can increase your wellness focus by being sure to identify client strengths and to use those strengths in working to relieve the client's problems. Mrs. Sanchez's strengths are that she is able to communicate adequately, has a healthy lifestyle, is well educated, and understands and complies with treatment regimens. Realizing this, her nurse could use discussion, pamphlets, and diagrams as nursing interventions. Because Mrs. Sanchez has a stable family situation and finances, a special discharge plan is probably not needed.

Clients have health-promotion and illness-prevention needs beyond their admitting medical diagnoses. Sometime before dismissal, the nurse might assess whether Mrs. Sanchez's health practices include regular exercise, eating balanced meals, and performing breast self-exams. Notice, though, that the nurses must first focus on Mrs. Sanchez's more basic and immediate needs—adequate oxygenation, hydration, anxiety, and potential complications of pneumonia. This illustrates the difficulty of addressing wellness needs in an acute-care setting. Still, such an assessment could help Mrs. Sanchez to follow through on her own to improve her health-style after dismissal.

ETHICAL CONSIDERATIONS

Some would say that because nursing affects people when they are most vulnerable, everything a nurse does has a moral aspect. Following this line of reasoning, the act of creating patient-care plans has a moral dimension.

Conventional ethical principles are those that are widely held, expressed in practice, and enforced by sanctions. Among the basic conventional principles held by nurses are the following:

1. Nurses have an obligation to be competent in their work.
2. The good of the patient should be the nurse's primary concern.

Date @ 0700:

Category Discharge Outcomes	Admission	Day 3	Day 4
Exercise/Rest Patient will ambulate independently &/or c̄ minimal assist.	Chair for meals c̄ assist --------→ BRP/BSC c̄ assist -------------→ Assess the need for PT/OT for strengthening -----------→	Chair for meals ---------------→ BRP/BSC c̄ assist --------------→ Amb. in halls c̄ help bid ------→	------------------------------→ ------------------------------→ Amb. in halls independently &/or c̄ assist tid --------------→
Nutrition/Fluid Patient will tolerate prescribed diet s̄ n/v.	Prescribed diet ---------------→ I&O ---------------------------→ IVF ---------------------------→	Prescribed diet ---------------→ I&O ---------------------------→ IVF ---------------------------→	------------------------------→ ------------------------------→ DC IVF/convert to SL.
Elimination Patient will have a soft non-distended abdomen c̄ bowel sounds. Patient will void s̄ difficulty.	GI assessment q̄ 12 hrs -------→ GU assessment q̄ 12 hrs ------→	GI assessment q̄ 12 hrs -------→ If no BM > 72 hrs, Rx --------→ GU assessment q̄ 12 hrs -----→	------------------------------→ ------------------------------→
Oxygenation Patient will have improved lung sounds & cough c̄ minimal dyspnea.	Pulm. assessment q̄ 12 hrs ---→ RC to eval. & implement O₂ protocol ► Portable/ext. tubing as needed ------------------→ RC to eval. & implement bronchodilator protocol -------→	Pulm. assessment q̄ 12 hrs ---→ RC to follow O₂ protocol -----→ RC to follow bronchodilator protocol ►	------------------------------→ ------------------------------→ DC O₂. ------------------------------→
Circulation Patient will have warm/dry skin of normal color.	Assess VS q̄ 4 hrs -----------→ Assess skin for color/warmth ----→	Assess VS q̄ 12 hrs ----------→ Assess skin for color/warmth q̄ 12 hrs ---------------------→	------------------------------→ ------------------------------→
Skin Integrity/ Infection Control Patient's IV/SL sites will be free of redness, drainage &/or swelling. Patient will have no skin breakdown.	Assess skin integrity q̄ 12 hrs --→ IV antibiotics ----------------→ Assess IV site q̄ 12 hrs ------→	Assess skin integrity q̄ 12 hrs --→ IV antibiotics ----------------→ Assess IV site q̄ 12 hrs ------→ Rotate IV site q̄ 72 hrs ------→	------------------------------→ Start p.o. antibiotics --------→ Assess SL site q̄ 12 hrs -----→ ------------------------------→

Date @ 0700: _____

Pneumonia - Kardex/Overview
Integrated Plan of Care - Admission Day - Day 2
© Shawnee Mission Medical Center 1993 - 01/11/95
9100 W. 74th Street
Shawnee Mission, KS 66204-4019

Figure 9–10. Expected Pathway for Client with Pneumonia. Courtesy Shawnee Mission Medical Center, Merriam, KS.

Category Discharge Outcomes	Admission Day	Day 3	Day 4
Sensory/Neuro Patient will be oriented to person, place & time.	Assess orientation q̄ 12 hrs ------------▶ Observe hrly from 2300-0600 for safety status ------------------▶	Assess orientation q̄ 12 hrs -----------▶ Observe hrly from 2300-0600 for safety status --------------------▶	---------------------------------------▶ ---------------------------------------▶
Pain Management Patient will verbalize/indicate comfort or tolerance of pain.	Assess pain rating & need for analgesia q̄ 4 hrs w/a --------------▶	Assess pain rating & need for analgesia q̄ 4 hrs w/a ---------------▶	---------------------------------------▶
Endocrine Patient will have no s/s of hypo/hyperglycemia.	Monitor for s/s of hypo/ hyperglycemia -------------------------▶	Monitor for s/s of hypo/ hyperglycemia ---------------------------▶	---------------------------------------▶
Psych/Emotional Patient/s.o. will indicate ability to cope c̄ ongoing health care needs.	Assess patient coping abilities ---------▶	Assess patient coping abilities ---------▶	---------------------------------------▶
Discharge Plan/Education Patient/s.o. will verbalize understanding of entire pneumonia discharge instructions.	Initiate ancillary consults. Give patient/s.o. pneumonia PIPOC --▶		Initiate discharge instructions -------------------------▶
Other	CXR.		CXR.
R = Reviewed I = Individualized	Date: _____ Time: _____ I / R Signature: _____ Date: _____ Time: _____ I / R Signature: _____	Date: _____ Time: _____ I / R Signature: _____ Date: _____ Time: _____ I / R Signature: _____	Date: _____ Time: _____ I / R Signature: _____ Date: _____ Time: _____ I / R Signature: _____

a:pneumon.ia

Date @ 0700: _____

Pneumonia - Kardex/Overview
Integrated Plan of Care - Admission Day - Day 4
© Shawnee Mission Medical Center 1993 - 01/11/95
9100 W. 74th Street
Shawnee Mission, KS 66204-4019

Figure 9–10. (concluded)

A nurse who is careless and uncaring violates both principles. Other nurses on the unit may sanction her by avoiding her or perhaps even by reporting her behavior to a supervisor. These ethical principles suggest that nurses have a moral duty to promote client healing. A good nursing care plan aids healing by assuring that the client's needs are communicated and met. When all caregivers understand her needs and preferences, the client is reassured and less anxious and can conserve energy needed for healing.

Although not a conventional principle of nursing, the moral principle of **justice** (in the sense of fairness) is also supported by good planning. In this era of cost-containment and limited health care resources, it is important not to misuse human and material resources. A written care plan makes efficient use of the nurse's time, assuring that efforts will not be duplicated or time wasted in ineffective interventions. As previously mentioned, critical pathways have been shown to conserve resources by decreasing the length of hospital stays. However, nurses must always be careful not to overlook individual needs in their zeal to keep patients "on the pathway."

SUMMARY

A comprehensive care plan
- ✓ is a written guide for goal-oriented nursing action.
- ✓ provides the written framework necessary for individualized care and third-party reimbursement.
- ✓ includes a client profile, instructions for meeting basic needs, aspects of the medical plan to be implemented by the nurse, and a nursing care plan for the client's nursing diagnoses and collaborative problems.
- ✓ may combine both standardized and individualized approaches.
- ✓ supports conventional ethical principles of nursing and the moral principle of justice.
- ✓ is replaced by a critical pathway for frequently occurring conditions in some institutions.

Everyone must know and use various kinds of information. For example, we must know certain information to unlock a combination lock. To use this kind of lock you must remember a pattern of numbers and which direction to turn the dial on the lock. You must know the combination exactly; if you make any mistakes, the lock will not open. In nursing you must know and use many different types of information. There are many ways to know and use information. One way is to remember the information (you know your telephone number by memory). Another way is to be able to identify incorrect information. This skill is related to the skill of remembering, but it is somewhat different.

Practice in Critical Thinking: Recognizing Correct Information

Learning the Skill

Sometimes when we do not remember how to spell a word, we try writing it out in different spellings until we recognize the correct spelling. Even when you are not sure you can remember the correct spelling, you can recognize the difference between the correct and incorrect spellings. You can also recognize incorrect grammar, even though you certainly have not memorized all possible sentences. We often recognize an incorrect sentence and then try to think of the grammar rule that applies to the situation.

Example A Some of the following sentences contain grammar errors. Indicate whether the grammar is correct or incorrect. If it is incorrect, tell why you think so.

1. Marta and Luis, both good athletes, runs every day.

2. My nursing class is so interesting that I think about it often!

3. The dean of our school told Jason and me to be sure to complete our program plans.

Example B In this activity you will be given a physician's order for IV fluids. There *may* be a mistake in some of this information. Your task is to recognize whether the information is correct or incorrect. If it is incorrect, you are to correct the mistake and explain briefly why the original information is incorrect.

Orders: Intravenous fluids, 5% Dextrose, 1000 mg to run over 8 hours

Applying the Skill

1. Some of the information in the following examples of norms contains errors. Make changes where you need to in order to make the information correct. Indicate your reasons for making the changes.

    a. The average B/P in the young adult is 120/80 mm H_2O.

    b. A normal pulse rate is 60–100 beats per minute.

    c. A normal white-blood-cell count is in the range of 4,500–11,000/mg.

    d. A normal red-blood-cell count for men is 4.6–6.2/mL.

    e. Normal range of pH for urine is 4.6–8.0.

2. In this activity, some of the information about the NANDA diagnostic labels may be incorrect. Make changes as needed to correct the information. Give your reasons for making the changes.

    a. Altered Nutrition: Less Than Body Requirements is the state in which an individual is experiencing an intake of nutrients that exceeds metabolic needs.

    b. Risk for Infection has no defining characteristics.

    c. Hypothermia is the state in which an individual's body temperature is reduced below normal range.

    d. The major defining characteristic for Hyperthermia is an increase in body temperature above normal range.

    e. The major defining characteristics for Perceived Constipation are decreased frequency; hard, dry stool; straining at stool; painful defecation; abdominal distention; palpable mass.

Adapted from *Critical Thinking Worksheets,* a Supplement of *Addison-Wesley Chemistry,* by Wilbraham et al. (Menlo Park, CA: Addison-Wesley Publishing Company, 1990).

Applying
Nursing Process

1. On the following form, construct a care plan (for one problem only) by placing the defining characteristics, nursing diagnosis, predicted outcomes, and nursing orders in the correct columns. Choose from the following scrambled list of items:

Verbally denies he is ill.
Pt. will adhere to activity limitations.
Observed out of bed in spite of medical order for bed rest.
Encourage to express feelings and concerns about being hospitalized.
Give positive reinforcement for compliance (e.g., staying in bed, taking meds).
Refused to take his 3 P.M. medication.
Patient will acknowledge consequences of not complying with treatment regimen.
Patient will agree to follow plans for care (e.g., medications, bed rest).
Noncompliance (medical treatment plan) r/t denial of illness.
Develop a written contract with patient regarding bed rest and meds.
Evaluate patient's support system and need for emotional support from staff.

Defining Characteristics	Nursing Diagnosis	Predicted Outcomes	Nursing Orders

2. Use the "Guidelines for Writing Comprehensive Care Plans" in Box 9–2 on page 318 to evaluate the nursing care plan in Figure 9–9 on pages 326-328. Use the following form. Comment on whether the care plan meets each of the guidelines (met/not met), or whether the guideline does not apply. If the guideline is not met, discuss or give an example to show how you arrived at that conclusion.

For Figure 9–9: Care Plan for Luisa Sanchez

Guideline 1:
Guideline 2:
Guideline 3:
Guideline 4:
Guideline 5:
Guideline 6:
Guideline 7:
Guideline 8:
Guideline 9:
Guideline 10:
Guideline 11:

3. Create a care plan for Mr. Cain, using the information in (*a*) through (*f*) and the instructions that follow (*f*).

    a. Use the Patient Kardex (Figure 9–11 on page 340) for the patient profile, basic care needs, and collaborative aspects of care.

    b. Use the blank Nursing Care Plan (Figure 9–12 on page 341) for your patient's complete problem list.

    c. You have the following information from the patient's data base.

Name: Harvey Cain   Age: 83   Birth date: 1/25/13
Marital Status: Married
Home Phone: 631-1098   Religion: Catholic: Wife's Name: Mildred Cain
                    Father Wise, 842-0097   Vital Signs: Temp 100°F
Allergies: Codeine; states no   No special rites.   BP 100/60, Pulse 90,
     food allergies   Resp. 20

Mr. Cain is a thin, elderly male being admitted to Room 426 for an intestinal obstruction and dehydration. He has not had a bowel movement for five days. His abdomen is distended and painful; bowel sounds are absent. He has been vomiting large amounts of green fluid. His skin turgor is poor; his sacrum and heels are reddened, but the skin is intact. His tongue and mouth are dry, and he complains he is a little bit thirsty. He says, "I really feel awful. Am I going to die?" He appears too weak to manage his own hygiene needs. He is oriented to place and person and able to follow second-level commands, but is drowsy and lethargic.

---

    d. The physician, Elton Hobbs, M.D., has left the following orders:

IV D₅Lactated Ringers, 125 mL/hr	Lab: CBC, Electrolytes, SMA12
NPO	X ray: Flat plate of Abdomen, Barium enema
Nasoenteric tube to Gomco suction	Call Dr. Martin Botha for consult
Foley catheter to dependent drainage	Save any stools
Hourly urine measurements	Bedrest
Upper GI	

    e. Your nursing unit has the following resources available:

Standards of Care:	*Standardized Care Plans:*
Anorectal Abscess	Altered Oral Mucous Membrane
Appendicitis	Bowel Incontinence
Cholecystitis	Impaired Verbal Communication
Intestinal Obstruction	Pain
Peritonitis	

Protocols for Care of Patients having:
   Barium Enema
   Cholecystography
   Fiberoptic Colonoscopy
   Liver Biopsy
   Paracentesis

Policies and Procedures:
   Intravenous Therapy
   Nasoenteric Intubation and Suction

f. Mr. Cain's complete problem list has already been developed for you:

Potential Complications of Bowel Obstruction:
   Dehydration
   Electrolyte Imbalance
   Hypovolemic Shock
   Necrosis → Infection
Risk for Altered Tissue Integrity (Pressure Ulcer) r/t decreased mobility, poor nutritional status, and poor skin turgor 2° dehydration
Abdominal Pain r/t abdominal distention
Altered Oral Mucous Membrane r/t fluid loss from vomiting 2° intestinal obstruction
Possible Fear of Dying r/t unknown outcome of illness and lack of information
Possible Fear or Anxiety r/t hospital environment, diagnostic tests, equipment & procedures
Potential Complications of IV Therapy: Phlebitis, Infiltration
Potential Complications of Nasoenteric Intubation: Ulceration → Hemorrhage
Potential Complications of Upper GI: Perforation, Aspiration
Potential Complications of Barium Enema

INSTRUCTIONS FOR PREPARING THE NURSING CARE PLAN

(Refer to "Content of the Comprehensive Care Plan" and Step 5 of the Care Planning Guide.)

1. Put the client profile information on the Kardex (Figure 9–11).

2. Put the instructions for meeting basic needs (hygiene, etc.) on the Kardex.

3. Incorporate the medical orders on the Kardex.

4. On the blank form (Figure 9–12), write the problems in the appropriate columns. Write them in order of priority, the most urgent one first, or assign priority numbers, with 1 being most urgent.

5. Indicate where the nursing interventions for each problem are to be found (review Table 9–1 on page 323 to see how this is done). Some of the problems would require the nurse to write the goals and nursing interventions. You do not need to do this; just write "Nurse will develop plan" beside those problems.

SHAWNEE MISSION MEDICAL CENTER

Date ord.	Radiology	Date Sch	DONE	Date ord.	Laboratory	Date Sch	DONE	Date ord.	Special Procedures	Date Sch	DONE
									Daily Tests		
	Ancillary Consults										
									Daily Weight		

Diet:

Food Allergies:

Hold:

Feeding/Fluids

- ☐ Self
- ☐ Assist
- ☐ Feeder
- ☐ Force
- ☐ Restrict

	meal	Ext	IV
7-3			
3-11			
11-7			

- ☐ I&O
- ☐ IV
- ☐ Other_____

Safety Measures

- ☐ Siderails
- ☐ Restraints
- ☐ Other_____

Activities

- ☐ Bedrest
- ☐ BRP
- ☐ Dangle
- ☐ Chair
- ☐ Commode
- ☐ Up ad Lib
- ☐ Turn
- ☐ Ambulate

Transportation

per _____

Hygiene

- ☐ Bedbath
- ☐ Assist
- ☐ Self Bath
- ☐ Shower
- ☐ Tub
- ☐ Vanity
- ☐ Oral Care

Bowel/Bladder

- ☐ Foley IN _____ OUT _____
- ☐ Cath care Bid
- ☐ Incontinent
- ☐ Colostomy
- ☐ Ileostomy
- ☐ Urostomy

Communication

Physical Therapy	Date	Treatments
Cardio-Pulmonary		

Drug Allergies: _____

Isolation: In _____ Out _____

Emergency Instructions:

Relatives:

Phone:

Clergy:

Religion:

Religious Rites:

Code Blue

Diagnosis:

Surgery & Dates:

Consults & Dates:

Room	Name	Adm Date	Age	Physician

Figure 9–11. Patient Kardex. Courtesy of Shawnee Mission Medical Center, Merriam, KS.

340

PROBLEM LIST FOR HARVEY CAIN		
Date and Initials	Nursing Diagnoses/Problems	Source for Goals and Nursing Orders

Figure 9–12. Nursing Care Plan (Problem List) Form.

REFERENCES

Carpenito, L. (1991). *Nursing Care Plans and Documentation: Nursing Diagnoses and Collaborative problems.* Philadelphia: J. G. Lippincott.

Carpenito, L. (1993). *Nursing Diagnosis: Application to Clinical Practice.* 5th ed. Philadelphia: Lippincott.

Gage, M. (1994). The patient-driven interdisciplinary care plan. *Journal of Nursing Administration,* 24(4):26–35.

Hampton, D. (1993). Implementing a managed care framework through care maps. *Journal of Nursing Administration,* 23 (5):21–27.

Zander, K. (1988). Managed care within acute care settings: Design and implementation via nursing case management. *Health Care Supervisor,* 6(2):27–43.

Appendix A
American Nurses Association Code for Nurses

1. The nurse provides services with respect for human dignity and the uniqueness of the client, unrestricted by considerations of social or economic status, personal attributes, or the nature of health problems.

2. The nurse safeguards the client's right to privacy by judiciously protecting information of a confidential nature.

3. The nurse acts to safeguard the client and the public when health care and safety are affected by the incompetent, unethical, or illegal practice of any person.

4. The nurse assumes responsibility and accountability for individual nursing judgments and actions.

5. The nurse maintains competence in nursing.

6. The nurse exercises informed judgment and uses individual competence and qualifications as criteria in seeking consultation, accepting responsibilities, and delegating nursing activities to others.

7. The nurse participates in activities that contribute to the ongoing development of the profession's body of knowledge.

8. The nurse participates in the profession's efforts to implement and improve standards of nursing.

9. The nurse participates in the profession's efforts to establish and maintain conditions of employment conducive to high-quality nursing care.

10. The nurse participates in the profession's effort to protect the public from misinformation and misrepresentation and to maintain the integrity of nursing.

11. The nurse collaborates with members of the health professions and other citizens in promoting community and national efforts to meet the health needs of the public.

From *Code for Nurses with Interpretive Statements,* © 1985 by American Nurses Association, Kansas City, MO. Reprinted with permission.

Nursing Assessment Form Based on Roy's Adaptation Model

PATIENT HISTORY

PLEASE COMPLETE THE FOLLOWING QUESTIONS.

1. What are the reasons or symptoms that brought you to the hospital?
_____
_____

2. What major illnesses, previous hospitalizations & surgeries have you had?
_____
_____
_____
_____
_____

3. Has there been any recent stress or crisis in your life (death, illness, divorce, family problems)? _____
_____
_____

4. Are you allergic to any drugs, foods, tapes, environmental substances?
No _____ Yes _____

List allergies	Describe Reactions

5. List all medications that you are currently taking. Include prescription, over-the-counter, and recreational drugs such as marijuana, cocaine, etc.

Medications	Amount Taken	Time Last Taken

6. What is your occupation? _____
Are you: ___ Married ___ Single ___ Separated ___ Widowed ___ Divorced

7. Do you have any children? _____

8. To what race or ethnic group do you belong? _____

9. Who can help you when you return home? _____
Do you plan to return to your present address after hospitalization?
_____

10. Who can we contact in case of emergency? _____
Phone number: _____

11. Do you have any religious practices that will affect your care while in the hospital? _____

12. Do you feel you will require post-discharge assistance? _____

13. Is there any additional information that would assist us in caring for you?
_____

PLEASE CONTINUE ON BACK OF PAGE

ADMISSION DATA (TO BE COMPLETED BY NURSE)

Date: _____ Arrive Time on Unit: _____
Accompanied by: _____
Mode of Transport: _____

Valuables: Sent home _____ Retained _____
List _____
Informed of Valuable Policy: Yes _____ No _____

Assistive Devices:
Contact Lenses _____ Glasses _____
Dentures: Upper _____ Lower _____ Partial _____
Hearing Aid: _____
Other _____ None _____

Ambulating Device:
Cane _____ Crutches _____
Walker _____ W/C _____
Brace _____
Other _____ None _____

Oriented to:
Call light _____
Bathroom _____
Bed Control _____
Patient Information Booklet _____

ID Bracelet: Correct _____ Replaced _____

VS: Temp _____ P _____ R _____ BP _____
Height _____ Weight _____

NURSING ASSESSMENT

Appears:
Calm _____ Oriented _____ Confused _____
Fearful _____ Cooperative _____ Anxious _____
Agitated _____ Withdrawn _____ Well-
Language Combative _____ groomed _____
Barrier_____
Other _____

Self Care Needs: None _____ Needs help with:
_____
_____
_____

Family Present: Yes _____ No _____
Who:_____
Potential Problems: Yes _____ No _____
Describe:_____

Discharge Planning Needs Identified:
Yes _____ No _____ Describe: _____
_____

Shawnee Mission Medical Center
NURSING ASSESSMENT FORM

Courtesy of Shawnee Mission Medical Center, Merriam, KS.

IF YOU ARE EXPERIENCING A PROBLEM IN THE AREAS BELOW, PLEASE CHECK ( ) APPROPRIATE BLANK(S). IF YOU HAVE NO PROBLEMS, CHECK THE NO PROBLEM BLANK.

EXERCISE/REST:
Walking _____ Pain with exercise _____
Weakness _____ Insomnia _____
Breathlessness with exertion _____
Use of sleeping aids: _____
No Problems _____

NUTRITION/FLUIDS:
Special Diet: _____
Recent weight gain _____ weight loss _____
Swallowing/chewing difficulty _____
Food dislikes/likes _____
Alcohol use: Type _____
How often _____
No Problem _____

ELIMINATION:
Constipation _____ Diarrhea _____
Ostomy _____ Type: _____
Use of laxatives/stool softeners/enemas _____
Urinary frequency _____ Burning _____
Blood in urine _____ Urinary infection _____
Urinating during night _____
No problem _____

OXYGENATION:
Shortness of breath _____ Wheeze _____ Cough _____
Pain with breathing _____ Blood in sputum _____
Home oxygen _____
Smoking: Packs/day _____ How long have you smoked? _____
Have you quit recently? _____
No problem _____

CIRCULATORY:
Heart Problems _____ Chest pain _____
High blood pressure _____ Varicose Veins _____
Swelling _____ Pacemaker _____ Shunts _____
Catheters _____
Have you ever had a blood transfusion: Yes _____ No _____
When? _____
No Problem _____

TEMPERATURE/SKIN:
With this illness, do you have:
Chills _____ Fever _____ Rashes _____ Bruises _____
Cuts _____ Open Sores _____
Have you travelled out of the USA in the last year?
Yes _____ No _____
No problem _____

NEURO/SENSORY:
Pain _____ Location: _____
Dizziness _____ Fainting _____ Seizures _____
Numbness/tingling _____ Difficulty with speech _____
Sight _____ Hearing _____ Taste _____
Memory loss _____
No Problem _____

ENDOCRINE/REPRODUCTIVE:
Menstrual problems _____ Bleeding _____ Cramping _____
Abnormal vaginal/penile discharge _____
Pelvic infection _____ Genital Lesions _____
Thyroid disorder _____
Diabetes _____ Duration of Diabetes _____
No Problem _____

Patient/Family Signature: _____

PHYSICAL ASSESSMENT: (TO BE COMPLETED BY NURSE)
No Problems Identified _____
Unsteady Gait _____ Paralysis _____ Limited ROM _____
Joint Deformity _____
Describe: _____
_____

No Problems Identified _____
Nausea _____ Vomiting _____
Describe last food/drink & time taken _____
Describe problems: _____

No Problems Identified _____
Incontinence _____ Foley in place _____ Diversions _____
Stomas _____
Bowel Sounds: Present _____ Absent _____
Abdomen: Soft _____ Tender _____ Flat _____ Distended _____
Date of last bowel movement: _____
Describe: _____

No Problems Identified _____
Irregular respirations _____ SOB _____ Using oxygen _____
Breath Sounds: Clear _____ Crackles _____ Wheezes _____
Cough: Productive _____ Non-productive _____
Describe: _____
_____

No Problems Identified _____
Peripheral Pulses: Normal _____ Slightly Impaired _____
Moderately Impaired _____ Absent _____
Edema: Present _____ Where _____
Heart Sounds: _____
C-V Devices Present _____ Where _____
Describe: _____

No Problems Identified _____
Skin Color: Pink _____ Pale _____ Flushed _____ Mottled _____
Cyanotic _____ Jaundiced _____ Other _____
Temperature: Warm _____ Hot _____ Cool _____ Dry _____
Moist _____ Diaphoretic _____
Condition: Bruises _____ Rash _____ Open Sores _____
Describe: _____

No Problems Identified _____
LOC: Alert _____ Lethargic _____ Unresponsive _____
Disoriented _____ Unconscious _____ Memory Deficit _____
Speech: Slurred _____ Aphasic _____
Pain: Type _____ Severity _____ Duration _____
Pupil Reaction _____ Hand Grip _____
Describe: _____

No Problems Identified _____
Vaginal Bleeding _____ Amount _____
Pregnancy _____ gravida _____ Para _____
Blood Sugar Monitoring _____
Describe: _____

RN Signature: _____ Time: _____

DR. notified: Date _____ Time _____

Patient Admission Assessment

Name: _____ Age:_____

Prefer to be called: _____ Date:_____

Next of Kin: _____ Relationship: _____ Phone:_____

Other contact person: _____ Phone:_____

Primary Language, if other than English: _____ Person completing form:_____

Why are you being admitted to the hospital?_____

NO NEED TO COMPLETE THIS SECTION IF THE PRE-OPERATIVE QUESTIONNAIRE IS COMPLETED

List any previous hospitalizations and/or surgeries:_____
_____
_____

Do you have any of these health problems (please check)

___Alzheimers	___Dizziness	___Hepatitis	___Asthma	___Chest Pain
___Epilepsy	___High Blood Pressure	___Hiatal Hernia	___Cough	___Heart Flutter
___Seizures	___Diabetes	___Arthritis	___Mucous Production	___Congestive Heart Failure
___Numbness	___Thyroid	___Back Injury	___Shortness of Breath on Activity	___Heart Pounding
___Tingling	___Swelling		___Difficulty Breathing	___Pacemaker
			___Emphysema	___No Problems

If yes, please explain:_____

Are there any other medical problems of which we should be aware?_____
_____

Do you have any eyesight and/or hearing difficulties? Yes ☐   No ☐

If yes, indicate use of: glasses   contacts   hearing aid   other: _____

Do you wear dentures? Yes ☐   No ☐   If yes, what kind?   Upper   Lower   Partial   Full

Are you on a special diet? Yes ☐   No ☐   If yes, what kind: _____

ALLERGIES

Do you have any allergies to: Food: _____ Type of Reaction:_____

Medications: _____ Type of Reaction:_____

Anesthesia: _____ Type of Reaction:_____

Other (wool, tape, pollens): _____ Type of Reaction:_____

It is important that we are aware of the use of any of the following substances in order to keep you comfortable and to avoid interaction with other medication/anesthetic that might be prescribed. Do you use any of the following? (Please circle)

Alcohol	Tobacco	Amphetamines (uppers)	Barbiturates (downers)	Tranquilizers
Marijuana	Heroin	Cocaine	Caffeine (tea, coffee, pop)	Other:_____

Are you currently taking _any_ medications? Yes ☐ No ☐   Did you bring them with you? Yes ☐ No ☐

Are you taking your medications as ordered by your physician? Yes ☐ No ☐

Please list below, any medications you are taking (including prescription and over the counter medications)

MEDICATIONS

MEDICATION	DOSE	HOW OFTEN	REASON	PRESCRIBING PHYSICIAN

Form No. 102A   (Revised 9/89)   PATIENT ADMISSION ASSESSMENT

Courtesy of Bronson Methodist Hospital, Kalamazoo, MI.

**PATIENT ADMISSION
ASSESSMENT**
continued—Page 2

NUTRITION/ METABOLIC

Any recent weight loss or gain?: Yes ☐ No ☐   If yes, how much:_____ ☐ Gain ☐ Loss

Do you have?: (Please circle)   Nausea/Vomiting   Stomach Pains   Poor Appetite

Difficulty Chewing or Swallowing   Heartburn   No Problems

Comments:_____

_____

ELIMINATION

Last bowel movement: _____

What is your usual bowel pattern?   Daily   Twice a day   Every other day   Other:_____

Do you have?   Constipation   Diarrhea   Hemorrhoids Other: _____

Indicate any laxatives/enemas or "home remedies" that you use:_____

Have you been experiencing any urinary problems?:   Burning   Frequency   Urgency

Bed Wetting   Bloody Urine   Problems holding urine   Difficulty starting to urinate   Last void: _____

No Problems   Other:_____

How often do you urinate?:_____   Describe color: _____

Comments:_____

SEXUAL/ REPRODUCTIVE

FEMALE: Have you been through menopause?: Yes ☐ No ☐   Please explain your normal menstrual pattern:_____

Any recent problems or changes in your menstrual pattern?: Yes ☐ No ☐   If yes, please explain:_____

Date of last normal period:_____   Could you be pregnant?: Yes ☐ No ☐

Do you take birth control pills?: Yes ☐ No ☐   Do you perform a monthly breast exam?: Yes ☐ No ☐

MALE: Have you experienced any?: (Please circle) Prostate problems   Sores on your penis Testicular problems   Bleeding   Discharge

Do you perform a monthly testicular exam?: Yes ☐ No ☐   No problems

SLEEP

How long do you sleep?:_____ p.m. to _____ a.m.   Is it adequate?: Yes ☐ No ☐   Do you nap? Yes ☐   No ☐

Do you have difficulty sleeping?:   Yes ☐ No ☐   If yes, what do you do to help yourself fall asleep?:_____

COGNITIVE/ PERCEPT

Do you have a history of chronic pain?:   Yes ☐ No ☐   If yes, please explain:_____

What do you do to relieve pain?:_____

How do you learn best?: (Please circle)   Reading   Listening   Demonstration

SELF-PERCEPT

How are you feeling about being hospitalized?:   Frightened   Calm   Angry   Worried   Relieved   Sad   Hopeful

Other:_____

ROLE/ RELATIONSHIP

Marital status: (Please circle)   Single   Married   Separated   Divorced   Widowed

Do you have children?:   Yes ☐   No ☐   List ages:_____

Are you presently employed?:   Yes ☐   No ☐   Occupation:_____

Are you presently in school?:   Yes ☐   No ☐   Will illness interfere?   Yes ☐ No ☐

Upon discharge, if needed, will you be able to afford: Medicine Yes ☐ No ☐   Supplies Yes ☐ No ☐   Medical Care Yes ☐ No ☐

COPING/ STRESS

Are you experiencing any stressful situations other than your illness/hospitalization?:   Yes ☐   No ☐

If yes, please describe:_____

How do you usually cope with tension or stress?:_____

VALUE/ BELIEF

Will illness/hospitalization interfere with any of the following?: (Please circle)

Spiritual or Religious Practice   Family Traditions   Cultural Beliefs or Practice   Will not interfere

If yes, please explain:_____

Would you like your Clergy or Hospital Chaplain to be contacted?:   Yes ☐   No ☐

If yes, state name and number:_____

347

Appendix D
Collaborative Problems Organized by Body System

Potential Complication: Gastrointestinal-Hepatic

PC: Paralytic Ileus/Small-Bowel Obstruction
PC: Hepatorenal Syndrome
PC: Hyperbilirubinemia
PC: Evisceration
PC: Hepatosplenomegaly
PC: Curling's Ulcer
PC: Ascites
PC: G.I. Bleeding

Potential Complication: Metabolic/Immune

PC: Hypoglycemia
PC: Hyperglycemia
PC: Negative Nitrogen Balance
PC: Electrolyte Imbalances
PC: Thyroid Dysfunction
PC: Hypothermia (severe)
PC: Hyperthermia (severe)
PC: Sepsis
PC: Acidosis/Alkalosis
PC: Diabetes
PC: Anasarca
PC: Hypo/Hyperthyroidism
PC: Allergic Reaction
PC: Donor-Tissue Rejection
PC: Adrenal Insufficiency

Potential Complication: Neurologic/Sensory

PC: Increased Intracranial Pressure
PC: Stroke
PC: Seizures
PC: Spinal Cord Compression
PC: Autonomic Dysreflexia
PC: Birth Injuries
PC: Hydrocephalus
PC: Microcephalus
PC: Meningitis
PC: Cranial Nerve Impairment
PC: Paresis/Paresthesia/Paralysis
PC: Peripheral Nerve Impairment
PC: Increased Intraocular Pressure
PC: Corneal Ulceration
PC: Neuropathies

Potential Complication: Cardiovascular

PC: Dysrhythmias
PC: Congestive Heart Failure
PC: Thromboemboli/Deep-Vein Thrombosis
PC: Hypovolemic Shock
PC: Peripheral Vascular Insufficiency
PC: Hypertension
PC: Congenital Heart Disease
PC: Thrombocytopenia
PC: Polycythemia
PC: Anemia
PC: Compartmental Syndrome
PC: Disseminated Intravascular Coagulation
PC: Endocarditis
PC: Sickling Crisis
PC: Embolism (air, fat)
PC: Spinal Shock
PC: Ischemic Ulcers

Potential Complication: Respiratory

PC: Atelectasis/Pneumonia
PC: Asthma
PC: COPD
PC: Pulmonary Embolism
PC: Pleural Effusion
PC: Tracheal Necrosis
PC: Ventilator Dependency
PC: Pneumothorax
PC: Laryngeal Edema

Potential Complication: Renal/Urinary

PC: Acute Urinary Retention
PC: Renal Failure
PC: Bladder Perforation

Potential Complication: Reproductive

PC: Fetal Compromise
PC: Uterine Atony
PC: Pregnancy-Induced Hypertension
PC: Eclampsia
PC: Hydramnios
PC: Hypermenorrhea
PC: Polymenorrhea
PC: Syphilis
PC: Tetanic Uterine Contractions
PC: Placenta Previa; Abruptio Placenta
PC: Uterine Rupture
PC: Dysfunctional Labor

Potential Complication: Muscular/Skeletal

PC: Stress Fractures
PC: Osteoporosis
PC: Joint Dislocation
PC: Joint Inflammation
PC: Muscle Atrophy
PC: Osteomyelitis

Adapted with permission from L. J. Carpenito (1993), *Nursing Diagnosis: Application to Clinical Practice,* 5th ed (Philadelphia: J. B. Lippincott), pp. 1025–1027.

Acute Confusion
Altered Family Process: Alcoholism
Chronic Confusion
Decreased Adaptive Capacity: Intracranial
Disorganized Infant Behavior
Effective Management of Therapeutic Regimen: Individual
Energy Field Disturbance
Impaired Environmental Interpretation Syndrome
Impaired Memory
Ineffective Management of Therapeutic Regimen: Community
Ineffective Community Coping
Ineffective Management of Therapeutic Regimen: Families
Potential for Enhanced Community Coping
Potential for Enhanced Organized Infant Behavior
Potential for Enhanced Spirtual Well-Being
Risk for Altered Parent/Infant/Child Attachment
Risk for Loneliness
Risk for Perioperative Positioning Injury
Risk for Disorganized Infant Behavior

Source: *NANDA Nursing Diagnoses: Definitions and Classification, 1995–1996.*
Philadelphia: North American Nursing Diagnosis Association, 1994.

Appendix F
Interviewing Elderly Patients

In addition to the general interview guidelines in Box 3–4 on page 64, consider the following suggestions when interviewing elderly clients:

1. *Proceed slowly.* Speak slowly and clearly, giving the client plenty of time to form an answer.

2. *Check for sensory deficits at the beginning of the interview.* Don't wait until you come to that area of the data collection form. Until you have checked the patient's hearing, look at him as you speak, to allow for lip reading.

3. *Don't assume all elderly people are deaf or unable to understand your meaning.* The fact that you need to speak slowly does not mean that you need to speak loudly.

4. *Be aware that appropriate affect and articulate speech do not always go together.* Also, inappropriate affect and incoherent speech do not necessarily indicate lack of understanding. A patient may be speaking coherently and making sense as she tells you about her loss of appetite, and then begin crying for no apparent reason. Nevertheless, the information about her appetite may be credible. Another patient may laugh appropriately at something funny and yet have difficulty speaking clearly or finding the words to express what he means.

5. *Rely more than usual on body language.* Be aware of nonverbal communication, such as quivering of the lips, tears in the eyes, or movements of the hands and feet. As noted in #4, some elderly patients have difficulty finding the words to express their ideas and feelings.

6. *Be alert for intermittent confusion.* Some elderly clients are confused at one time and not another. A client may be giving you credible information and then, as the interview progresses, begin to lose track of the topic or introduce irrelevant material. When the patient seems confused, use focused assessment to determine his mental status. If you conclude that the patient's answers may be unreliable, you can return later to finish the interview when he is no longer confused.

7. *Try to get data directly from the client when it is possible.* Some clients are reluctant to answer questions. Also, families are sometimes very protective of clients, and tend to answer for them. Explain to them that it is important for you to hear what the client has to say.

These suggestions apply in some degree to people of all ages, but they are especially important in meeting the challenges that occur when the aging process is superimposed on a disease process.

This *Nursing Diagnosis Guide* provides a quick reference in the clinical setting. The diagnostic labels, definitions, defining characteristics, and risk and related factors in this guide are from NANDA *Nursing Diagnoses: Definitions and Classification,* 1995–1996 unless otherwise specified. The author's discussion and recommendations for using diagnoses are identified by the phrase *Author's Note.* If your cue cluster does not completely fit the label you have chosen, consider the suggested alternative labels indicated by "See also" and the pointing-finger symbol (☛).

Choosing a problem label: To use this guide, first identify your client's problem and its cue cluster (signs and symptoms). Using the list of NANDA labels organized by your chosen framework (inside front and back cover of your text), locate the labels that seem to describe the problem. Find these labels in this guide. Use the label that has defining characteristics that best match your client's cue cluster to describe the *problem* part of your nursing diagnosis.

Writing the etiology: A complete nursing diagnosis consists of *Problem + Etiology.* You may find the etiology under "related factors" or "risk factors," or it may be one of the other diagnostic labels. Because etiologies vary greatly among individuals, you will often need to write the etiology in your own words.

Alphabetical organization: Diagnostic labels are listed in the guide in alphabetical order. Look for the noun, or main thought, rather than the modifier. For example, Ineffective Airway Clearance is found under *A* rather than *I*. The client has an *airway* problem, not an *ineffective* problem.

ACTIVITY DEFICIT, DIVERSIONAL
(*see* Diversional Activity Deficit)

ACTIVITY INTOLERANCE
Definition: A state in which an individual has insufficient physiological or psychological energy to endure or complete required or desired daily activities.

Defining Characteristics: Abnormal heart rate or blood pressure in response to activity; exertional discomfort or dyspnea; electrocardiographic changes reflecting arrhythmias or ischemia. **Critical**—Verbal report of fatigue or weakness.
Related Factors: Bedrest/immobility; generalized weakness; sedentary lifestyle; imbalance between oxygen supply/demand.
Author's Note: Use this label only if the client has verbally reported fatigue or weakness in response to activity. Activity Intolerance is often caused by medical conditions (e.g., heart disease or peripheral arterial disease); however, a diagnostic statement such as Activity Intolerance r/t coronary artery disease is not useful for planning nursing care, since the nurse cannot effect change on either side of the statement.

Activity Intolerance is often the etiology of other problems, such as Self-Care Deficit, Social Isolation, or Sexual Dysfunction, and it is probably used most effectively in this manner. Gordon (1987, p. 147) suggests that Activity Intolerance be specified by levels of endurance:

Level I: Walks regular pace on level ground but becomes more short of breath than normal when climbing one or more flights of stairs.
Level II: Walks one city block 500 feet on level or climbs one flight of stairs slowly without stopping.
Level III: Walks no more than 50 feet on level without stopping and is unable to climb one flight of stairs without stopping.
Level IV: Dyspnea and fatigue at rest.

An example of a resulting diagnostic statement is Self-care Deficit (Total) r/t Activity Intolerance (Level IV). Do not use Activity Intolerance if it is not possible to increase the client's endurance.
☛ *See also* Fatigue, Self-Care Deficit.

ACTIVITY INTOLERANCE, RISK FOR
Definition: A state in which an individual is at risk of experiencing insufficient physiological or psychological energy to endure or complete required or desired daily activities.

Defining Characteristics: Presence of risk factors such as history of previous intolerance; deconditioned status; presence of circulatory/respiratory problems; inexperience with the activity.
Related Factors: *See* the risk factors listed in Defining Characteristics.
Author's Note: Discriminate between Activity Intolerance, Fatigue, and Self-Care Deficit. Do not use Activity Intolerance if it is not possible to increase the client's endurance. *See* the note for Activity Intolerance.

ADJUSTMENT, IMPAIRED

Definition: The state in which the individual is unable to modify his/her lifestyle/behavior in a manner consistent with a change in health status.

Defining Characteristics: *Major*—Verbalization of non-acceptance of health status change; nonexistent or unsuccessful ability to be involved in problem solving or goal setting. *Minor*—Lack of movement toward independence; extended period of shock, disbelief, or anger regarding health-status change; lack of future-oriented thinking.

Related Factors: Disability requiring change in lifestyle; inadequate support systems; impaired cognition; sensory overload; assault to self-esteem; altered locus of control; incomplete grieving.

☛ *See also* Coping, Ineffective Individual.

AIRWAY CLEARANCE, INEFFECTIVE

Definition: A state in which an individual is unable to clear secretions or obstructions from the respiratory tract to maintain airway patency.

Defining Characteristics: Abnormal breath sounds (crackles, wheezes); changes in rate or depth of respiration; tachypnea; cough, effective/ineffective, with or without sputum; cyanosis; dyspnea.

Related Factors: Decreased energy/fatigue; tracheobronchial infection, obstruction, secretion; perceptual/cognitive impairment; trauma.

☛ Discriminate between this label and Impaired Gas Exchange, Ineffective Breathing Pattern, and Risk for Aspiration.

ANTICIPATORY GRIEVING

(*see* Grieving, Anticipatory)

ANXIETY

Definition: A vague uneasy feeling whose source is often nonspecific or unknown to the individual.

Defining Characteristics: *Subjective*—Increased tension; apprehension; painful and persistent increased helplessness; uncertainty; fearful; scared; regretful; overexcited; rattled; distressed; jittery; feelings of inadequacy; shakiness; fear of unspecific consequences; expressed concerns regarding change in life events; worried; anxious. *Objective*—Restlessness; insomnia; glancing about; poor eye contact; trembling/hand tremors; extraneous movement (foot shuffling, hand/arm movements); facial tension; voice quivering; focus on self; increased wariness; increased perspiration. *Critical*—Sympathetic stimulation: cardiovascular excitation, superficial vasoconstriction, pupil dilation.

Related Factors: Unconscious conflict about essential values/goals of life; threat to self-concept; threat of death; threat to or change in health status; threat to or change in role functioning; threat to or change in environment; threat to or change in interaction patterns; situational/maturational crises; interpersonal transmission/contagion; unmet needs.

Author's Note: Anxiety must be clearly differentiated from Fear because the nursing interventions are different. When a client is fearful, the focus is on removing or helping him to deal with the specific fear. When a client is anxious, the nurse helps him identify the cause of the anxiety; because the source of Anxiety cannot always be identified, however, nursing care may also focus on helping the client explore and express anxious feelings—not an effective approach when dealing with Fear.

The Anxious person cannot define, or does not know, the source of his anxiety. The only critical defining characteristic is stimulation of the sympathetic nervous system. A variety of other subjective and objective signs and symptoms can be used to help identify Anxiety (e.g., increased tension, worry, restlessness, poor eye contact, trembling). In contrast, Fear is specifically defined as "a feeling of dread related to an identifiable source which the person validates." People experience any number of physical and psychological reactions to fear; however, the only defining characteristic needed to make the diagnosis is *ability to identify the object of fear.*

Because the level of anxiety determines the nursing interventions, you should indicate whether anxiety is moderate, severe, or panic-level. Panic may require collaborative interventions, such as medication. Mild Anxiety should not be used at all, since it is a normal condition present in all human beings. Diagnose Anxiety only for clients who require special nursing interventions. Mild anxiety before surgery is a normal, healthy response. You would, in fact, wonder about the mental status of someone who felt absolutely no anxiety before surgery. Taylor et al. (1989, p. 137) use these four levels of anxiety:

Mild anxiety: Present in day-to-day living, mild anxiety increases alertness and perceptual fields. It motivates learning and growth.
Moderate anxiety: Narrows the person's perceptual fields so that the focus is on immediate concerns, with inattention to other communications and details.
Severe anxiety: Creates a very narrow focus on specific detail. All behavior is geared toward getting relief.

Panic: The person has loss of control and experiences dread and terror. The resulting disorganized state results in increased physical activity, distortion of perceptions and relationships, and loss of rational thought. This level of anxiety can lead to exhaustion and death.

Fear and Anxiety present diagnostic difficulty because they are not mutually exclusive. That is, a person who is afraid is usually anxious as well. Furthermore, many of the same signs and symptoms are present in both Fear and Anxiety, for example, increased heart and respiratory rate, dilated pupils, diaphoresis, muscle tension, and fatigue. Remember that in Fear the person can identify the threat; in Anxiety he usually cannot (Whitley, 1992a).

Anxiety	Fear
Vague uneasy feeling	Feeling of dread
Source of feeling unknown by person	Source of feeling is known by person
Threat is vague, nonspecific	Threat is specific, identifiable
Threat usually psychological (e.g., to self-image)	Threat often physical (e.g., to safety)
A variety of defining characteristics, both verbal and autonomic	Defining characteristic: Ability to identify object of fear

☛ Fear is a related diagnosis.

ASPIRATION, RISK FOR
Definition: The state in which an individual is at risk for entry of gastrointestinal secretions, oropharyngeal secretions, or solids or fluids into tracheobronchial passages.

Defining Characteristics: Presence of risk factors such as reduced level of consciousness; depressed cough and gag reflexes; presence of tracheostomy or endotracheal tube; incomplete lower esophageal sphincter; GI tubes; tube feedings; medication administration; situations hindering elevation of upper body; increased intragastric pressure; increased gastric residual; decreased GI motility; delayed gastric emptying; impaired swallowing; facial/oral/neck surgery or trauma; wired jaws.
Related Factors: *See* the risk factors above.
Author's Note: Use the most specific label for which the patient has the necessary defining characteristics.
☛ Related labels: Ineffective Airway Clearance, Risk for Suffocation, Risk for Injury, and Risk for Trauma.

BATHING/HYGIENE SELF-CARE DEFICIT
(*see* Self-Care Deficit, Bathing/Hygiene)

BODY IMAGE DISTURBANCE
Definition: Disruption in the way one perceives one's body image.

Defining Characteristics: Critical—*A or B* must be present to justify the diagnosis of Body Image Disturbance. (*A*) verbal response to actual or perceived change in structure and/or function; (*B*) nonverbal response to actual or perceived change in structure and/or function. *Other*—The following clinical manifestations may be used to validate the presence of *A* or *B. Objective:* Missing body part; actual change in structure and/or function; not looking at body part; not touching body part; hiding or overexposing body part (intentional or unintentional); trauma to nonfunctioning part; change in social involvement; change in ability to estimate spatial relationship of body to environment. *Subjective:* Verbalization of change in lifestyle; fear of rejection or of reaction by others; focus on past strength, function, or appearance; negative feelings about body; and feelings of helplessness, hopelessness, or powerlessness; preoccupation with change or loss; emphasis on remaining strengths, heightened achievement; extension of body boundary to incorporate environmental objects; personalization of part or loss by name; depersonalization of part or loss by impersonal pronouns; refusal to verify actual change.
Related Factors: Biophysical; cognitive/perceptual; psychosocial; cultural or spiritual.
Author's Note: This label is related to Self-Esteem Disturbance and includes negative feelings about one's body or body parts. While Body Image Disturbance is often caused by loss of a body part or actual body changes, the change in structure or function can be perceived rather than actual. Clients on prolonged bedrest or who are dependent on machines (e.g., dialysis, respirator) may experience distortion of body image.
☛ *See also* Self-Esteem Disturbance.

BODY TEMPERATURE, RISK FOR ALTERED
Definition: The state in which the individual is at risk for failure to maintain body temperature within normal range.

Defining Characteristics: Presence of risk factors such as extremes of age; extremes of age or weight; exposure to cold/cool or warm/hot environments; dehydration; inactivity or vigorous activity; medications causing vasoconstriction/

vasodilation; altered metabolic rate; sedation; inappropriate clothing for environmental temperature; illness or trauma affecting temperature regulation.

Related Factors: *See* risk factors above.

☛ Differentiate between Altered Body Temperature, Hypo- or Hyperthermia, and Ineffective Thermoregulation.

BOWEL INCONTINENCE
(*see* Incontinence, Bowel)

BREASTFEEDING, EFFECTIVE (POTENTIAL FOR ENHANCED)

Definition: The state in which a mother-infant dyad/family exhibits adequate proficiency and satisfaction with breastfeeding process.

Defining Characteristics: *Major*—Mother able to position infant at breast to promote a successful latch-on response; infant is content after feeding; regular and sustained suckling/swallowing at the breast; appropriate infant weight patterns for age; effective mother/infant communication patterns (infant cues, maternal interpretation and response). *Minor*—Signs and/or symptoms of oxytocin release (let down or milk ejection reflex); adequate infant elimination patterns for age; eagerness of infant to nurse; maternal verbalization of satisfaction with the breastfeeding process.

Related Factors: Basic breastfeeding knowledge; normal breast structure; normal infant oral structure; infant gestational age greater than 34 weeks; support sources; maternal confidence.

BREASTFEEDING, INEFFECTIVE

Definition: The state in which a mother, infant, or child experiences dissatisfaction or difficulty with the breastfeeding process.

Defining Characteristics: *Major*—Unsatisfactory breastfeeding process. *Minor*—Actual or perceived inadequate milk supply; infant inability to attach onto maternal breast correctly; no observable signs of oxytocin release; observable signs of inadequate infant intake; nonsustained suckling at the breast; insufficient emptying of each breast per feeding; persistence of sore nipples beyond the first week of breastfeeding; insufficient opportunity for suckling at the breast; infant exhibiting fussiness and crying within the first hour after breastfeeding; unresponsive to other comfort measures; infant arching and crying at the breast; resisting latching on.

Related Factors: Prematurity; infant anomaly; maternal breast anomaly; previous breast surgery; previous history of breastfeeding failure; infant receiving supplemental feedings with artificial nipple; poor infant sucking reflex; nonsupportive partner/family; knowledge deficit; interruption in breastfeeding; maternal anxiety or ambivalence.

BREASTFEEDING, INTERRUPTED

Definition: A break in the continuity of the breastfeeding process as a result of inability or inadvisability to put baby to breast for feeding.

Defining Characteristics: *Major*—Infant does not receive nourishment at the breast for some or all of feedings. *Minor*—Maternal desire to maintain lactation and provide (or eventually provide) breast milk for her infant's nutritional needs; lack of knowledge regarding expression and storage of breast milk; separation of mother and infant.

Related Factors: Abrupt weaning of infant; engorgement; maternal medications that are contraindicated for the infant; maternal obligations outside the home; maternal or infant illness; prematurity; sore/cracked nipples.

Author's Note: Discriminate among this label and the suggested alternative diagnoses. This label does not focus on the mother's satisfaction with the feeding process nor with the adequacy of her milk supply.

Diagnosis	*Cues (Defining Characteristics)*
Ineffective Breastfeeding	Dissatisfaction with feeding process
Ineffective Infant Feeding Pattern	Inability of infant to suck or poorly coordinated suck-swallow response
Interrupted Breastfeeding	Mother wishes to maintain lactation; unable to put baby to breast for some feedings (e.g., illness or work)

Interrupted Breastfeeding actually represents a situation rather than a response, so there is little the nurse can do to correct the interruption (e.g., the need for the mother to work). Therefore, this label might function best as an etiology (e.g., Risk for Ineffective Breastfeeding related to Interrupted Breastfeeding secondary to mother's employment).

☛ Compare this label to Ineffective Breastfeeding and Ineffective Infant Feeding Pattern.

BREATHING PATTERN, INEFFECTIVE

Definition: The state in which an individual's inhalation and/or exhalation pattern does not enable adequate pulmonary inflation or emptying.

Defining Characteristics: Dyspnea, shortness of breath, tachypnea, fremitus, abnormal arterial blood gas, cyanosis, cough, nasal flaring, respiratory depth changes, assumption of 3-point position, pursed-lip breathing/prolonged expiratory phase, increased anteroposterior diameter, use of accessory muscles, altered chest excursion.

Related Factors: Neuromuscular impairment; pain, musculoskeletal impairment; perception/cognitive impairment; anxiety; decreased energy/fatigue.

Author's Note: Use this label with caution. If the condition cannot be treated by independent nursing actions, write it as a collaborative problem. Consider, too, that the ineffective breathing pattern may be merely a symptom of another problem, such as Anxiety.

☛ Compare this label to Activity Intolerance, Ineffective Airway Clearance, and Impaired Gas Exchange.

CARDIAC OUTPUT, DECREASED

Definition: A state in which the blood pumped by an individual's heart is sufficiently reduced that it is inadequate to meet the needs of the body's tissues.

Defining Characteristics: Variations in blood-pressure readings; arrhythmias; fatigue; jugular vein distention; color changes, skin and mucous membranes; oliguria; decreased peripheral pulses; cold, clammy skin; rales; dyspnea, orthopnea; restlessness. *Other Possible Characteristics:* Change in mental status; shortness of breath; syncope; vertigo; edema; cough; frothy sputum; gallop rhythm; weakness.

Author's Note: Author recommends that you do not use this label. The nurse can neither conclusively diagnose nor definitively treat this problem. When the client has Actual Decreased Cardiac Output, use a statement in which the problem is described as a human response to this pathophysiology (e.g., Activity Intolerance r/t decreased cardiac output). If the client is at risk of developing complications, write them as collaborative problems (e.g., Potential Complication of M.I.: Cardiogenic Shock).

☛ Activity Intolerance, Self-Care Deficit.

CAREGIVER ROLE STRAIN (ACTUAL AND RISK)

Definition (Actual): A caregiver's felt difficulty in performing the family caregiver role.

Definition (Risk): A caregiver is vulnerable for felt difficulty in performing the family caregiver role

Defining Characteristics: *Major*—Does not have sufficient resources to provide the care needed; feels that caregiving interferes with other important roles in life; feels loss because the care receiver is a different person than before caregiving began or, in the case of a child, that the care receiver was never the child the caregiver expected; feels family conflict around issues of providing care; feels stress or nervousness in the relationship with the care receiver; feels depressed; finds it hard to perform specific caregiving activities; worries about the care receiver's health and emotional state, having to put the care receiver in an institution, and who will care for the care receiver if something should happen to the caregiver.

Related/Risk Factors: *Developmental*—Caregiver not developmentally ready for caregiver role, e.g., young adult needing to provide care for a middle-aged parent; developmental delay or retardation of the care receiver or caregiver. *Pathophysiological*—Addiction or codependency; caregiver health impairment; discharge of family member with significant home care needs; illness severity of the care receiver; premature birth/congenital defect; unpredictable illness course or instability in the care receiver's health. *Psychosocial*—Care receiver exhibits deviant, bizarre behavior; caregiver is female; caregiver is spouse; caregiver's marginal coping patterns; marginal family adaptation or dysfunction prior to the caregiving situation; past history of poor relationship between caregiver and care receiver; psychological or cognitive problems in care receiver. *Situational*—Caregiver's competing role commitments; complexity/amount of caregiving tasks; duration of required caregiving, inadequate physical environment for providing care, e.g., housing, transportation, community services, equipment; family/caregiver isolation; inexperience with/lack of knowledge of caregiving skills; lack of respite and recreation for caregiver; presence of abuse or violence; presence of situational stressors that normally affect families, such as significant loss, disaster or crisis, poverty or economic vulnerability; major life events, e.g., birth, hospitalization, leaving home, returning home, marriage, divorce, employment, retirement, death.

Author's Note: This diagnosis provides a different perspective from Altered Family Processes and Ineffective Family Coping. Altered Family Processes refers to the inability to provide care in the presence of altered family dynamics (such as divorce); Ineffective Family Coping refers to the inability to cope with the diagnosis given to a loved one. Caregiver Role Strain is specific to the situation in which a family member must give care and is unable to do so (Burns et al., 1993)

☛ *See also* Coping (Family): Ineffective; and Family Processes, Altered.

CHRONIC LOW SELF-ESTEEM
(*see* Self-Esteem, Chronic Low)

CHRONIC PAIN
(*see* Pain, Chronic)

COMMUNICATION, IMPAIRED VERBAL
Definition: The state in which an individual experiences a decreased or absent ability to use or understand language in human interaction.

Defining Characteristics: Critical—Unable to speak dominant language; speaks or verbalizes with difficulty; does not or cannot speak. *Other*—Stuttering; slurring; difficulty forming words or sentences; difficulty expressing thought verbally; inappropriate verbalization; dyspnea; disorientation.
Related Factors: Decrease in circulation to brain; brain tumor; physical barrier (tracheostomy, intubation); anatomical defect, cleft palate; psychological barriers (psychosis, lack of stimuli); cultural difference; developmental or age-related.
Author's Note: This label should be used for those who desire to communicate but are having difficulty (Carpenito, 1993).

CONFLICT, DECISIONAL
(*see* Decisional Conflict)

CONSTIPATION
Definition: A state in which an individual experiences a change in normal bowel habits characterized by a decrease in frequency and/or passage of hard, dry stools.

Defining Characteristics: Decreased activity level; frequency less than usual pattern; hard, formed stools; palpable mass; reported feeling of pressure in rectum; reported feeling of rectal fullness; straining at stool. Other possible characteristics: Abdominal or back pain; decreased appetite; headache; interference with daily living; use of laxatives.
☞ Other labels to consider: Colonic Constipation, Perceived Constipation.

CONSTIPATION, COLONIC
Definition: The state in which an individual's pattern of elimination is characterized by hard, dry stool that results from a delay in passage of food residue.

Defining Characteristics: *Major*—Decreased frequency; hard, dry stool; straining at stool; painful defecation; abdominal distention; palpable mass. *Minor*—Rectal pressure; headache, decreased appetite; abdominal pain.
Related Factors: Less than adequate dietary, fluid, or fiber intake; inadequate physical activity; immobility; lack of privacy; emotional disturbances; chronic use of laxatives and/or enemas; stress; change in daily routine; metabolic problems (e.g., hypothyroidism, hypocalcemia, hypokalemia).
☞ *See also* Constipation and Perceived Constipation.

CONSTIPATION, PERCEIVED
Definition: The state in which an individual makes a self-diagnosis of constipation and ensures a daily bowel movement through abuse of laxatives, enemas, and suppositories.

Defining Characteristics: *Major*—Expectation of a daily bowel movement with the resulting overuse of laxatives, enemas, and suppositories; expected passage of stool at same time every day.
Related Factors: Cultural/family health beliefs; faulty appraisal; impaired thought processes.
☞ *See also* Constipation and Colonic Constipation.

COPING, DEFENSIVE
Definition: The state in which an individual repeatedly projects falsely positive self-evaluation based on a self-protective pattern which defends against underlying perceived threats to positive self-regard.

Defining Characteristics: *Major*—Denial of obvious problems/weaknesses; projection of blame/responsibility; rationalizes failures; hypersensitive to slight/criticism; grandiosity. *Minor*—Superior attitude toward others; difficulty establishing/maintaining relationships; hostile laughter or ridicule of others; difficulty in reality-testing perceptions; lack of follow-through or participation in treatment or therapy.
☞ Related labels: Ineffective Individual Coping, Ineffective Denial, Impaired Adjustment.

COPING, INEFFECTIVE FAMILY: COMPROMISED

Definition: A usually supportive primary person (family member or close friend) is providing insufficient, ineffective, or compromised support, comfort, assistance, or encouragement that may be needed by the client to manage or master adaptive tasks related to his or her health challenge.

Defining Characteristics: *Subjective*—Client expresses or confirms a concern or complaint about significant other's response to his or her health problem; significant person describes preoccupation with personal reaction (e.g., fear, anticipatory grief, guilt, anxiety) to client's illness, disability, or to other situational or developmental crises; significant person describes or confirms an inadequate understanding or knowledge base, which interferes with effective assistive or supportive behaviors. *Objective*—Significant person attempts assistive or supportive behaviors with less than satisfactory results; significant person withdraws or enters into limited or temporary personal communication with the client at the time of need; significant person displays protective behavior disproportionate (too little or too much) to the client's abilities or need for autonomy.

Related Factors: Inadequate or incorrect information or understanding by a primary person; temporary preoccupation by a significant person who is trying to manage emotional conflicts and personal suffering and is unable to perceive or act effectively in regard to client's needs; temporary family disorganization and role changes; other situational or developmental crises or situations the significant person may be facing; little support provided by client, in turn, for primary person; prolonged disease or disability progression that exhausts supportive capacity of significant people.
☛ *See also* Ineffective Family Coping: Disabling, Altered Family Processes, Altered Parenting, and Parental Role Conflict.

COPING, INEFFECTIVE FAMILY: DISABLING

Definition: Behavior of significant person (family member or other primary person) that disables his or her own capacities and the client's capacities to effectively address tasks essential to either person's adaptation to the health challenge.

Defining Characteristics: Neglectful care of the client in regard to basic human needs and/or illness treatment; distortion of reality regarding the client's health problem, including extreme denial about its existence or severity;

intolerance; rejection; abandonment; desertion; carrying on usual routines, disregarding client's needs; psychosomaticism; taking on illness signs of client; decisions and actions by family that are detrimental to economic or social well-being; agitation, depression, aggression, hostility; impaired restructuring of a meaningful life for self, impaired individualization, prolonged overconcern for client; neglectful relationships with other family members; client's development of helpless, inactive dependence.

Related Factors: Significant person with chronically unexpressed feelings of guilt, anxiety, hostility, despair, etc.; dissonant discrepancy of coping styles for dealing with adaptive tasks by the significant person and client or among significant people; highly ambivalent family relationships; arbitrary handling of family's resistance to treatment, which tends to solidify defensiveness as it fails to deal adequately with underlying anxiety.
☛ *See also* Ineffective Family Coping: Compromised, Altered Family Processes, Altered Parenting.

COPING, FAMILY: POTENTIAL FOR GROWTH

Definition: Effective managing of adaptive tasks by family member involved with the client's health challenge, who now is exhibiting desire and readiness for enhanced health and growth in regard to self and in relation to the client.

Defining Characteristics: Family member attempting to describe growth impact of crisis on his or her own values, priorities, goal, or relationships; family member moving in direction of health-promoting and enriching lifestyle that supports and monitors maturational processes, audits and negotiates treatment programs, and generally chooses experiences that optimize wellness; individual expressing interest in making contact on a one-to-one basis or on a mutual-aid group basis with another person who has experienced a similar situation.

Related Factors: Needs sufficiently gratified and adaptive tasks effectively addressed to enable goals of self-actualization to surface.

COPING, INEFFECTIVE INDIVIDUAL

Definition: Impairment of adaptive behaviors and problem-solving abilities of a person in meeting life's demands and roles.

Defining Characteristics: *Major*—Verbalization of inability to cope or inability to ask for help; inability to problem-solve. *Other*—Inability to meet role expectations; inability to meet basic needs; alteration in societal participation; destructive behavior toward self or others; inappropriate use of defense mechanisms; change in usual communication patterns; verbal manipulation; high illness rate; high rate of accidents.

Related Factors: Situational crises; maturational crises; personal vulnerability.

☞ Related labels: Defensive Coping, Impaired Adjustment.

DECISIONAL CONFLICT (SPECIFY)

Definition: The state of uncertainty about a course of action to be taken when the choice among competing actions involves risk, loss, or challenge to personal life values.

Defining Characteristics: *Major*—Verbalized uncertainty about choices; verbalization of undesired consequences of alternative actions being considered; vacillation between alternative choices; delayed decision making. *Minor*—Verbalized feeling of distress while attempting a decision; self-focusing; physical signs of distress or tension (increased heart rate, increased muscle tension, restlessness, etc.); questioning personal values and beliefs while attempting a decision.

Related Factors: Unclear personal values/beliefs; perceived threat to value system; lack of experience or interference with decision making; lack of relevant information; support system deficit; multiple or divergent sources of information.

Author's Note: Differentiate between this label, Spiritual Distress, and the inability to problem-solve associated with Ineffective Individual Coping.

DEFENSIVE COPING

(*see* Coping, Defensive)

DENIAL, INEFFECTIVE

Definition: The state of a conscious or unconscious attempt to disavow the knowledge or meaning of an event to reduce anxiety/fear to the detriment of health.

Defining Characteristics: *Major*—Delays seeking or refuses health-care attention to the detriment of health; does not perceive personal relevance of symptoms or danger. *Minor*—Uses home remedies (self-treatment) to relieve symptoms; does not admit fear of death or invalidism;

minimizes symptoms; displaces source of symptoms to other organs; unable to admit impact of disease on life pattern; makes dismissive gestures or comments when speaking of distressing events; displaces fear of impact of the condition; displays inappropriate affect.

Author's Note: Do not use to describe the denial that occurs as a part of the normal grief process.

☞ Discriminate between this label and Ineffective Individual Coping, Altered Health Maintenance, Noncompliance, and Dysfunctional Grieving.

DIARRHEA

Definition: A state in which an individual experiences a change in normal bowel habits characterized by the frequent passage of loose, fluid, unformed stools.

Defining Characteristics: Abdominal pain; cramping; increased frequency; increased frequency of bowel sounds; loose liquid stools; urgency. *Other Possible Characteristics:* Change in color.

☞ *See also* Bowel Incontinence.

DISUSE SYNDROME, RISK FOR

Definition: A state in which an individual is at risk for deterioration of body systems as the result of prescribed or unavoidable musculoskeletal inactivity. (Complications from immobility can include pressure ulcer, constipation, stasis of pulmonary secretions, thrombosis, urinary tract infection/retention, decreased strength/endurance, orthostatic hypotension, decreased range of joint motion, disorientation, body image disturbance, and powerlessness.)

Defining Characteristics: Presence of risk factors such as paralysis; mechanical immobilization; prescribed immobilization; severe pain; altered level of consciousness.

Related Factors: *See* risk factors above.

Author's Note: This label describes potential complications of immobility. It is not necessary to write separate risk diagnoses such as Risk for Impaired Skin Integrity or Risk for Activity Intolerance when the risk factor is immobility. These more specific labels should be used only if an actual problem develops (Carpenito, 1993) or if the risk factor is other than immobility.

DIVERSIONAL ACTIVITY DEFICIT

Definition: The state in which an individual experiences a decreased stimulation from or interest or engagement in recreational or leisure activities.

Defining Characteristics: Patient's statements regarding boredom, wish there was something to do, to read, etc.; usual hobbies cannot be undertaken in hospital.

Related Factors: Environmental lack of diversional activity, as in long-term hospitalization, frequent lengthy treatments.

DRESSING-GROOMING SELF-CARE DEFICIT
(*see* Self-Care Deficit, Dressing-Grooming)

DYSFUNCTIONAL GRIEVING
(*see* Grieving, Dysfunctional)

DYSREFLEXIA
Definition: The state in which an individual with a spinal cord injury at T7 or above experiences a life-threatening, uninhibited sympathetic response of the nervous system to a noxious stimulus.

Defining Characteristics: *Major*—Paroxysmal hypertension (sudden periodic elevated B/P, where systolic pressure is over 140 mm Hg and diastolic is above 90 mm Hg); bradycardia or tachycardia (pulse rate < 60 or > 100 beats per minute); diaphoresis (above the injury); red splotches on skin (above the injury); pallor (below the injury); headache (a diffuse pain in different portions of the head and not confined to any nerve-distribution area). *Minor*— Chilling; conjunctival congestion; Horner's Syndrome (contraction of the pupil, partial ptosis of the eyelid, enophthalmos and sometimes loss of sweating over the affected side of the face); paresthesia; pilomotor reflex (gooseflesh formation when skin is cooled); blurred vision; chest pain; metallic taste in mouth; nasal congestion.

Related Factors: Bladder distention; bowel distention; skin irritation; lack of patient and caregiver knowledge.

Author's Note: Dysreflexia exists as a potential problem for the patient with high spinal cord injury. If it occurs as an actual problem, and nursing interventions do not immediately resolve it, medical treatment is necessary. It cannot continue as an actual nursing diagnosis. Therefore, Risk for Dysreflexia is a more useful label (Carpenito, 1993).

ELIMINATION, URINARY
(*see* Urinary Elimination, Altered Patterns)

FAMILY COPING, INEFFECTIVE
(*see* Coping, Ineffective Family)

FAMILY COPING, POTENTIAL FOR GROWTH
(*see* Coping, Family; Potential for Growth)

FAMILY PROCESSES, ALTERED
Definition: The state in which a family that normally functions effectively experiences a dysfunction.

Defining Characteristics: Family system unable to meet physical, emotional, or spiritual needs of its members; parents do not demonstrate respect for each other's views on child-rearing practices; inability to express/accept wide range of feelings; inability to express/accept feelings of members; family unable to meet security needs of its members; inability of the family members to relate to each other for mutual growth and maturation; family uninvolved in community activities; inability to accept/receive help appropriately; rigidity in function and roles; a family not demonstrating respect for individuality and autonomy of its members; family unable to adapt to change/deal with traumatic experience constructively; family failing to accomplish current/past developmental task; unhealthy family decision-making process; failure to send and receive clear messages; inappropriate boundary maintenance; inappropriate/poorly communicated family rules, rituals, symbols; unexamined family myths; inappropriate level and direction of energy.

Related Factors: Situation transition and/or crises; developmental transition and/or crisis.

Author's Note: This label describes a family that normally functions effectively but is experiencing a stressor that alters its functioning. The stressors causing Altered Family Processes tend to be situational or developmental transitions and crises like the following:

Serious illness of a family member	Loss of job
Death of a family member	Divorce
Infidelity	

This label is different from Ineffective Family Coping: Compromised, in which the stressor is withdrawal of support by a significant other. The family coping problem is caused by a change in the relationship between the family members—not necessarily by an external stressor such as death or divorce. Compromised Family Coping involves the client and a significant other, whereas Altered Family Processes involves the entire family.

Altered Family Processes describes a family that has the resources for effectively coping with stressors, in contrast with Ineffective Family Coping: Disabling, which describes a family that demonstrates destructive behaviors. If stressors are not effectively resolved, Altered Family Processes can progress to Ineffective Family Coping.

To differentiate among these three labels, carefully examine the defining characteristics and related factors of each in your *Nursing Diagnosis Guide*.

☛ *See also* Ineffective Family Coping, Parental Role Conflict, and Altered Parenting.

FATIGUE

Definition: An overwhelming sustained sense of exhaustion and decreased capacity for physical and mental work.

Defining Characteristics: *Major*—Verbalization of an unremitting and overwhelming lack of energy; inability to maintain usual routines. *Minor*—Perceived need for additional energy to accomplish routine tasks; increase in physical complaints; emotionally labile or irritable; impaired ability to concentrate; decreased performance; lethargic or listless; disinterest in surroundings/introspection; decreased libido; accident-prone.

Related Factors: Decreased/increased metabolic energy production; overwhelming psychological or emotional demands; increased energy requirements to perform activity of daily living; excessive social and/or role demands; states of discomfort; altered body chemistry (e.g., medications, drug withdrawal, chemotherapy).

Author's Note: Do not use this label to describe temporary tiredness resulting from lack of sleep. Fatigue describes a chronic condition; the client's previous energy levels and capabilities cannot be restored.

☛ *See also* Activity Intolerance, Self-Care Deficit, and Sleep Pattern Disturbance.

FEAR

Definition: Feeling of dread related to an identifiable source which the person validates.

Defining Characteristics: Ability to identify object of fear.
Author's Note: Differentiate between Fear and Anxiety (Whitley, 1992b).

☛ *See* Anxiety note.

FEEDING SELF-CARE DEFICIT
(*see* Self-Care Deficit, Feeding)

FLUID VOLUME DEFICIT (1)
Definition: The state in which an individual experiences vascular, cellular, or intracellular dehydration.

Defining Characteristics: *Major*—Dilute urine; increased urine output; sudden weight loss. *Minor*—Possible weight gain; hypotension; decreased venous filling; increased pulse rate; decreased skin turgor; decreased pulse volume/pressure; increased body temperature; dry skin; dry mucous membranes; hemoconcentration; weakness; edema; thirst.
Related Factors: Failure of regulatory mechanisms.
Author's Note: Use this label for clients experiencing vascular, cellular, or intracellular dehydration. Use cautiously, because many problems with fluid balance require a collaborative approach. Do not use this label routinely, even as a potential problem, for patients who are NPO. Independent nursing treatments for Fluid Volume Deficit aim to prevent fluid loss (e.g., diaphoresis) and encourage oral fluids. For a diagnosis such as Risk for Fluid Volume Deficit r/t NPO order, there are no independent nursing actions to prevent or treat either side of the diagnostic statement.

Do not use Risk for Fluid Volume Deficit to describe clients who are hemorrhaging or at risk of hemorrhaging; these situations usually represent collaborative problems.

> *Incorrect:* Risk for Fluid Volume Deficit r/t postpartum hemorrhage
> *Correct:* Potential Complication of Childbirth: Postpartum Hemorrhage; Risk for Postpartum Hemorrhage r/t retained placental fragments

This label can sometimes be used effectively as a nursing diagnosis; for example, Fluid Volume Deficit r/t decreased desire for fluids 2° altered taste caused by chemotherapy. An *actual* fluid volume deficit may be the etiology for other nursing diagnoses, such as Altered Oral Mucous Membranes r/t fluid volume deficit 2° fluid loss from severe vomiting and diarrhea.

☛ Differentiate between this label and Fluid Volume Deficit (2).

FLUID VOLUME DEFICIT (2)
Definition: The state in which an individual experiences vascular, cellular, or intracellular dehydration.

Defining Characteristics: *Major*—Decreased urine output; concentrated urine; output greater than intake; sudden weight loss; decreased venous filling; hemoconcentration, increased serum sodium. *Minor*—Hypotension; thirst; increased pulse rate; decreased skin turgor; decreased pulse volume/pressure; change in mental state; increased body temperature; dry skin; dry mucous membranes; weakness.

Related Factors: Active loss.

Author's Note: *See* note for Fluid Volume Deficit (1).
☛ Differentiate between this label and Fluid Volume Deficit (1).

FLUID VOLUME DEFICIT, RISK FOR

Definition: The state in which an individual is at risk of experiencing vascular, cellular, or intracellular dehydration.

Defining Characteristics: Presence of risk factors such as extremes of age or weight; excessive losses through normal routes (e.g., diarrhea); loss of fluid through abnormal routes (e.g., indwelling tubes); deviations affecting access to or intake or absorption of fluids (e.g., physical immobility); factors influencing fluids needs (e.g., hypermetabolic state); knowledge deficit related to fluid volume; medications (e.g., diuretics).

Related Factors: *See* risk factors above.

Author's Note: *See* note for Fluid Volume Deficit (1). Do not use routinely for patients who are NPO.

FLUID VOLUME EXCESS

Definition: The state in which an individual experiences increased fluid retention and edema.

Defining Characteristics: Edema; effusion; anasarca; weight gain; shortness of breath, orthopnea; intake greater than output; S_3 heart sound; pulmonary congestion (chest X ray); abnormal breath sounds, crackles; change in respiratory pattern; change in mental status; decreased hemoglobin and hematocrit; blood-pressure changes; central venous pressure or pulmonary artery pressure changes; jugular vein distention; positive hepatojugular reflex; oliguria; specific gravity changes; azotemia; altered electrolytes; restlessness and anxiety.

Related Factors: Compromised regulatory mechanism; excess fluid intake; excess sodium intake.

Author's Note: Be sure you use this label to describe a condition that nurses can prevent or treat with independent actions. The main type of Fluid Volume Excess that nurses can treat independently is peripheral, dependent edema, which can be symptomatically relieved by elevating the client's affected limbs. If the client requires medical intervention to resolve the fluid imbalance, use a collaborative problem such as Potential Complication of Renal Failure: Generalized Edema. Fluid Volume Excess can also be the cause of complications, such as Potential Complication of Fluid Volume Excess: Pulmonary Edema.

Examples:

Incorrect: Fluid Volume Excess r/t decreased cardiac output

Correct: Potential Complication of Decreased Cardiac Output: Fluid Volume Excess

Correct: Potential Complication of Heart Failure: Pulmonary Edema

Correct: Risk for Impaired Skin Integrity r/t fluid volume excess A.M.B. generalized edema

☛ This label is related to Decreased Cardiac Output, which also tends to be a collaborative problem rather than a nursing diagnosis.

FUNCTIONAL INCONTINENCE (URINARY)
(*see* Incontinence, Functional Urinary)

GAS EXCHANGE, IMPAIRED

Definition: The state in which the individual experiences a decreased passage of oxygen and/or carbon dioxide between the alveoli of the lungs and the vascular system.

Defining Characteristics: Confusion; somnolence; restlessness; irritability; inability to move secretions; hypercapnea; hypoxia.

Related Factors: Ventilation perfusion imbalance.

Author's Note: Author does not recommend using this label. Decreased passage of gases between the alveoli of the lungs and the vascular system can only be discovered by means of a medically prescribed diagnostic test: blood gas analysis. The defining characteristics offer little help. A client might easily have most of them without actually having impaired alveolar gas exchange. Since nurses can neither diagnose nor treat this condition, you should use a diagnostic statement that describes oxygen-related problems the nurse *can* treat (e.g., Activity Intolerance). If the client is *at risk* for Impaired Gas Exchange, you should write a collaborative problem, such as Potential Complication of Thrombophlebitis: Pulmonary Embolus.
☛ *See also* Activity Intolerance, Ineffective Airway Clearance, Ineffective Breathing Pattern.

GRIEVING, ANTICIPATORY

Definition: Intellectual and emotional responses and behaviors by which individuals work through the process of modifying self-concept based on the perception of potential loss.

Defining Characteristics: Potential loss of significant object; expression of distress at potential loss; denial of potential loss; guilt; anger; sorrow; choked feelings; changes in eating habits; alterations in sleep patterns; alterations in activity level; altered libido; altered communication patterns.

Related Factors: To be developed.

Author's Note: Anticipatory Grieving may be a normal, not necessarily maladaptive, response. It occurs *before* the loss.
☛ *See also* Dysfunctional Grieving.

GRIEVING, DYSFUNCTIONAL

Definition: Extended, unsuccessful use of intellectual and emotional responses by which individuals attempt to work through the process of modifying self-concept based upon the perception of loss.

Defining Characteristics: Verbal expression of distress at loss; denial of loss; expression of guilt; expression of unresolved issues; anger; sadness; crying; difficulty in expressing loss; alterations in eating habits, sleep patterns, dream patterns, activity level, libido; idealization of lost object; reliving of past experiences; interference with life functioning; developmental regression; labile affect; alterations in concentration and/or pursuits of tasks.

Related Factors: Actual or perceived object loss (object loss is used in the broadest sense); objects may include people, possessions, a job, status, home, ideals, parts and processes of the body.

Author's Note: Most of the defining characteristics may also be present in the normal grief process. Grieving is dysfunctional only if it is prolonged (perhaps a year after the loss), or if the symptoms are unusually numerous or severe.

GROWTH AND DEVELOPMENT, ALTERED

Definition: The state in which an individual demonstrates deviations in norms from his/her age group.

Defining Characteristics: *Major*—Delay or difficulty in performing skills (motor, social, or expressive) typical of age group; altered physical growth; inability to perform self-care or self-control activities appropriate for age. *Minor*—Flat affect; listlessness, decreased responses.

Related Factors: Inadequate caretaking; indifference, inconsistent responsiveness, multiple caretakers; separation from significant others; environmental and stimulation deficiencies; effects of physical disability; prescribed dependence.

Author's Note: Author does not recommend use of this label. It is too broad to suggest nursing interventions. There are many nursing diagnoses that could be considered alterations in growth and development or that could be caused by altered growth and development (e.g., Self-Care Deficit, Urinary Incontinence, Impaired Verbal Communication, and Altered Parenting). When possible, these more specific labels should be used. Because growth and development are routinely assessed in nursing care of children, a diagnostic statement is usually not required for that application (it is usually included in pediatric standards of care).

HEALTH MAINTENANCE, ALTERED

Definition: Inability to identify, manage, and/or seek out help to maintain health.

Defining Characteristics: Demonstrated lack of knowledge regarding basic health practices; demonstrated lack of adaptive behaviors to internal/external environmental changes; reported or observed inability to take responsibility for meeting basic health practices in any or all functional pattern areas; history of lack of health-seeking behavior; expressed interest in improving health behaviors; reported or observed lack of equipment, financial and/or other resources; reported or observed impairment of personal support systems.

Related Factors: Lack of or significant alteration in communication skills (written, verbal, and/or gestural); lack of ability to make deliberate and thoughtful judgments; perceptual/cognitive impairment (complete/partial lack of gross and/or fine motor skills); ineffective individual coping; dysfunctional grieving; unachieved developmental tasks; ineffective family coping; disabling spiritual distress; lack of material resources.

Author's Note: Altered Health Maintenance should be used for clients who *wish* to change an unhealthy lifestyle or who *lack knowledge* of their disease or condition. It should not be used to describe clients who are not motivated to change or learn.
☛ *See also* Impaired Adjustment, Health-Seeking Behaviors, Knowledge Deficit, Noncompliance.

HEALTH-SEEKING BEHAVIORS (SPECIFY)

Definition: A state in which an individual in stable health is actively seeking ways to alter personal health habits and/or the environment in order to move toward a higher level of health. (Stable health status is defined as age-appropriate illness-prevention measures achieved, client reports good or excellent health, and signs and symptoms of disease, if present, are controlled.)

Defining Characteristics: *Major*—Expressed or observed desire to seek a higher level of wellness. *Minor*—Expressed or observed desire for increased control of health practice; expression of concern about current environmental conditions on health status; stated or observed unfamiliarity with wellness community resources; demonstrated or observed lack of knowledge in health-promotion behaviors.

Author's Note: This label should be used for well clients who wish information about disease prevention or health promotion.

☞ *See also* Altered Health Maintenance.

HOME MAINTENANCE MANAGEMENT, IMPAIRED

Definition: Inability to independently maintain a safe, growth-promoting immediate environment.

Defining Characteristics: Critical—Household members express difficulty in maintaining their home in a comfortable fashion; household requests assistance with home maintenance; household members describe outstanding debts or financial crises; unwashed or unavailable cooking equipment, clothes, or linen; accumulation of dirt, food wastes, or hygienic wastes; overtaxed family members (e.g., exhausted, anxious; repeated hygienic disorders, infestations, or infections). *Other*—Disorderly surroundings; offensive odors; inappropriate household temperature; presence of vermin or rodents.

Related Factors: Individual/family member disease or injury; insufficient family organization or planning; insufficient finances; unfamiliarity with neighborhood resources; impaired cognitive or emotional functioning; lack of knowledge; lack of role modeling; inadequate support system.

☞ *See also* Risk for Injury.

HOPELESSNESS

Definition: A subjective state in which an individual sees limited or no alternatives or personal choices available and is unable to mobilize energy on own behalf.

Defining Characteristics: *Major*—Passivity, decreased verbalization; decreased affect; verbal cues (despondent content, "I can't," sighing). *Minor*—Lack of initiative; decreased response to stimuli; decreased affect; turning away from speaker; closing eyes; shrugging in response to speaker; decreased appetite; increased/decreased sleep; lack of involvement in care/passively allowing care.

Related Factors: Prolonged activity restriction creating isolation; failing or deteriorating physiological condition; long-term stress; abandonment; lost belief in transcendent values/God.

Author's Note: Differentiate between this label and Powerlessness. Hopelessness implies that the person believes there *is* no solution to his problem ("no way out"). In Powerlessness, the person may know of a solution to his problem, but believe it is beyond his control to achieve the solution.

HYPERTHERMIA

Definition: A state in which an individual's body temperature is elevated above his/her normal range.

Defining Characteristics: *Major*—Increase in body temperature above normal range. *Minor*—Flushed skin, warm to touch, increased respiratory rate, tachycardia, seizures/convulsions.

Related Factors: Exposure to hot environment; vigorous activity; medications/anesthesia; inappropriate clothing; increased metabolic rate; illness or trauma; dehydration; inability or decreased ability to perspire.

Author's Note: If written as risk nursing diagnosis, the nurse can prescribe interventions to prevent and monitor for development of this condition. As an actual diagnosis, it presents difficulties. For many patients, an elevated temperature is not a problem, but merely a symptom of a disease process, which is treated by a medication such as acetaminophen or aspirin. Many (maybe most) hyperthermias require no independent nursing actions. Mild sustained elevation or reduction of body temperature because of external factors (*actual* Hyper- or Hypothermia) can be treated by nursing interventions such as adding or removing clothing. However, severe Hyper- or Hypothermia is a life-threatening condition requiring both medical and nursing intervention; it would be a collaborative problem, not a nursing diagnosis.

☞ *See also* Risk for Altered Body Temperature, Ineffective Thermoregulation.

HYPOTHERMIA

Definition: The state in which the individual's temperature is reduced below normal range.

Defining Characteristics: *Major*—Reduction in body temperature below normal range; shivering (mild); cool skin; pallor (moderate). *Minor*—Slow capillary refill; tachycardia; cyanotic nail beds; hypertension; piloerection.

Related Factors: Exposure to cool or cold environment; illness or trauma; damage to hypothalamus; inability or decreased ability to shiver; malnutrition; inadequate clothing; consumption of alcohol; medications causing vasodilation; evaporation from skin in cool environment; decreased metabolic rate, inactivity; aging.

Author's Note: *See* Hyperthermia note.
☛ *See also* Risk for Altered Body Temperature, Ineffective Thermoregulation.

IDENTITY DISTURBANCE, PERSONAL

(*see* Personal Identity Disturbance)

INCONTINENCE, BOWEL

Definition: A state in which an individual experiences a change in normal bowel habits characterized by involuntary passage of stool.

Defining Characteristics: Involuntary passage of stool.
Related Factors: To be developed.
☛ Discriminate between this label and Diarrhea.

INCONTINENCE, FUNCTIONAL (URINARY)

Definition: The state in which an individual experiences an involuntary, unpredictable passage of urine.

Defining Characteristics: *Major*—Urge to void or bladder contractions sufficiently strong to result in loss of urine before reaching an appropriate receptacle.
Related Factors: Altered environment; sensory, cognitive, or mobility deficits.
☛ *See also* Reflex Incontinence, Stress Incontinence, Total Incontinence, Urge Incontinence, and Altered Patterns of Urinary Elimination.

INCONTINENCE, REFLEX (URINARY)

Definition: The state in which an individual experiences an involuntary loss of urine, occurring at somewhat predictable intervals when a specific bladder volume is reached.

Defining Characteristics: *Major*—No awareness of bladder filling; no urge to void or feelings of bladder fullness; uninhibited bladder contraction/spasm at regular intervals.
Related Factors: Neurological impairment (e.g., spinal cord lesion that interferes with conduction of cerebral messages above the level of the reflex arc).
☛ *See also* Functional Incontinence, Stress Incontinence, Total Incontinence, Urge Incontinence, and Altered Patterns of Urinary Elimination.

INCONTINENCE, STRESS (URINARY)

Definition: The state in which an individual experiences a loss of urine of less than 50 mL occurring with increased abdominal pressure.

Defining Characteristics: *Major*—Reported or observed dribbling with increased abdominal pressure. *Minor*—Urinary urgency; urinary frequency (more often than every 2 hours).
Related Factors: Degenerative changes in pelvic muscles and structural supports associated with increased age; high intra-abdominal pressure (e.g., obesity, gravid uterus); incompetent bladder outlet; overdistention between voidings; weak pelvic muscles and pelvic supports.
☛ *See also* Functional Incontinence, Total Incontinence, Reflex Incontinence, Urge Incontinence, and Altered Patterns of Urinary Elimination.

INCONTINENCE, TOTAL (URINARY)

Definition: The state in which an individual experiences a continuous and unpredictable loss of urine.

Defining Characteristics: *Major*—Constant flow of urine occurs at unpredictable times without distention or uninhibited bladder contractions/spasm; unsuccessful incontinence refractory treatments; nocturia. *Minor*—Lack of perineal or bladder-filling awareness; unawareness of incontinence.
Related Factors: Neuropathy preventing transmission of reflex indicating bladder fullness; neurological dysfunction causing triggering of micturition at unpredictable times; independent contraction of detrusor reflex due to surgery; trauma or disease affecting spinal cord nerves; anatomic (fistula).
☛ *See also* Functional Incontinence, Stress Incontinence, Reflex Incontinence, Urge Incontinence, and Altered Patterns of Urinary Elimination.

INCONTINENCE, URGE (URINARY)

Definition: The state in which an individual experiences involuntary passage of urine occurring soon after a strong sense of urgency to void.

Defining Characteristics: *Major*—Urinary urgency; frequency (voiding more often than every 2 hours); bladder contracture/spasm. *Minor*—Nocturia (more than two times per night); voiding in small amounts (less than 100 mL) or in large amounts (more than 550 mL); inability to reach toilet in time.

Related Factors: Decreased bladder capacity (e.g., history of PID, abdominal surgeries, indwelling urinary catheter); irritation of bladder stretch receptors causing spasm (e.g., bladder infection); alcohol; caffeine; increased fluids; increased urine concentration; overdistention of bladder.

☞ *See also* Functional Incontinence, Reflex Incontinence, Stress Incontinence, Total Incontinence, and Altered Patterns of Urinary Elimination.

INDIVIDUAL COPING, INEFFECTIVE

(*see* Coping, Ineffective Individual)

INFANT FEEDING PATTERN, INEFFECTIVE

Definition: A state in which an infant demonstrates an impaired ability to suck or coordinate the suck-swallow response.

Defining Characteristics: Inability to coordinate sucking, swallowing, breathing; inability to initiate or sustain an effective suck.

Related Factors: Anatomical abnormalities; neurological impairment/delay; oral hypersensitivity; prematurity; prolonged NPO.

Author's Note: This label describes a baby with sucking or swallowing difficulties. It focuses on the nutritional needs of the infant. The goal of nursing activities is to prevent weight loss or promote weight gain. Discriminate among this label and the suggested alternative diagnoses. The following are defining characteristics that can be used to differentiate between these related diagnostic labels.

	Key Defining Characteristics
Ineffective Breastfeeding	Dissatisfaction with feeding process
Ineffective Infant Feeding Pattern	Inability of infant to suck or poorly coordinated suck-swallow response
Interrupted Breastfeeding	Mother wishes to maintain lactation; unable to put baby to breast for some feedings (e.g., because of working)

☞ Breastfeeding, Ineffective; Breastfeeding, Interrupted; Nutrition, Altered: Less Than Body Requirements

INFECTION, RISK FOR

Definition: The state in which an individual is at increased risk for being invaded by pathogenic organisms.

Defining Characteristics: Presence of risk factors such as inadequate primary defenses (broken skin, traumatized tissue, decrease in ciliary action, stasis of body fluids, change in pH secretions, altered peristalsis); inadequate secondary defenses (e.g., decreased hemoglobin, leukopenia, suppressed inflammatory response) and immunosuppression; inadequate acquired immunity; tissue destruction and increased environmental exposure; chronic disease; invasive procedures; malnutrition; pharmaceutical agents; trauma; rupture of amniotic membranes; insufficient knowledge to avoid exposure to pathogens.

Related Factors: *See* risk factors above.

☞ *See also* Altered Protection.

INJURY, RISK FOR

Definition: A state in which the individual is at risk of injury as a result of environmental conditions interacting with the individual's adaptive and defensive resources.

Defining Characteristics: Presence of risk factors such as the following. *Internal*—biochemical, regulatory function (sensory dysfunction, integrative dysfunction, effector dysfunction, tissue hypoxia); malnutrition; immune/autoimmune; abnormal blood profile (leukocytosis/leukopenia; altered clotting factors; thrombocytopenia; sickle cell, Thalassemia; decreased hemoglobin); physical (broken skin, altered mobility); developmental age (physiological, psychosocial); psychological (affective, orientation). *External*—biological (immunization level of community, microorganism); chemical (pollutants, poisons, drugs, pharmaceutical agents, alcohol, caffeine, nicotine, preservative, cosmetics and dyes); nutrients (vitamins, food types); physical (design, structure, and arrangement of community, building, and/or equipment); mode of transport/transportation; people/provider (nosocomial agents, staffing patterns, cognitive, affective, and psychomotor factors).

Related Factors: *See* risk factors above.

Author's Note: This is a broad title that includes internal risk factors such as altered clotting factors and decreased hemoglobin. NANDA has not identified any critical defining characteristics for this title, so it is important to identify only those clients who are at risk for this problem. Everyone has at least some risk for accidents and injury, but the label should be used only for those who require nursing intervention to prevent injury.

This label consists of five subcategories that describe *injury* more specifically: Risk for Suffocation, Poisoning, Trauma, Aspiration, and Disuse Syndrome. When possible, use these more specific labels instead of Risk for Injury, because they provide clearer direction for nursing care. None of the subcategories needs further specification except Risk for Trauma, which includes wounds, burns, and fractures, and an unlimited number of risk factors.

☞ Related labels: Risk for Aspiration, Poisoning, Suffocation, Trauma, Infection, or Altered Protection.

KNOWLEDGE DEFICIT (SPECIFY)

Definition: Absence or deficiency of cognitive information related to specific topic.

Defining Characteristics: Verbalization of the problem; inaccurate follow-through of instruction; inaccurate performance of test; inappropriate or exaggerated behaviors (e.g., hysterical, hostile, agitated, apathetic).

Related Factors: Lack of exposure; lack of recall; information misinterpretation; cognitive limitation; lack of interest in learning; unfamiliarity with information resources.

Author's Note: Author does not recommend use of this label, except as an etiology. Although this label was accepted in 1980, NANDA has not yet developed a definition or critical defining characteristics for it. At least two studies show Knowledge Deficit is one of the diagnoses most frequently used by nurses (Gordon, 1985; Lambert and Jones, 1989). This seems to be due at least in part to premature diagnosing: it is easy to recognize a knowledge deficit, label it as a problem, and not look beyond that to the human *response* to the lack of knowledge. It also happens because of the mistaken belief that information-giving is effective in changing human behavior.

For the following reasons, Knowledge Deficit should not, as a rule, be used to label the problem side of your diagnostic statement:

1. Knowledge Deficit is not truly a human response. *Response* suggests a behavior or action; Knowledge Deficit is simply a state of being.

2. Knowledge Deficit does not necessarily describe a *health* state.

3. Knowledge Deficit does not necessarily describe a *problem*. Nursing diagnoses should reflect altered functioning; but Knowledge Deficit simply means the person does not have some needed knowledge, not that his functioning is changed as a result of that. A client might not have any knowledge at all about the Food Guide Pyramid; but that does not necessarily mean he has impaired nutritional status.

Knowledge Deficit can contribute to any number of responses, including Anxiety, Altered Parenting, Self-Care Deficit, or Impaired Coping. Therefore, it may be used effectively as the etiology of a nursing diagnosis.

Examples: Risk for Injury (Trauma) r/t lack of knowledge of proper application of seat-belts when pregnant

Anxiety r/t lack of knowledge of procedures involved in bone marrow aspiration.

If Knowledge Deficit is used as a problem, the goal must be "Patient will acquire knowledge about . . ." This causes the nurse to focus on giving information rather than on the behaviors caused by the patient's lack of knowledge. Using Knowledge Deficit as a problem label reinforces the belief that giving information will change behavior and solve the problem. On the other hand, when Knowledge Deficit is used as the etiology, it focuses attention on behaviors that indicate self-doubt, decisional conflict, anxiety, and so on. Note the different nursing care suggested by these statements:

Knowledge Deficit (Bone Marrow Aspiration) r/t lack of prior experience

Anxiety r/t knowledge deficit (bone marrow aspiration)

Patient teaching is an important intervention for most patients and for all the diagnostic labels (e.g., Constipation, Ineffective Breastfeeding, Altered Nutrition). It is not necessary, or even desirable, to have a Knowledge/Deficit diagnosis on every patient's care plan. You should simply include teaching as one of the nursing interventions for the other diagnoses you have made.

Some patients, such as a newly diagnosed diabetic, require a great deal of teaching in order to acquire necessary self-care skills. Such special teaching plans should be a part of the routine care on standardized care plans for these patients and should not require an individualized diagnosis. However, if the agency does not use standardized care plans or protocols, you would need to write individualized orders for the teaching. If so, the best approach is still to use Knowledge Deficit as the etiology rather than the problem. If the patient does not have the necessary knowledge, she may not be able to manage her own health-care needs. The human response is not lack of knowledge, but risk for decreased ability for maintaining health.

Example: Risk for Altered Health Maintenance (Diabetes Management) r/t knowledge deficit (medication, diet, exercise, and skin care) r/t new diagnosis

Knowledge Deficit, if used, should describe conditions in which the patient needs new or additional knowledge. It should not be used for problems involving the patient's ability to learn (as in Knowledge Deficit r/t severe anxiety about outcome of surgery). Rakel and Bulechek (1990) propose a diagnosis of "Situational Learning Disability: Impaired Ability to Learn" or "Situational Learning Disability: Lack of Motivation to Learn" for such conditions; however, these are not yet NANDA-approved labels.

LOW SELF-ESTEEM, CHRONIC
(*see* Self-Esteem, Chronic Low)

LOW SELF-ESTEEM, SITUATIONAL
(*see* Self-Esteem, Situational Low)

MOBILITY, IMPAIRED PHYSICAL
Definition: A state in which the individual experiences a limitation of ability for independent physical movement.

Defining Characteristics: Inability to purposefully move within the physical environment, including bed mobility, transfer, and ambulation; reluctance to attempt movement; limited range of motion; decreased muscle strength, control, and/or mass; imposed restrictions of movement, including mechanical, medical protocol; impaired coordination.

Related Factors: Intolerance to activity/decreased strength and endurance; pain/discomfort; perceptual/cognitive impairment; neuromuscular impairment; musculoskeletal impairment; depression/severe anxiety.

Suggested Functional-Level Classification:

   0 = Completely independent
   1 = Requires use of equipment or device
   2 = Requires help from another person for assistance, supervision, or teaching.
   3 = Requires help from another person and equipment or device.
   4 = Dependent; does not participate in activity.

The preceding code is adapted from E. Jones et al., *Patient Classification for Long-Term Care: Users' Manual,* HEW, Publication No. HRA-74-3107, November 1974, as quoted in NANDA Taxonomy I—Revised, 1990.

Author's Note: Use this label for individuals with limited ability for independent physical movement, such as decreased ability to move arms or legs or generalized muscle weakness, when nursing interventions will focus on restoring mobility and function or preventing further deterioration.

> *Example:* Impaired Physical Mobility r/t ineffective management of chronic pain 2° rheumatoid arthritis

Do not use Impaired Physical Mobility to describe temporary immobility that cannot be changed by the nurse (e.g., traction, prescribed bedrest, or permanent paralysis). It can, in these and many other instances, be used effectively as the etiology of other problems.

> *Examples:* Impaired Tissue Integrity (Decubitis Ulcer) r/t impaired physical mobility +4
>
> Diversional Activity Deficit r/t prescribed bedrest

☛ *See also* Risk for Disuse Syndrome, Risk for Injury, and Self-Care Deficit.

MUCOUS MEMBRANE, ALTERED ORAL
(*see* Oral Mucous Membrane, Altered)

NONCOMPLIANCE (SPECIFY)
Definition: A person's informed decision not to adhere to a therapeutic recommendation.

Defining Characteristics: Critical—Behavior indicative of failure to adhere (by direct observation or by statements of patient or significant others). *Other*—Objective tests (physiological measures, detection of markers); evidence of development of complications; evidence of exacerbation of symptoms; failure to keep appointments; failure to progress.

Related Factors: Patient value system: health beliefs, cultural influences, spiritual values; client-provider relationships.

Author's Note: According to NANDA, Noncompliance should be diagnosed when a client makes an informed decision *not* to adhere to a therapeutic recommendation; for instance, when a medication has unpleasant side effects. Nursing intervention might then be directed at convincing the client of the value of continuing with the therapy, but the nurse should balance this with respect for the client's autonomy when a truly informed decision has been made. Remember that a decision to refuse therapy can be as rational as a decision to have therapy.

> *Example:* Noncompliance with Low-Calorie Diet r/t desire not to change eating habits A.M.B. "I realize being overweight is bad for my heart, but I'm far too old to change my ways. If eating what I like means I don't live as long, that's okay; these last few years won't be much fun anyway if I have to eat boiled eggs and lettuce."

The client in the above example knows the relationship between calories, obesity, and heart problems and has *chosen* not to comply with the prescribed diet. It is not clear how the nurse should intervene in this type of diagnosis.

You could try to persuade the client that she may enjoy life even more if she is thin, or that low-calorie foods can taste just as good as her usual diet; however, it may be that neither of these is true.

Gordon's (1987) definition is more useful. She defines Noncompliance as failure to adhere to a therapeutic recommendation after have made an informed decision *to* do so, and after expressing intention to do so. If the client is informed and *intends* to follow instructions, then nursing intervention can be directed at finding and removing the factors that keep him from doing so. In the following example, the client would like to comply with her diet, but situational factors are making it difficult. This diagnosis does suggest nursing intervention.

> ***Example:*** Noncompliance with Low-Calorie Diet r/t inconvenience of preparing special foods A.M.B. "My husband doesn't need to lose weight, and he loves fried food and pastries. He just won't eat the diet foods, and I really don't have time to cook one meal for myself and one for the rest of the family."

Following is a comparison of the NANDA and Gordon definitions of Noncompliance:

NANDA Definition of Noncompliance
    Client has the necessary information
    Client chooses not to comply
Gordon's Definition of Noncompliance
    Client has the necessary information
    Client has said he intends to comply
    Does not comply

Noncompliance should not be used in cases where the client is unable to follow instructions (e.g., too weak, cognitive disability) or lacks necessary information. If lack of ability or information is causing the noncompliance, Altered Health Maintenance is preferred.

Some nurses feel Noncompliance has a negative connotation. When using this label, be sure to express the etiology in neutral, nonjudgmental terms. You might prefer to use the term Nonadherence (Geissler, 1991), although it is not a NANDA-approved label.
☛ *See* Altered Health Maintenance.

NUTRITION, ALTERED: LESS THAN BODY REQUIREMENTS

Definition: The state in which an individual experiences an intake of nutrients insufficient to meet metabolic needs.

Defining Characteristics: Loss of weight with adequate food intake; body weight 20% or more under ideal; reported inadequate food intake less than recommended daily allowance; weakness of muscles required for swallowing or mastication; reported or evidence of lack of food; aversion to eating; reported altered taste sensation; satiety immediately after ingesting food; abdominal pain with or without pathology; sore, inflamed buccal cavity; capillary fragility; abdominal cramping; diarrhea and/or steatorrhea; hyperactive bowel sounds; lack of interest in food; perceived inability to ingest food; pale conjunctival and mucous membranes; poor muscle tone; excessive loss of hair; lack of information, misinformation; misconceptions.

Related Factors: Inability to ingest or digest food or absorb nutrients due to biological, psychological, or economic factors.

Author's Note: Use this label for clients who are able to eat, but unable to ingest, digest, or absorb nutrients adequate to meet metabolic needs. Inadequate ingestion might occur because of decreased appetite, nausea, being too poor to buy food, or any number of situations. Examples of clients unable to digest food or absorb particular nutrients are those with allergies, diarrhea, lactose intolerance, or poorly fitting dentures. NANDA does not specify which defining characteristics must be present in order to use this label. The author recommends using this label only if one of the following cues is present:

> Body weight 20% under ideal
> Observed or reported food intake less than recommended daily allowance (RDA)—either total calories or specific nutrients
> Observed or reported food intake less than metabolic needs—either total calories or specific nutrients
> Weight loss with adequate food intake

Do not use this label routinely for persons who are NPO or for those completely unable to ingest food for other reasons (e.g., unconscious patients). Nurses cannot prescribe independent nursing interventions for a diagnosis such as Altered Nutrition: Less Than Body Requirements r/t NPO—they cannot give the missing nutrients, and they cannot change the NPO order. Additionally, the patient is often NPO for only a short time before and after surgery; thus, any lack of nutrients is temporary and is resolved without nursing intervention. Long-term NPO status is a risk factor for other nursing diagnoses, such as Risk for Fluid Volume Deficit or Risk for Altered Oral Mucous Membrane, and for collaborative problems such as Potential Electrolyte Imbalance.

The client can have a total nutritional deficit, or she might be deficient in only one nutrient. When the deficit is less than total, it should be specified as follows:

> ***Example:*** Altered Nutrition: Less Than Body Requirements *for Protein* r/t lack of knowledge of Food Guide Pyramid and limited budget for food

NUTRITION, ALTERED: MORE THAN BODY REQUIREMENTS

Definition: The state in which an individual is experiencing an intake of nutrients that exceeds metabolic needs.

Defining Characteristics: Weight 10% over ideal for height and frame; sedentary activity level; reported or observed dysfunctional eating pattern: pairing food with other activities; concentrating food intake at the end of day; eating in response to external cues such as time of day, social situation; eating in response to internal cues other than hunger (e.g., anxiety). **Critical**—Weight 20% over ideal for height and frame; triceps skin fold greater than 15 mm in men, 25 mm in women.

Related Factors: Excessive intake in relation to metabolic need.

NUTRITION, ALTERED: POTENTIAL FOR MORE THAN BODY REQUIREMENTS

Definition: The state in which an individual is at risk of experiencing an intake of nutrients that exceeds metabolic needs.

Defining Characteristics: Presence of risk factors such as: Reported use of solid food as major food source before 5 months of age; observed use of food as reward or comfort measure; reported or observed higher baseline weight at beginning of each pregnancy; dysfunctional eating patterns: pairing food with other activities; concentrating food intake at end of day; eating in response to external cues such as time of day, social situation; eating in response to internal cues other than hunger, such as anxiety. **Critical**—Reported or observed obesity in one or both parents; rapid transition across growth percentiles in infants or children.

Related Factors: *See* risk factors above.

ORAL MUCOUS MEMBRANE, ALTERED

Definition: The state in which an individual experiences disruptions in the tissue layers of the oral cavity.

Defining Characteristics: Oral pain/discomfort; coated tongue; xerostomia (dry mouth); stomatitis; oral lesions or ulcers; lack of or decreased salivation; leukoplakia; edema; hyperemia; oral plaque; desquamation; vesicles; hemorrhagic gingivitis, carious teeth, halitosis.

Related Factors: Pathological conditions—oral cavity (radiation to head or neck); dehydration; trauma (chemical, e.g., acidic foods, drugs, noxious agents, alcohol; mechanical, e.g., ill-fitting dentures, braces, endotracheal/nasogastric tubes, surgery in oral cavity); NPO for more than 24 hours; ineffective oral hygiene; mouth breathing; malnutrition; infection; lack of or decreased salivation; medication.

☛ *See also* Impaired Tissue Integrity.

PAIN

Definition: A state in which an individual experiences and reports the presence of severe discomfort or an uncomfortable sensation.

Defining Characteristics: *Subjective*—Communication (verbal or coded) of pain descriptors. *Objective*—Guarding behavior, protective; self-focusing; narrowed focus (altered time perception, withdrawal from social contact, impaired thought process); distraction behavior (moaning, crying, pacing, seeking out other people and/or activities; restlessness); facial mask of pain (eyes lack luster, "beaten look," fixed or scattered movement, grimace); alteration in muscle tone (may span from listless to rigid); autonomic responses not seen in chronic stable pain (diaphoresis, blood pressure and pulse change, pupillary dilation, increased or decreased respiratory rate).

Related Factors: Injury agents (biological, chemical, physical, psychological).

Author's Note: There are no critical defining characteristics, but Pain can be diagnosed on the patient's verbal report alone, since that is sometimes the only sign of pain. None of the other defining characteristics taken alone would be sufficient to diagnose Pain. The related factors that NANDA lists, injury agents (biological, chemical, physical, psychological), indicate that a client can suffer both physical and psychological pain. The diagnosis is more useful if you use qualifiers to indicate the severity, location, and nature of the pain.

> **Examples:** Severe, stabbing chest **Pain** r/t fractured ribs
>
> Mild frontal **headache** r/t sinus congestion
>
> Moderate chronic **Pain** in knee joints (aching) r/t exercise 2° arthritis

It is important to differentiate between Pain and Chronic Pain because the nursing focus is different for each. Acute Pain, such as postoperative incision pain, is usually a collaborative problem that is managed primarily by administering narcotic analgesics. There are a few helpful independent nursing interventions, such as supporting the client during ambulation or teaching the client to splint the incision while moving about, but these alone would not provide adequate pain relief. The nurse can take a more active role in teaching the client self-management of Chronic Pain. When Pain is acute or caused by a stressor that is not amenable to nursing intervention (e.g., a surgical incision), you may prefer to use it as an etiology rather than a problem.

> *Examples:* Ineffective Airway Clearance r/t weak cough r/t **pain** 2° chest incision
>
> Risk for Disuse Syndrome r/t **severe pain** 2° metastasized cancer
>
> Sexual Dysfunction r/t partner's **severe chronic pain** 2° arthritis
>
> Sleep-Pattern Disturbance r/t **aching pain** in legs

☞ *See also* Pain, Chronic.

PAIN, CHRONIC
Definition: A state in which the individual experiences pain that continues for more than 6 months in duration.

Defining Characteristics: *Major*—Verbal report or observed evidence of pain experienced for more than 6 months. *Minor*—Fear of reinjury; physical and social withdrawal; altered ability to continue previous activities; anorexia; weight changes; changes in sleep patterns; facial mask; guarded movement.
Related Factors: Chronic physical-psychosocial disability.
☞ *See also* Pain.

PARENTAL ROLE CONFLICT
Definition: The state in which a parent experiences role confusion and conflict in response to crisis.

Defining Characteristics: *Major*—Parent(s) express(es) concerns/feelings of inadequacy to provide for child's physical and emotional needs during hospitalization or in the home; demonstrated disruption in caretaking routines; parent(s) express(es) concerns about changes in parental role, family functioning, communication, or health. *Minor*—Expresses concern about perceived loss of control over decisions relating to the child; reluctant to participate in usual caretaking activities even with encouragement and support; verbalizes, demonstrates feelings of guilt, anger, fear, anxiety and/or frustrations about effect of child's illness on family process.
Related Factors: Separation from child due to chronic illness; intimidation with invasive or restrictive modalities (e.g., isolation, intubation), specialized care centers, policies; home care of a child with special needs (e.g., apnea monitoring, postural drainage, hyperalimentation); change in marital status; interruptions of family life due to home-care regimen (treatments, caregivers, lack of respite).

Author's Note: This label should be used when a situation, such as the child's illness, causes unsatisfactory role performance by previously effective parents.
☞ *See also* Altered Parenting, Risk for Altered Parenting, Altered Family Processes.

PARENTING, ALTERED
(It is important to state as a preface to this diagnosis that adjustment to parenting in general is a normal maturational process that elicits nursing behaviors of prevention of potential problems and health promotion.)
Definition: The state in which a nurturing figure(s) experience(s) an inability to create an environment that promotes the optimum growth and development of another human being.

Defining Characteristics: Critical—Inattentive to infant/child needs; inappropriate caretaking behavior (toilet training, sleep/rest, feeding); history of child abuse or abandonment by primary caretaker. *Other*—Abandonment; runaway; verbalization, cannot control child; incidence of physical and psychological trauma; lack of parental attachment behaviors; inappropriate visual, tactile, auditory stimulation; negative identification of infant/child's characteristics; negative attachment of meanings to infant/child's characteristics; constant verbalization of disappointment in gender or physical characteristics of the infant/child; verbalization of resentment towards the infant/child; verbalization of role inadequacy; verbal disgust at body functions of infant/child; noncompliance with health appointments for self and/or infant/child; inappropriate or inconsistent discipline practices; frequent accidents; frequent illness; growth and development lag in the child; verbalizes desire to have child call him/herself by first name versus traditional cultural tendencies; child receives care from multiple caretakers without consideration for the needs of the infant/child; compulsively seeking role approval from others.
Related Factors: Lack of available role model; ineffective role model; physical and psychosocial abuse of nurturing figure; lack of support between/from significant other(s); unmet social/emotional maturation needs of parenting figures; interruption in bonding process (i.e., maternal, paternal, other); unrealistic expectation for self, infant, partner; perceived threat to own survival, physical and emotional; mental and/or physical illness; presence of stress (financial, legal, recent crisis, cultural move); lack of knowledge; limited cognitive functioning; lack of role identity; lack of or inappropriate response of child to relationship; multiple pregnancies.
Author's Note: This label represents a less healthy level of functioning than Parental Role Conflict.

☛ *See also* Risk for Altered Parenting, Altered Family Processes, Ineffective Family Coping, and Parental Role Conflict.

PARENTING, RISK FOR ALTERED

(It is important to state as a preface to this diagnosis that adjustment to parenting in general is a normal maturational process that elicits nursing behaviors of prevention of potential problems and health promotion.)

Definition: The state in which a nurturing figure(s) is (are) at risk to experience an inability to create an environment that promotes the optimum growth and development of another human being.

Defining Characteristics: Critical—Inattentive to infant/child needs; inappropriate caretaking behavior (toilet training, sleep/rest, feeding); history of child abuse or abandonment by primary caretaker. *Other*—Lack of parental attachment behaviors; inappropriate visual, tactile, auditory stimulation; negative identification of infant/child's characteristics; negative attachment of meanings to infant/child's characteristics; constant verbalization of disappointment in gender or physical characteristics of the infant/child; verbalization of resentment towards the infant/child; verbalization of role inadequacy; verbal disgust at body functions of infant/child; noncompliance with health appointments for self and/or infant/child; inappropriate or inconsistent discipline practices; frequent accidents; frequent illness; growth and development lag in the child; verbalizes desire to have child call him/herself by first name versus traditional cultural tendencies; child receives care from multiple caretakers without consideration for the needs of the infant/child; compulsively seeking role approval from others.

Related Factors: Lack of available role model; ineffective role model; physical and psychosocial abuse of nurturing figure; lack of support between/from significant other(s); unmet social/emotional maturation needs of parenting figures; interruption in bonding process (i.e., maternal, paternal, other); unrealistic expectation for self, infant, partner; perceived threat to own survival, physical and emotional; mental and/or physical illness; presence of stress (financial, legal, recent crisis, cultural move); lack of knowledge; limited cognitive functioning; lack of role identity; lack of or inappropriate response of child to relationship; multiple pregnancies.

Author's Note: Critical Defining Characteristics are identical to *actual* Altered Parenting. If they are present, use Altered Parenting instead of this diagnosis.

☛ *See also* Altered Parenting, Altered Family Processes, Ineffective Family Coping, and Parental Role Conflict.

PERIPHERAL NEUROVASCULAR DYSFUNCTION: RISK FOR

Definition: A state in which an individual is at risk of experiencing a disruption in circulation, sensation, or motion of an extremity.

Defining Characteristics: Presence of risk factors such as: Burns; fractures; immobilization; mechanical compression, e.g., tourniquet, cast, brace, dressing, or restraint; orthopedic surgery; trauma; vascular obstruction.

Related/Risk Factors: *See* Defining Characteristics.

Author's Note: Use this label for situations nurses can prevent by reducing or eliminating causative factors (e.g., Risk for Peripheral Neurovascular Dysfunction r/t compression from restraints). For situations requiring medical treatment (e.g., thrombophlebitis), use a collaborative problem such as Potential Complication of Thrombophlebitis in Left Leg: Peripheral Neurovascular Dysfunction.

PERSONAL IDENTITY DISTURBANCE

Definition: Inability to distinguish between self and nonself.

Defining Characteristics: To be developed.

PHYSICAL MOBILITY, IMPAIRED

(*see* Mobility, Impaired Physical)

POISONING, RISK FOR

Definition: Accentuated risk of accidental exposure to or ingestion of drugs or dangerous products in doses sufficient to cause poisoning.

Defining Characteristics: Presence of risk factors such as the following. *Internal* (*individual*)—Reduced vision; verbalization of occupational setting without adequate safeguards; lack of safety or drug education; lack of proper precaution; cognitive or emotional difficulties; insufficient finances. *External* (*environmental*)—Large supplies of drugs in house; medicines stored in unlocked cabinets accessible to children or confused persons; availability of illicit drugs potentially contaminated by poisonous additives; flaking, peeling paint or plaster in presence of young children; chemical contamination of food and water; unprotected contact with heavy metals or chemicals; paint, lacquer, etc., in poorly ventilated areas or without effective protection; presence of poisonous vegetation; presence of atmospheric pollutants.

Related Factors: *See* risk factors above.

Author's Note: Use the most specific label for which defining characteristics are present.

☛ *See* Risk for Injury, Impaired Home Maintenance Management, and Risk for Trauma.

POST-TRAUMA RESPONSE

Definition: The state of an individual experiencing a sustained painful response to an overwhelming traumatic event(s).

Defining Characteristics: *Major*—Reexperience of the traumatic event, which may be identified in cognitive, affective, and/or sensory motor activities (flashbacks, intrusive thoughts, repetitive dreams or nightmares, excessive verbalization of the traumatic event, verbalization of survival guilt or guilt about behavior required for survival). *Minor*—Psychic/emotional numbness (impaired interpretation of reality, confusion, dissociation or amnesia, vagueness about traumatic event, constricted affect); altered lifestyle (self-destructiveness, such as substance abuse, suicide attempt, or other acting-out behavior, difficulty with interpersonal relationship, development of phobia regarding trauma, poor impulse control/irritability and explosiveness).

Related Factors: Disasters, wars, epidemics, rape, assault, torture, catastrophic illness or accident.

☛ *See also* Rape-Trauma Syndrome.

POWERLESSNESS

Definition: Perception that one's own action will not significantly affect an outcome; a perceived lack of control over a current situation or immediate happening.

Defining Characteristics: *Severe*—Verbal expressions of having no control or influence over situation; verbal expressions of having no control or influence over outcome; verbal expressions of having no control over self-care; depression over physical deterioration that occurs despite patient compliance with regimens; apathy. *Moderate*—Nonparticipation in care or decision making when opportunities are provided; expressions of dissatisfaction and frustration over inability to perform previous tasks and/or activities; does not monitor progress; expression of doubt regarding role performance; reluctance to express true feelings; fearing alienation from caregivers; passivity; inability to seek information regarding care; dependence on others that may result in irritability, resentment, anger, and guilt; does not defend self-care practices when challenged. *Low*—Expressions of uncertainty about fluctuating energy levels; passivity.

Related Factors: Health-care environment; interpersonal interaction; illness-related regimen; lifestyle of helplessness.

Author's Note: Differentiate between this label and Hopelessness. Hopelessness implies that the person believes there *is* no solution to his problem ("no way out"). In Powerlessness, the person may know of a solution to his problem, but believe it is beyond his control to achieve the solution.

☛ *See also* Risk for Disuse Syndrome.

PROTECTION, ALTERED

Definition: The state in which an individual experiences a decrease in the ability to guard the self from internal or external threats such as illness or injury.

Defining Characteristics: *Major*—Deficient immunity; impaired healing; altered clotting; maladaptive stress response; neuro-sensory alteration. *Minor*—Chilling; perspiring; dyspnea; cough; itching; restlessness; insomnia; fatigue; anorexia; weakness; immobility; disorientation; pressure sores.

Related Factors: Extremes of age; inadequate nutrition; alcohol abuse; abnormal blood profiles (leukopenia, thrombocytopenia, anemia, coagulation); drug therapies (antineoplastic, corticosteroid, immune, anticoagulant, thrombolytic); treatments (surgery, radiation), and diseases such as cancer and immune disorders.

Author's Note: When possible, use a more specific label, such as Risk for Infection, Impaired Skin Integrity, Impaired Tissue Integrity, Altered Oral Mucous Membrane, or Fatigue.

☛ *See also* Risk for Injury.

RAPE-TRAUMA SYNDROME

Definition: Forced, violent sexual penetration against the victim's will and consent. The trauma syndrome that develops from this attack or attempted attack includes an acute phase of disorganization of the victim's lifestyle and a long-term process of reorganization of lifestyle.

Defining Characteristics: *Acute Phase*—Emotional reactions (anger, embarrassment, fear of physical violence and death, humiliation, revenge, self-blame); multiple physical symptoms (gastrointestinal irritability, genitourinary discomfort, muscle tension, sleep-pattern disturbance). *Long-Term Phase*—Changes in lifestyle (change in residence; dealing with repetitive nightmares and phobias; seeking family support; seeking social network support).

☛ *See also* Rape-Trauma Syndrome: Compound Reaction and Rape-Trauma Syndrome: Silent Reaction.

RAPE-TRAUMA SYNDROME: COMPOUND REACTION

Definition: Forced, violent sexual penetration against the victim's will and consent. The trauma syndrome that develops from this attack or attempted attack includes an acute phase of disorganization of the victim's lifestyle and a long-term process of reorganization of lifestyle.

Defining Characteristics: *Acute Phase*—Emotional reactions (anger, embarrassment, fear of physical violence and death, humiliation, revenge, self-blame); multiple physical symptoms (gastrointestinal irritability, genitourinary discomfort, muscle tension, sleep-pattern disturbance); reactivated symptoms of such previous conditions (i.e., physical illness, psychiatric illness; reliance on alcohol and/or drugs). *Long-Term Phase*—Changes in lifestyle (change in residence; dealing with repetitive nightmares and phobias; seeking family support; seeking social network support).
☞ *See also* Rape-Trauma Syndrome and Rape-Trauma Syndrome: Silent Reaction.

RAPE-TRAUMA SYNDROME: SILENT REACTION

Definition: Forced, violent sexual penetration against the victim's will and consent. The trauma syndrome that develops from this attack or attempted attack includes an acute phase of disorganization of the victim's lifestyle and a long-term process of reorganization of lifestyle.

Defining Characteristics: Abrupt changes in relationships with men; increase in nightmares; increased anxiety during interview (i.e., blocking of associations, long periods of silence, minor stuttering, physical distress); pronounced changes in sexual behavior; no verbalization of the occurrence of rape; sudden onset of phobic reactions.
☞ *See also* Rape-Trauma Syndrome and Rape-Trauma Syndrome: Compound Reaction.

REFLEX INCONTINENCE
(*see* Incontinence, Reflex)

RELOCATION STRESS SYNDROME

Definition: Physiological and/or psychosocial disturbances as a result of transfer from one environment to another.

Defining Characteristics: *Major*—Anxiety; apprehension; increased confusion (elderly population); loneliness; change in environment/location; depression. *Minor*—Increased verbalization of needs; unfavorable comparison of post-/pretransfer staff; verbalization of being concerned/upset about transfer; verbalization of unwillingness to relocate; change in eating habits; dependency; gastrointestinal disturbances; insecurity; lack of trust; restlessness; sad affect; sleep disturbance; vigilance; weight change; withdrawal.

Related Factors: Decreased physical status; feeling of powerlessness; history and types of previous transfers; impaired psychosocial health status; lack of adequate support system; little or no preparation for the impending move; losses involved with decision to move; moderate to high degree of environmental change; past, concurrent, and recent losses.

RESPIRATORY FUNCTION
(*see* Airway Clearance, Ineffective; Breathing Patterns, Ineffective; Gas Exchange, Impaired)

ROLE CONFLICT, PARENTAL
(*see* Parental Role Conflict)

ROLE PERFORMANCE, ALTERED

Definition: Disruption in the way one perceives one's role performance.

Defining Characteristics: Change in self-perception of role; denial of role; change in others' perception of role; conflict in roles; change in physical capacity to resume role; lack of knowledge of role; change in usual patterns of responsibility.

Related Factors: To be developed.

Author's Note: This label is not well developed. When applicable, use the more specific Parental Role Conflict, Sexual Dysfunction, or Altered Family Processes. Carpenito (1993) recommends considering role-performance disruptions as the etiology of other problems, such as Self-Concept Disturbance or Risk for Impaired Home Maintenance Management.

SELF-CARE DEFICIT

Author's Note: This label describes a state in which a person experiences impaired ability to perform self-care activities. If the person is unable to perform any self-care activities, this is described as Total Self-Care Deficit. However the label is subdivided into more specific problems, each with its own critical defining characteristics, which can exist in various combinations:

    Feeding Self-Care Deficit
    Bathing/Hygiene Self-Care Deficit
    Dressing/Grooming Self-Care Deficit
    Toileting Self-Care Deficit

Self-Care Deficits are frequently caused by Activity Intolerance, Impaired Physical Mobility, Pain, Anxiety, or Perceptual or Cognitive Impairment (e.g., Feeding Self-Care Deficit +2 r/t hyperactivity). As an etiology, Self-Care Deficit can cause Depression, Fear of becoming dependent, and Powerlessness (e.g., Fear of Becoming Totally Dependent r/t Total Self-Care Deficit +2 secondary to residual weakness from CVA).

In order to promote efforts to restore functioning, classify the patient's functional level using the following scale:

0 = Completely independent
1 = Requires use of equipment or device
2 = Requires help from another person for assistance, supervision, or teaching
3 = Requires help from another person and equipment or device
4 = Dependent, does not participate in activity

This code adapted from E. Jones et al., *Patient Classification for Long-Term Care: Users' Manual,* HEW Publication No. HRA-74-3107, November 1974; as it appears in NANDA Taxonomy I—Revised, 1990.

☞ Related diagnostic labels: Activity Intolerance, Impaired Physical Mobility, Sensory/Perceptual Alterations, Altered Thought Processes. These are often etiologies of Self-Care Deficit.

SELF-CARE DEFICIT, BATHING/HYGIENE (SPECIFY LEVEL)

Definition: A state in which the individual experiences an impaired ability to perform or complete bathing/hygiene activities for self.

Defining Characteristics: Critical—Inability to wash body or body parts. *Other*—Inability to obtain or get to water source; inability to regulate temperature or flow.
Related Factors: Intolerance to activity, decreased strength and endurance; pain; discomfort; perceptual or cognitive impairment; neuromuscular impairment; musculoskeletal impairment; depression, severe anxiety.
Author's Note: Classify functional level (*see* Self-Care Deficit).

SELF-CARE DEFICIT, DRESSING/GROOMING (SPECIFY LEVEL)

Definition: A state in which the individual experiences an impaired ability to perform or complete dressing and grooming activities for self.

Defining Characteristics: Critical—Impaired ability to put on or take off necessary items of clothing. *Other*—

Impaired ability to obtain or replace articles of clothing; impaired ability to fasten clothing; inability to maintain appearance at a satisfactory level.
Related Factors: Intolerance to activity, decreased strength and endurance; pain, discomfort; perceptual or cognitive impairment; neuromuscular impairment; musculoskeletal impairment; depression, severe anxiety.
Author's Note: Classify functional level (*see* Self-Care Deficit).

SELF-CARE DEFICIT, FEEDING (SPECIFY LEVEL)

Definition: A state in which the individual experiences an impaired ability to perform or complete feeding activities for self.

Defining Characteristics: Inability to bring food from a receptacle to the mouth.
Related Factors: Intolerance to activity, decreased strength and endurance; pain, discomfort; perceptual or cognitive impairment; depression, severe anxiety.
Author's Note: Classify functional level (*see* Self-Care Deficit).

SELF-CARE DEFICIT, TOILETING (SPECIFY LEVEL)

Definition: A state in which the individual experiences an impaired ability to perform or complete toileting activities for self.

Defining Characteristics: Critical—Unable to get to toilet or commode; unable to sit on or rise from toilet or commode; unable to manipulate clothing for toileting; unable to carry out proper toilet hygiene. *Other*—Unable to flush toilet or commode.
Related Factors: Impaired transfer ability; impaired mobility status; intolerance to activity, decreased strength and endurance; pain, discomfort; perceptual impairment; depression, severe anxiety.
Author's Note: Classify functional level (*see* Self-Care Deficit).

SELF-CARE DEFICIT, TOTAL

Author's Note: Use this label when patient has a self-care deficit in all areas: bathing/hygiene, dressing/grooming, feeding, and toileting. Specify level 0–4 (*see* Self-Care Deficit).

SELF-ESTEEM, CHRONIC LOW

Definition: Long-standing negative self-evaluation/feelings about self or own capabilities.

Defining Characteristics: *Major*—Self-negating verbalization; expressions of shame/guilt; evaluates self as unable to deal with events; rationalizes away/rejects positive feedback and exaggerates negative feedback about self; hesitant to try new things/situations. *Minor*—Frequent lack of success in work or other life events; overly conforming; dependent on others' opinions; lack of eye contact; nonassertive/passive; indecisive; excessively seeks reassurance.

☛ *See also* Situational Low Self-Esteem, Self-Esteem Disturbance, Hopelessness, Powerlessness.

SELF-ESTEEM DISTURBANCE

Definition: Negative self-evaluation/feelings about self or own capabilities, which may be directly or indirectly expressed.

Defining Characteristics: Self-negating verbalization; expressions of shame/guilt; evaluates self as unable to deal with events; rationalizes away/rejects positive feedback and exaggerates negative feedback about self; hesitant to try new things/situations; denial of problems obvious to others; projection of blame/responsibility for problems; rationalizing personal failures; hypersensitive to slight or criticism; grandiosity.

Author's Note: When you have adequate supporting clinical data, use the more specific labels, such as Chronic Low Self-Esteem.

☛ *See also* Body Image Disturbance, Personal Identity Disturbance, Chronic Low Self-Esteem, Situational Low Self-Esteem, Hopelessness, and Powerlessness.

SELF-ESTEEM, SITUATIONAL LOW

Definition: Negative self-evaluation/feelings about self that develop in response to a loss or change in an individual who previously had a positive self-evaluation.

Defining Characteristics: *Major*—Episodic occurrence of negative self-appraisal in response to life events in a person with previous positive self-evaluation; verbalization of negative feelings about the self (helplessness, uselessness). *Minor*—Self-negating verbalizations; expressions of shame/guilt; evaluates self as unable to handle situations/events; difficulty making decisions.

☛ *See also* Body Image Disturbance, Personal Identity Disturbance, Chronic Low Self-Esteem, Hopelessness, and Powerlessness.

SELF-MUTILATION, RISK FOR

Definition: A state in which an individual is at high risk to perform an act on the self to injure, not kill, which produces tissue damage and possible tension relief.

Defining Characteristics: Presence of risk factors, such as: Command hallucinations; drug/alcohol abuse; dysfunctional family; feelings of depression, rejection, self-hatred, separation anxiety, guilt, and depersonalization; fluctuating emotions; inability to cope with increased psychological/physiological tension in a healthy manner; need for sensory stimuli; parental emotional deprivation.

Groups at Risk: Emotionally disturbed and/or battered children; mentally retarded and autistic children; patients in psychotic state—frequently males in young adulthood; patients with a history of self-injury; patients with Borderline Personality Disorder, especially females 16–25 years of age; patients with history of physical, emotional, or sexual abuse; patients with Multiple Personality Disorder.

Related/Risk Factors: *See* Defining Characteristics

Author's Note: Risk for Self-Mutilation is a more specific diagnosis than Risk for Self-Directed Violence, although they have some of the same defining characteristics (risk factors). Self-Directed Violence includes such actions as drug and alcohol abuse and high-risk lifestyle (e.g., driving fast), which are not included in Self-Mutilation.

☛ *See also* Suicide: Risk for; Violence, Self-Directed: Risk

SENSORY/PERCEPTUAL ALTERATIONS (SPECIFY): Auditory, Gustatory, Kinesthetic, Olfactory, Tactile, Visual

Definition: A state in which an individual experiences a change in the amount or patterning of incoming stimuli accompanied by a diminished, exaggerated, distorted, or impaired response to such stimuli.

Defining Characteristics: Disoriented in time, in place, or with persons; altered abstraction; altered conceptualization; change in problem-solving abilities; reported or measured change in sensory acuity; change in behavior pattern; anxiety; apathy; change in usual response to stimuli; indication of body-image alteration; restlessness; irritability; altered communication patterns. *Other Possible Characteristics*—Complaints of fatigue; alteration in posture; change in muscular tension; inappropriate responses; hallucinations.

Related Factors: Excessive or insufficient environmental stimuli; altered sensory reception, transmission and/or integration; chemical alterations: endogenous (electrolyte), exogenous (drugs, etc.); psychological stress.

Author's Note: This label may be more useful as the etiology of other problems. When Risk for Sensory/Perceptual Alteration exists as a result of Immobility, consider using Risk for Disuse syndrome.

When stated as a problem, the etiology is often a medical condition or pathophysiology that cannot be changed by nursing intervention. For Sensory/Perceptual Alteration (Auditory) r/t intracranial lesion, the nurse can do little to affect either the problem or the etiology. It would be better to diagnose something like Social Isolation r/t hearing loss. When possible, identify the client's specific response to the sensory/perceptual alteration.

> *Examples:* Risk for Trauma (Burns) r/t **Tactile Alteration** A.M.B. numbness in fingers
>
> Self-Care Deficit (Total) r/t **Sensory/Perceptual Alteration** (Visual) A.M.B. ability to distinguish only light and dark.

☞ *See also* Altered Thought Processes and Unilateral Neglect.

SEXUAL DYSFUNCTION

Definition: The state in which an individual experiences a change in sexual function that is viewed as unsatisfying, unrewarding, or inadequate.

Defining Characteristics: Verbalization of problem; alterations in achieving perceived sex role; actual or perceived limitation imposed by disease and/or therapy; conflicts involving values; alteration in achieving sexual satisfaction; inability to achieve desired satisfaction; seeking confirmation of desirability; alteration in relationship with significant other; change of interest in self and others.

Related Factors: Biopsychosocial alteration of sexuality: ineffectual or absent role models; physical abuse; psychosocial abuse (e.g., harmful relationships); vulnerability; values conflict; lack of privacy; lack of significant other; altered body structure or function (pregnancy, recent childbirth, drugs, surgery, anomalies, disease process, trauma, radiation); misinformation or lack of knowledge.

Author's Note: If client data does not fit defining characteristics, consider the more general label, Altered Sexuality Patterns.

SEXUALITY PATTERNS, ALTERED

Definition: The state in which an individual expresses concern regarding his/her sexuality.

Defining Characteristics: *Major*—Reported difficulties, limitations, or changes in sexual behaviors or activities.

Related Factors: Knowledge/skill deficit about alternative responses to health-related transitions; altered body function or structure, illness or medical; lack of privacy; lack of significant other; ineffective or absent role models; conflicts with sexual orientation or variant preferences; fear of pregnancy or of acquiring a sexually transmitted disease; impaired relationship with a significant other.

☞ *See also* Sexual Dysfunction, a more specific label.

SITUATIONAL LOW SELF-ESTEEM

(*see* Self-Esteem, Situational Low)

SKIN INTEGRITY, IMPAIRED

Definition: A state in which the individual's skin is adversely altered.

Defining Characteristics: Disruption of skin surface; destruction of skin layers; invasion of body structures.

Related Factors: *External (environmental)*—Hyper- or hypothermia; chemical substance; mechanical factors (shearing forces, pressure, restraint); radiation; physical immobilization; humidity. *Internal (somatic)*—Medication; altered nutritional state (obesity, emaciation); altered metabolic state; altered circulation; altered sensation; altered pigmentation; skeletal prominence; developmental factors; immunological deficit; alterations in turgor (change in elasticity).

Author's Note: Impaired Skin Integrity is rather nonspecific, even though it is at the sixth level of the taxonomy. A disruption of the skin surface might be a surgical incision, abrasion, blisters, or decubitus ulcers—to name only a few. When this label is used, the type of disruption should be specified in the problem, not the etiology. Note in the following example that dermal ulcer is a specific *type* of impaired skin integrity, not a cause of impairment.

> *Example:*
>
> *Correct:* Impaired Skin Integrity: **dermal ulcer** r/t complete immobility
>
> *Incorrect:* Impaired Skin Integrity r/t **dermal ulcer**

When an ulcer is deeper than the epidermis, use Impaired Tissue Integrity instead of Impaired Skin Integrity. Deeper ulcers may require a collaborative approach (e.g., surgical treatment).

Do not use Impaired Skin Integrity as a label for a surgical incision, since there are no independent nursing actions to treat this condition, and the condition is usually self-limiting. The usual nursing care for a surgical incision is to prevent and detect infection; therefore, a diagnosis of Risk for Infection of Surgical Incision might be used instead of Impaired Skin Integrity. (Recall, also, that high-risk problems should be diagnosed only when the client is at higher risk than the general population; thus, even Risk for Infection should not be used routinely for all surgery patients.)

SKIN INTEGRITY, RISK FOR IMPAIRED

Definition: A state in which the individual's skin is at risk of being adversely altered.

Defining Characteristics: *External (environmental)*— Hyper- or hypothermia; chemical substance; mechanical factors (shearing forces, pressure, restraint); radiation; physical immobilization; excretions; humidity. *Internal (somatic)*—Medication; altered nutritional state (obesity, emaciation); altered metabolic state; altered circulation; altered sensation; altered pigmentation; skeletal prominence; developmental factors; immunological deficit; alterations in turgor (change in elasticity).

Author's Note: This label should be used for clients who have no symptoms, but who are at risk of developing disruption of skin surface or destruction of skin layers. The presence of more than one risk factor increases the likelihood of skin damage. When Risk for Impaired Skin Integrity occurs as a result of Immobility, and when other body systems are also at risk for impairment, Carpenito (1993) recommends using Risk for Disuse Syndrome.

SLEEP-PATTERN DISTURBANCE

Definition: Disruption of sleep time causes discomfort or interferes with desired lifestyle.

Defining Characteristics: Critical—Verbal complaints of difficulty falling asleep; awakening earlier or later than desired; interrupted sleep; verbal complaints of not feeling well-rested. *Other*—Changes in behavior and performance (increasing irritability, restlessness, disorientation, lethargy, listlessness); physical signs (mild fleeting nystagmus, slight hand tremor, ptosis of eyelid, expressionless face, dark circles under eyes, frequent yawning, changes in posture); thick speech with mispronunciation and incorrect words.

Related Factors: Sensory alterations—internal (illness, psychological stress); external (environmental changes, social cues).

Author's Note: This label is used when disruption of sleep causes discomfort or interferes with the client's desired lifestyle. Do not confuse it with Fatigue.

Sleep-Pattern Disturbance is a rather general label. The etiological factors can sometimes make it specific enough to direct nursing intervention, as in *Sleep-Pattern Disturbance related to frequent awakening of infant during the night*. When possible, the specific type of Sleep-Pattern Disturbance should be identified in order to better direct care.

> ***Examples:*** Sleep-Pattern Disturbance (**Early Awakening**) r/t depression
>
> Sleep-Pattern Disturbance (**Delayed Onset of Sleep**) r/t overstimulation prior to bedtime.

☛ *See also* Fatigue and Activity Intolerance.

SOCIAL INTERACTION, IMPAIRED

Definition: The state in which an individual participates in an insufficient or excessive quantity or ineffective quality of social exchange.

Defining Characteristics: *Major*—Verbalized or observed discomfort in social situations; verbalized or observed inability to receive or communicate a satisfying sense of belonging, caring, interest, or shared history; observed use of unsuccessful social interaction behaviors; dysfunctional interaction with peers, family and/or others. *Minor*— Family report of change of style or pattern of interaction.

Related Factors: Knowledge/skill deficit about ways to enhance mutuality; communication barriers; self-concept disturbance; absence of available significant others or peers; limited physical mobility; therapeutic isolation; sociocultural dissonance; environmental barriers; altered thought processes.

☛ *See also* Altered Thought Processes, Impaired Communication, and Social Isolation.

SOCIAL ISOLATION

Definition: Aloneness experienced by the individual and perceived as imposed by others and as a negative or threatened state.

Defining Characteristics: Critical—Absence of supportive significant other(s) (family, friends, group); expresses feelings of aloneness imposed by others; expresses feelings of rejection. *Other*—Sad, dull affect; inappropriate or immature interests/activities for developmental age/stage; uncommunicative, withdrawn, no eye contact; preoccupation with own thoughts; repetitive meaningless actions; projects hostility in voice, behavior; seeks to be alone, or exists in a subculture; evidence of physical/mental handicap or altered state of wellness; shows behavior unaccepted by dominant cultural group; experiences feelings of difference from others; inadequacy in or absence of significant purpose in life; inability to meet expectations of others; insecurity in public; expresses values acceptable to the subculture but· unacceptable to the dominant cultural group; expresses interests inappropriate to the developmental age/stage.

Related Factors: Factors contributing to the absence of satisfying personal relationships, such as delay in accomplishing developmental tasks; immature interests; alterations in physical appearance; alterations in mental status; unaccepted social behavior; unaccepted social values; altered state of wellness; inadequate personal resources; inability to engage in satisfying personal relationships.

☛ *See also* Altered Thought Processes, Impaired Communication, and Impaired Social Interaction.

SPIRITUAL DISTRESS (DISTRESS OF THE HUMAN SPIRIT)

Definition: Disruption in the life principle that pervades a person's entire being and that integrates and transcends one's biological and psychosocial nature.

Defining Characteristics: Critical—Expresses concern with meaning of life/death and/or belief systems. *Other*—anger toward God; questions meaning of suffering; verbalizes inner conflict about beliefs; verbalizes concern about relationship with deity; questions meaning of own existence; unable to participate in usual religious practices; seeks spiritual assistance; questions moral/ethical implications of therapeutic regimen; gallows humor; displacement of anger toward religious representatives; description of nightmares/sleep disturbances; alteration in behavior/mood evidenced by anger, crying, withdrawal, preoccupation, anxiety, hostility, apathy, and so forth.

Related Factors: Separation from religious/cultural ties; challenged belief and value system (e.g., due to moral/ethical implications of therapy or intense suffering).

STRESS INCONTINENCE

(*see* Incontinence, Stress)

SUFFOCATION, RISK FOR

Definition: Accentuated risk of accidental suffocation (inadequate air available for inhalation).

Defining Characteristics: Presence of risk factors such as the following. *Internal (individual)*—Reduced olfactory sensation; reduced motor abilities; lack of safety education; lack of safety precautions; cognitive or emotional difficulties; disease or injury process. *External (environmental)*—Pillow placed in an infant's crib; propped bottle placed in an infant's crib; vehicle warming in closed garage; children playing with plastic bags or inserting small objects into their mouths or noses; discarded or unused refrigerators or freezers without removed doors; children left unattended in bathtubs or pools; household gas leaks; smoking in bed; use of fuel-burning heaters not vented to outside; low-strung clothesline; pacifier hung around infant's head; person who eats large mouthfuls of food.

Related Factors: *See* risk factors above.

Author's Note: Use the most specific label that matches the client's defining characteristics.

☛ *See also* Impaired Home Maintenance Management, Risk for Injury, and Risk for Trauma.

SWALLOWING, IMPAIRED

Definition: The state in which an individual has decreased ability to voluntarily pass fluids and/or solids from the mouth to the stomach.

Defining Characteristics: *Major*—Observed evidence of difficulty in swallowing (e.g., stasis of food in oral cavity, coughing/choking). *Minor*—Evidence of aspiration.

Related Factors: Neuromuscular impairment (e.g., decreased or absent gag reflex, decreased strength or excursion of muscles involved in mastication, perceptual impairment, facial paralysis); mechanical obstruction (e.g., edema, tracheostomy tube, tumor); fatigue; limited awareness; reddened, irritated oropharyngeal cavity.

☛ *See also* Risk for Aspiration.

TEMPERATURE, BODY, HIGH RISK FOR ALTERED

(*see* Body Temperature . . .)

THERAPEUTIC REGIMEN (INDIVIDUAL), INEFFECTIVE MANAGEMENT OF

Definition: A pattern of regulating and integrating into daily living a program for treatment of illness and the sequelae of illness that is unsatisfactory for meeting specific health goals.

Defining Characteristics: *Major*—Choices of daily living ineffective for meeting the goals of a treatment or prevention program. *Minor*—Verbalized desire to manage the treatment of illness and prevention of sequelae; verbalized difficulty with regulation/integration of one or more prescribed regimens for treatment of illness and its effects or prevention of complications; verbalized not taking action to include treatment regimens in daily routines; verbalized not taking action to reduce risk factors for progression of illness and sequelae; acceleration (expected or unexpected) of illness symptoms.

Related Factors: Complexity of health care system; complexity of therapeutic regimen; decisional conflict; economic difficulties; excessive demands made on individual or family; family conflict; family patterns of health care; inadequate number and types of cues to action; knowledge deficits; mistrust of regimen and/or health care personnel; perceived barriers; perceived benefits; perceived seriousness; perceived susceptibility; powerlessness; social support deficits.

Author's Note: Use this diagnosis for patients or families who wish to follow a therapeutic regimen and are motivated to do so, but who are having difficulty doing so. For example, the diagnosis would be appropriate for a patient who is trying to lose weight and has the necessary information, but finds it difficult to adhere to a low-calorie diet because her business requires her to entertain and eat out frequently. It would not be appropriate for an obese patient who is not interested in dieting or losing weight.

☛ *See also* Adjustment, Impaired; Health Maintenance, Altered; Noncompliance (specify).

THERMOREGULATION, INEFFECTIVE

Definition: The state in which the individual's temperature fluctuates between hypothermia and hyperthermia.

Defining Characteristics: *Major*—Fluctuations in body temperature above or below the normal range. See also major and minor characteristics present in hypothermia and hyperthermia.

Related Factors: Trauma or illness; immaturity; aging; fluctuating environmental temperature.

Author's Note: This label is most appropriate for those who are especially vulnerable to environmental conditions (i.e., newborns and the elderly).

☛ *See also* Risk for Altered Body Temperature, Hyperthermia, and Hypothermia.

THOUGHT PROCESSES, ALTERED

Definition: A state in which an individual experiences a disruption in cognitive operations and activities.

Defining Characteristics: Inaccurate interpretation of environment; cognitive dissonance; distractibility; memory deficit/problems; egocentricity; hyper- or hypovigilance. *Other Possible Characteristics:* Inappropriate non-reality-based thinking.

Related Factors: To be developed.

Author's Note: May be the etiology of other problems, such as Self-Care Deficit, Impaired Home Maintenance Management, or Impaired Social Interaction.

☛ *See also* Sensory/Perceptual Alterations.

TISSUE INTEGRITY, IMPAIRED

Definition: A state in which an individual experiences damage to mucous membrane, corneal, integumentary, or subcutaneous tissue.

Defining Characteristics: *Major*—Damaged or destroyed tissue (cornea, mucous membrane, integumentary, or subcutaneous).

Related Factors: Altered circulation; nutritional deficit/excess; fluid deficit/excess; knowledge deficit; impaired physical mobility; irritants, chemical (including body excretions, secretions, medications); thermal (temperature extremes); mechanical (pressure, shear, friction); radiation (including therapeutic radiation).

Author's Note: If tissue integrity is at risk because of immobility, and if other systems are also at risk, consider using Risk for Disuse Syndrome.

☛ *See also* Altered Oral Mucous Membrane and Impaired Skin Integrity.

TISSUE PERFUSION, ALTERED (SPECIFY): Cardiopulmonary, Cerebral, Gastrointestinal, Peripheral, Renal.

Definition: The state in which an individual experiences a decrease in nutrition and oxygenation at the cellular level due to a deficit in capillary blood supply.

Defining Characteristics:

A. Chances that characteristics will be present in given diagnosis.

B. Estimated sensitivities and specificities. Chances that characteristic will not be explained by any other diagnosis.

	A.	B.
Skin temperature: cold extremities	High	Low
Skin color, dependent: blue or purple	Moderate	Low
(**Critical**) Limb pale on elevation; color does not return on lowering of extremity	High	High
(**Critical**) Diminished arterial pulsations	High	High
Skin quality: shining	High	Low
Lack of lanugo	High	Moderate
Round scars covered with atrophied skin; gangrene	Low	High
Slow-growing, dry, brittle nails	High	Moderate
Claudication	Moderate	High
Blood-pressure changes in extremities; bruits	Moderate	Moderate
Slow healing of lesions	High	Low

Related Factors: Interruption of flow, arterial; interruption of flow, venous; exchange problems; hypovolemia; hypervolemia.

Author's Note: Further work and development are required for the subcomponents, specifically cerebral, renal, and gastrointestinal. Unlike Altered Peripheral Tissue Perfusion, the qualifying labels Renal, Cerebral, Cardiopulmonary, and Gastrointestinal require medical intervention to improve tissue perfusion; they are useful primarily as etiologies for other problems. Even if potential rather than actual, these conditions usually represent collaborative problems. Nursing care should focus on interventions for specific *responses* to impaired perfusion, such as the following:

> Altered Thought Processes r/t decreased cerebral tissue perfusion
>
> Activity Intolerance r/t decreased cardiopulmonary tissue perfusion
>
> Fluid Volume Excess r/t decreased renal tissue perfusion.

Altered *Peripheral* Tissue Perfusion is the only one of these labels that can be treated by independent nursing interventions. For that label, it is important to determine whether the altered tissue perfusion is venous or arterial. ☞ *See also* Risk for Injury and Risk for Disuse Syndrome.

TOILETING SELF-CARE DEFICIT
(*see* Self-Care Deficit, Toileting)

TOTAL INCONTINENCE
(*see* Incontinence, Total)

TRAUMA, RISK FOR
Definition: Accentuated risk of accidental tissue injury (e.g., wound, burn, fracture).

Defining Characteristics: Presence of risk factors such as the following. *Internal (individual)*—Weakness; poor vision; balancing difficulties, reduced temperature and/or tactile sensation; reduced large or small muscle coordination; reduced hand-eye coordination; lack of safety education; lack of safety precautions; insufficient finances to purchase safety equipment or effect repairs; cognitive or emotional difficulties; history of previous trauma. *External (environmental)*—Slippery floors (e.g., wet or highly waxed); snow or ice collected on stairs, walkways; unanchored rugs; bathtub without hand grip or antislip equipment; use of unsteady ladders or chairs; entering unlighted rooms; unsturdy or absent stair rails; unanchored electric wires; litter or liquid spills on floors or stairways; high beds; children playing without gates at the top of the stairs; obstructed passageways; unsafe window protection in homes with young children; inappropriate call-for-aid mechanisms for bed-resting client; pot handles facing toward front of stove; bathing in very hot water (e.g., unsupervised bathing of young children); potential igniting gas leaks; delayed lighting of gas burner or oven; experimenting with chemicals or gasoline; unscreened fires or heaters; wearing plastic apron or flowing clothes around open flame; children playing with matches, candles, cigarettes; inadequately stored combustibles or corrosives (e.g., matches, oily rags, lye); highly flammable children's toys or clothing; overloaded fuse boxes; contact with rapidly moving machinery, industrial belts, or pulleys; sliding on coarse bed linen or struggling within bed restraints; faulty electrical plugs, frayed wires, or defective appliances; contact with acids or alkalis; playing with fireworks or gunpowder; contact with intense cold; overexposure to sun, sun lamps, radiotherapy; use of cracked dishware or glasses; knives stored uncovered; guns or ammunition stored unlocked; large icicles hanging from the roof; exposure to dangerous machinery; children playing with sharp-edged toys; high-crime neighborhood and vulnerable clients; driving a mechanically unsafe vehicle; driving after partaking of alcoholic beverages or drugs; driving at excessive speeds; driving without necessary visual aids; children riding in the front seat in car; smoking in bed or near oxygen; overloaded electrical outlets; grease waste collected on stoves; use of thin or worn potholders; misuse of necessary headgear for motorized cyclists; young children carried on adult bicycles; unsafe road or road-crossing conditions; play or work near vehicle pathways (e.g., driveways, laneways, railroad tracks); nonuse or misuse of seat restraints.

Related Factors: *See* risk factors above.

☛ *See also* Risk for Injury, Risk for Aspiration, Risk for Poisoning, Risk for Suffocation, and Impaired Home Maintenance Management.

UNILATERAL NEGLECT

Definition: A state in which an individual is perceptually unaware of and inattentive to one side of the body.

Defining Characteristics: *Major*—Consistent inattention to stimuli on an affected side. *Minor*—Inadequate self-care; positioning and/or safety precautions in regard to the affected side; does not look toward affected side; leaves food on plate on the affected side.

Related Factors: Effects of disturbed perceptual abilities (e.g., hemianopsia; one-sided blindness); neurologic illness or trauma.

☛ *See also* Self-Care Deficit and Sensory/Perceptual Alterations.

URGE INCONTINENCE

(*see* Incontinence, Urge)

URINARY ELIMINATION, ALTERED

Definition: The state in which the individual experiences a disturbance in urine elimination.

Defining Characteristics: Dysuria; frequency; hesitancy; incontinence; nocturia; retention; urgency.

Related Factors: Multiple causality, including anatomical obstruction, sensory motor impairment, urinary tract infection.

Author's Note: Use a more specific label when possible.

☛ *See also* Urinary Incontinence (Functional, Reflex, Stress, Total, and Urge) and Urinary Retention.

URINARY INCONTINENCE, FUNCTIONAL

(*see* Incontinence, Functional Urinary)

URINARY INCONTINENCE, REFLEX

(*see* Incontinence, Reflex Urinary)

URINARY INCONTINENCE, STRESS

(*see* Incontinence, Stress Urinary)

URINARY INCONTINENCE, TOTAL

(*see* Incontinence, Total Urinary)

URINARY INCONTINENCE, URGE

(*see* Incontinence, Urge Urinary)

URINARY RETENTION

Definition: The state in which the individual experiences incomplete emptying of the bladder.

Defining Characteristics: *Major*—Bladder distention; small, frequent voiding or absence of urine output. *Minor*—Sensation of bladder fullness; dribbling; residual urine; dysuria; overflow incontinence.

Related Factors: High urethral pressure caused by weak detrusor; inhibition of reflex arc; strong sphincter; blockage.

Author's Note: Do not use for temporary conditions (e.g., postdelivery) for which the only treatment is catheterization.

☛ *See also* Altered Patterns of Urinary Elimination.

VENTILATION, INABILITY TO SUSTAIN SPONTANEOUS

Definition: A state in which the response pattern of decreased energy reserves results in an individual's inability to maintain breathing adequate to support life.

Defining Characteristics: *Major*—Dyspnea; increased metabolic rate. *Minor*—Increased restlessness; apprehension; decreased tidal volume; decreased PO_2; decreased cooperation; increased use of accessory muscles; increased heart rate; increased PCO_2; decreased PaO_2.

Related Factors: Metabolic factors (alkalemia, hypokalemia, hypochloremia, hypophosphatemia, anemia); respiratory muscle fatigue.

Author's Note: Impaired Gas Exchange is one of the defining characteristics for this label. When blood gases are altered, but the patient is able to breathe without mechanical assistance, a diagnosis of Impaired Gas Exchange should be made instead of Inability to Sustain Spontaneous Ventilation.

☛ *See also* Dysfunctional Ventilatory Weaning Response (DVWR); Gas Exchange, Impaired.

VENTILATORY WEANING RESPONSE (DYSFUNCTIONAL)

Definition: A state in which a patient cannot adjust to lowered levels of mechanical ventilator support, which interrupts and prolongs the weaning process.

Defining Characteristics: Nurses have defined three levels of Dysfunctional Ventilatory Weaning Response (DVWR), in which these defining characteristics occur in response to weaning (Logan and Jenny, 1990).

Mild DVWR

Major—Restlessness; slight increased respiratory rate from baseline. *Minor*—Responds to lowered levels of mechanical ventilator support with expressed feelings of increased need for oxygen, breathing discomfort, fatigue, warmth, queries about possible machine malfunction; responds to lowered levels of mechanical ventilator support with increased concentration on breathing.

Moderate DVWR

Major—Responds to lowered levels of mechanical ventilator support with baseline increase in respiratory rate < 5 breaths/minute; slight increase from baseline blood pressure < 20 mm Hg; slight increase from baseline heart rate < 20 beats/minute. *Minor*—Apprehension; color changes: pale, slight cyanosis; decreased air entry on auscultation; diaphoresis; eye widening ("wide-eyed" look); hypervigilance to activities; inability to cooperate; inability to respond to coaching; slight respiratory accessory muscle use.

Severe DVWR

Major—Responds to lowered levels of mechanical ventilatory support with agitation, deterioration in arterial blood gases from current baseline; increase from baseline blood pressure > 20 mm Hg; increase from baseline heart rate > 20 beats/minute; respiratory rate increases significantly from baseline. *Minor*—Adventitious breath sounds, audible airway secretions; cyanosis; decreased level of consciousness; discoordinated breathing with the ventilator; full respiratory accessory muscle use; paradoxical abdominal breathing; profuse diaphoresis; shallow, gasping breaths.

Related Factors: *Physical*—Inadequate nutrition; ineffective airway clearance; sleep-pattern disturbance; uncontrolled pain or discomfort. *Situational*—Adverse environment (noisy, active environment, negative events in the room, low nurse-patient ratio, extended nurse absence from bedside, unfamiliar nursing staff); history of multiple unsuccessful weaning attempts; history of ventilator dependence > 1 week; inadequate social support; inappropriate pacing of diminished ventilator support; uncontrolled episodic energy demands of problems. *Psychological*—Anxiety: moderate, severe; decreased motivation; decreased self-esteem; fear; hopelessness; insufficient trust in the nurse; knowledge deficit of the weaning process; patient perceived inefficacy about the ability to wean; patient role; powerlessness.

Author's Note: DVWR is concerned specifically with patient responses to separation from the mechanical ventilator. Other respiratory diagnoses may also occur during weaning, for example, Ineffective Airway Clearance, Ineffective Breathing pattern, and Impaired Gas Exchange. This label does not include the reasons for the weaning problems. If you do not know the etiology of the DVWR, use "unkown etiology."

☛ *See also* Airway Clearance, Ineffective; Breathing Pattern, Ineffective; Gas Exchange, Impaired; Respiratory Function, Altered (Risk for).

VERBAL COMMUNICATION, IMPAIRED
(*see* Communication, Impaired Verbal)

VIOLENCE, RISK FOR: SELF-DIRECTED OR DIRECTED AT OTHERS

Definition: A state in which an individual experiences behaviors that can be physically harmful either to the self or others.

Defining Characteristics: Presence of risk factors such as body language (e.g., clenched fists, tense facial expression, rigid posture, tautness indicating effort to control); hostile threatening verbalizations (e.g., boasting to or prior abuse of others); increased motor activity (e.g., pacing, excitement, irritability, agitation); overt and aggressive acts (e.g., goal-directed destruction of objects in environment); possession of destructive means (e.g., gun, knife, or other weapon); rage; self-destructive behavior, active aggressive suicidal acts; suspicion of others, paranoid ideation, delusions, hallucinations; substance abuse/withdrawal. *Other Possible Characteristics:* Increasing anxiety levels; fear of self or others; inability to verbalize feelings; repetition of verbalizations (continued complaints, requests, or demands); anger; provocative behavior (e.g., argumentative, dissatisfied, overreactive, hypersensitive); vulnerable self-esteem; depression (specifically active, aggressive, suicidal acts).

Related Factors: Antisocial character; battered women; catatonic excitement; child abuse; manic excitement; organic brain syndrome; panic states; rage reactions; suicidal behavior; temporal lobe epilepsy; toxic reactions to medications.

REFERENCES

Burns, et al. (1993). New diagnosis: Caregiver role strain. *Nursing Diagnosis,* 4(2):70–76.

Carpenito, L. J. (1993). *Handbook of Nursing Diagnosis,* 5th ed. Philadelphia: J. B. Lippincott.

Geissler, E. (1991). Transcultural nursing and nursing diagnoses. *Nursing and Health Care,* 12(4):190–92, 203.

Gordon, M. (1985). Practice based data set for a nursing information system. *Journal of Medical Systems, 9:*43–55.

Gordon, M. (1987). *Nursing Diagnosis: Process and Application.* 2nd ed. New York: McGraw-Hill.

Janken, J. and Cullinan, C. (1991). Validation of the nursing diagnosis sensory/perceptual alteration: Auditory. In Carrol-Johnson, R., ed., *Classification of Nursing Diagnoses: Proceedings of the Ninth Conference.* North American Nursing Diagnosis Association. Philadelphia: J. B. Lippincott.

Lambert, M., and Jones, P. (1989). Nursing diagnoses recorded in nursing situations encountered in a Department of Public Health. In Carroll-Johnson, R., ed., *Classification of Nursing Diagnoses: Proceedings of the Eighth Conference.* North American Nursing Diagnosis Association. Philadelphia: J. B. Lippincott, 364–67.

Logan, J. and Jenny, J. (1991). Analyzing expert nursing practice to develop a new nursing diagnosis: Dysfunctional ventilatory weaning response. In Carroll-Johnson, R., ed. *Classification of Nursing Diagnoses: Proceedings of the Ninth Conference.* Philadelphia: J. B. Lippincott, 133–140.

Rakel, B., and Bulechek, G. (1990). Development of alterations in learning: Situational learning disabilities. *Nursing Diagnosis, 1*(4):134–145.

Taylor, et al. (1989). *Fundamentals of Nursing.* Philadelphia: J. B. Lippincott.

Whitley, G. (1992a). Concept analysis of anxiety. *Nursing Diagnosis, 3*(3):107–116.

Whitley, G. (1992b). Concept analysis of fear. *Nursing Diagnosis, 3*(4):155–161.

ANSWER KEY for "Applying Nursing Process"

CHAPTER 1

1. The appropriate phenomena of concern for the nurse are that Mr. Callaway
- a. smokes two packs of cigarettes a day.
- b. coughs a lot.
- c. becomes short of breath when climbing stairs.

Lesions on his lungs are clearly a medical concern. Biopsy, too, is most directly a medical concern. Nursing would deal with any fears, anxieties, or knowledge deficits, and so forth that Mr. Callaway had about the biopsy or the lesions.

2.
1—c	4—d	7—d
2—a	5—d	8—e
3—c	6—a	9—b

3.
- a. Interpersonal skills
- b. Technical skills
- c. Intellectual skills
- d. Creativity and curiosity
- e. Adaptability

4a.
I—settled her comfortably in bed	P—set a goal
A—interviewed her	P—wrote nursing orders for skin care
A—obtained a temperature	I—bathed Ms. Boiko
A—examined Ms. Boiko's chart	E—observed that her coccygeal area was still red (This could also be *A* for ongoing assessment.)
I —applied oxygen	
A—performed the physical examination	
D—wrote a diagnosis	E—concluded the goal had not been met
	E—decided to change the care plan

4b. The client data is as follows: Temp 101°, pulse 120, resp. 32, B/P 100/68, reddened area over coccyx, unable to move about in bed, coccyx still red, a small area of skin was peeling off, there was some serous drainage. (Juan also obtained data that Ms. Boiko had been turned every 2 hours except for 6 hours each night. This is data about care that was given to Ms. Boiko, but it is not data about human responses.)

4c. You should have circled the following as examples of reexamination of the nursing process steps:
- *Juan concluded that the goal had not been met.* This shows that he went back and examined his original goal.
- *He was sure his data was adequate and that his nursing diagnosis was accurate.* This demonstrates reexamination of the data base and the original nursing diagnosis.
- *When asked, the other staff members assured Juan that the 2-hour turning schedule had been carried out.* This shows that Juan checked to see if the nursing orders were correctly implemented.
- *He decided to change the order on the care plan.* This shows revision of the care plan.

4d. The nursing orders are
- Orders for skin care
- A schedule for turning every 2 hours except at night
- Orders for frequent, continued observation
- An order to turn every 2 hours around the clock

Because your information states that Juan was bathing Ms. Boiko, you may have assumed he wrote a nursing order for that; however, the case study does not say this, and you must use only the information provided. Juan did perform some other nursing actions, such as settling the client in bed; however we do not know that they were written as nursing orders. Don't confuse nursing interventions (carried out) with nursing orders (written down).

4e. This is the most obvious example of overlapping of steps: "Two days later, when bathing Ms. Boiko, Juan observed that her coccygeal area was still red, a small area of skin was peeling off, and there was some serous drainage." In this example, Juan is implementing (bathing) at the same time he is assessing or evaluating (observing her coccygeal area).

You might also have chosen: "Juan Apodaca, RN, settled her comfortably in bed and briefly interviewed her about her symptoms." *Settling* is implementation, while *interviewed* is assessment. As written, it isn't 100% clear that these occurred at the same time; however, if you think they did, then this, too, is a case of overlapping steps.

4f. Juan demonstrated the nursing qualities of creativity and adaptability by not continuing to use the turning schedule that was the routine on his unit. He was not content to do what was usually done, but reasoned that in this case something more was needed.

4g. The answer is (3)—individualized care.
- (1) Any turning schedule assures continuity of care over shifts and caregivers. The pertinent information in the question is that this is not just any schedule. It is a special schedule.
- (2) See comment (1).
- (4) Nothing about the schedule encourages client participation.

CHAPTER 2

1. *Nursing is an applied discipline.* **C is correct**. The nurse applied principles of nursing to the care of a particular patient.

D may match, too. The nurse probably used principles to make the decisions, although the case doesn't say so. She might have based her decisions on what the other nurses had been doing, on habit, on some rules she was aware of, and on her emotions. This case doesn't clearly demonstrate application of principles.

In *A,* the nurse is active, but the case doesn't mention application of principles. In *B,* the nurse is acquiring knowledge but not applying it.

Nursing draws on knowledge from other subjects and fields. **B is correct**. The nurse is acquiring knowledge from other subjects and fields: psychology, pharmacology, and physiology.

In *A,* it appears the nurse will need knowledge from other subjects, but the case doesn't point out which fields, nor that such knowledge is actually being used.

C would be correct if the knowledge clearly came from a field other than nursing (such as physics). This case clearly demonstrates the application of principles, but it isn't clear which field the principles came from.

In *D,* the nurse may have used knowledge from other fields to make the decisions, although the case doesn't say so. She might have based her decisions on what the other nurses had been doing, on habit, on some rules she was aware of, on her emotions, etc.

Nurses deal with change in stressful environments. **A is the best example** of change: the client stopped breathing, he has 3 IVs to keep track of, the nurse had to interrupt her care to go to a meeting, the schedule for neuro checks was changed, and the patient's medication was changed. All of these changes are stressful, as would be the workload of 15-minute neuro checks and 3 IVs.

B does not necessarily indicate change or stress. This nurse may not find all that reading stressful. *C* indicates neither change or stress. Perhaps this is the only patient the nurse has to care for, and he finds it relaxing to deal with immobile patients.

D demonstrates that the nurse made several decisions, probably based on some principles. You might interpret these as stressful, but the situation doesn't make that clear. Nothing is said about change in the example.

Nurses make frequent, varied, and important decisions in their work. **D is correct.** It demonstrates a series of decisions the nurse made.

C represents only one decision made by the nurse, not "frequent and varied" decisions.

In *A* and *B* the nurse made no decisions.

2. *Nurse C* demonstrated critical thinking.

3. *Nurse A* did not have an attitude of inquiry. She blindly accepted the night nurse's advice for therapy (authority) without any evidence that Mr. Stewart was truly hypoglycemic. The description of Mr. Stewart given by the night nurse could have indicated almost anything—not necessarily diabetes. Nurse A may also have failed to be reflective, jumping to the conclusion that Mr. Stewart was hypoglycemic.
Nurse B made the same thinking errors as Nurse A—even more so, since she had no plans of her own to assess Mr. Stewart (as far as we can tell from the case). She did not look up diabetes in a text in order to make her own judgments about Mr. Stewart's symptoms. She appears to have no confidence in her ability to make judgments.
Nurse D did not reflect before giving the orange juice. She accepted the night nurse's advice to give orange juice without any evidence that it was needed. She certainly jumped to the conclusion that Mr. Stewart had a hypoglycemic reaction when she initiated a care plan without even assessing the patient.

4. a. Creative   c. Critical
   b. Directed   d. Associative

5. a. E   c. S
   b. E   d. P
   Actually, (*a*) and (*b*) might demonstrate practice wisdom. In the absence of ethical knowledge, the nurse in (*a*) might have said what she did because her nursing instructor told her this was the proper behavior, or because agency policies specify that patient data is confidential. The nurse in (*b*) might have heard another nurse say that families should not look at the charts; if her action is based on this, it is practice wisdom. If it is based upon her understanding of the principles of autonomy and confidentiality, it is ethical knowledge.

CHAPTER 3

1. These meet standards and should have check marks: *a* and *d.*
   a. Demonstrates that data collection is "systematic, accessible, communicated, and recorded."
   d. Demonstrates that data collection is "accessible, communicated, and recorded."
   These are incorrect: *b* and *c.*
   b. Data collection is not "continuous."
   c. Data collection is not "systematic."

2. a. C   d. I   f. C
   b. C   e. C   g. I
   c. I

3.

Subjective Data	*Objective Data*	*Primary Source*	*Secondary Source*
f, j, n, r	a, b, c, d, e, g, h, i, k, l, m, o, p, q	c, e, f, i, j, k, l, m, n, o, q, r	a, b, d, g, h, p

4. Either way is correct. If you chose to read the chart first, your reasons should include the following:
   a. It would give me at least some information about her, so I would feel more comfortable.
   b. It might help me to formulate my initial questions.
   c. It would prevent me from repeating examinations or topics that had already been covered.
   d. It would assure that I review the chart early in the data-collection process. I might forget to do it later.
   If you chose not to read the chart first, your reasons should probably be as follows:
   a. I prefer not to have any preconceived ideas or biases about her when I interview her. It would help me to be more objective.
   b. I might not have time to read the chart and still be sure of getting the interview and examination all finished in time for surgery.

5. a. The nurse who recorded the B/P on the chart used examination(*E*). The nurse reading the chart really used none of these; you could say she used observation, since she used her sense of sight to read the number on the chart.
   b. I   e. E   h. E
   c. O   f. O   i. I
   d. O   g. I
   j. E (Auscultation does use the sense of hearing, but it is a special examination skill that requires the use of a stethoscope to aid that sense.)
   k. I (In a sense, the nurse obtained the data by interview [I] from the anesthetist; the anesthetist used the sense of touch, or observation [O].)

6. a. C   d. O   g. O   I. O
   b. O   e. O   h. C   j. O
   c. C   f. C

7. Some examples of questions the nurse might ask follow:
   a. *Closed questions:* "Is it sharp or dull?" "Is it continuous, or does it come and go?" "How long have you had it?" "Do you take any medication for it?"
   b. *Open-ended questions:* "Tell me more about it." "Would you describe it for me?" "Tell me about how it began."

8. a. To *prepare* for the interview you should do the following:

(1) Form your goals for the interview.
(2) Decide on a time to do it. You will need 15–20 minutes when you do not have treatments and other tasks to do for other patients. You will need to be sure the patient isn't scheduled to leave the unit for tests or treatments, that it isn't too close to mealtime, and so on.
(3) Ask her family to leave.
(4) Ask her if she needs anything for pain, and allow enough time for the medication to work if you give it.
(5) Be sure she has water; ask if she needs to go to the bathroom.
(6) Assess her emotional status/anxiety level.
(7) Turn down TV; turn off phone.
(8) Pull the curtain around the bed.
(Note: You should not have listed "review her chart," because this had already been done.)

b. To elicit from Ms. Contini *her* understanding of "Reason for Hospitalization," you might say, "Tell me why you are here," or "Why did you come to the hospital?" Since the chart tells you she is here for knee surgery, it is more open and honest to say something like, "I see you're having knee surgery. I'd like to hear what brought you to that decision."

c. In a comprehensive assessment you should ask the questions about sexual functioning. You cannot assume she is celibate or uninterested in sex because she is too old, single, or in too much pain. In fact, if the patient does have a sexual partner, one of the nurse's roles is to help the patient adapt to diseases/disabilities in order to preserve sexual functioning. This might be important to this patient, if her arthritis pain is interfering with her sexual functioning.

9. The data that should be validated are as follows:
Because subjective and objective data do not match: *a, b, f*
The subjective information is not the same at both times: *d*
You will want to repeat the earlier data to be sure the client was giving reliable data. If he tells you the same thing both times, and he seems lucid, it is probably valid: *e*
The data in item *c* does *not* need to be validated. You would expect some staining of the fingers and teeth from a heavy smoker.

10. The judgments/conclusions you should draw a line through are: *c, e, f, h, k, l, m.*

11. a. Neither. This action contributes to the patient's autonomy. Both veracity and confidentiality can affect the patient's autonomy, but neither of those is involved in this instance.
b. Veracity
c. Veracity
d. Confidentiality
e. Both veracity and confidentiality: Confidentiality, because the nurse does not intend to keep the information confidential; veracity, because she is being honest with the client about what she intends to do with the information.

CHAPTER 4

1. You might discuss with her how nursing diagnosis can accomplish the following:

a. Help her to individualize her patient care
b. Actually make care planning easier for her instead of "more work"
c. Improve her care by providing a focus for planning goals and interventions
d. Help her define her job to patients and other health-care professionals
e. Help in staffing, budgeting, and work load
f. Improve communication between nurses
g. Increase her autonomy and accountability
h. Help her prepare for the time when patient records will be computerized
(Nursing diagnosis is also important for nursing education and research, but these are less relevant reasons to the staff nurse, whose most immediate concern is in providing quality patient care.)

2. The patient problems are *c, e, h,* and *i.*
a. Appendicitis is a medical diagnosis. (Recall that a medical diagnosis can be the cause of a patient problem.)
b. Catheter obstruction might be the etiology for a problem of urinary retention or infection. It is a nursing problem.
d. Asthma is a medical diagnosis.
f. Bowel resection surgery is a treatment. It may be the source of several patient problems.
g. NPO is a medical order. It may cause thirst, dry mouth, and various other human responses.
j. Skin care is stated as a need. The problem might be High risk for Impaired Skin Integrity.
k. Low white-blood-cell count is a lab test value. It might be the symptom of a problem.
l. Lack of cooperation is a problem for the nurse, not necessarily for the patient.
m. Contant need for attention is a problem for the nurse, not necessarily for the patient. The problem is whatever is causing the patient to need constant attention (a symptom).

3. Stressors
A blood clot in her right thigh.
Intravenous catheter.
Heparin drip. While this is a therapy for the blood clot, it is also a stressor in other ways because of its possible side effects.
Complete bedrest. (If you are not aware of the physiological and psychological effects of immobility, ask your instructor to recommend some reading, or look under "Hazards of Immobility" in a fundamentals of nursing book.)

Responses
Thigh was swollen and warm; also slightly red.
She rang for the nurse several times.
Asking to have her leg checked.
Requesting pain medication.
She was observed reading her Bible . . .
Twenty-four hours later, her clotting time returned to normal.

4.

Response	Level	Dimension
Thigh swollen	Organic	Physical
Thigh warm	Organic	Physical
Thigh red	Organic	Physical

Response	Level	Dimension
Rang for nurse several times	Whole-person	Interpersonal; probably caused by a psychological response (e.g., anxiety, fear)
Requesting pain medication	Whole-person	Interpersonal
Observed reading her Bible	Whole-person	Spiritual
Clotting time returned to normal	Systemic	Physical

5.

For a client with a medical diagnosis of

	Problem	r/t Etiology
Fractured femur	a. Acute Pain	*r/t edema and tissue trauma*
	b. Risk for Impaired Skin Integrity: pressure sores or excoriation	*r/t pressure from cast, immobility*
Pneumonia	a. Ineffective Breathing Patterns	*r/t obstructed airways and decreased chest excursion*
	b. Activity Intolerance	*r/t decreased oxygenation secondary to ineffective breathing patterns*

6.

a.	*c*	c.	*c*	e.	*n*	g. *c*
b.	*n*	d.	*c*	f.	*c*	h. *n*

7.
a. A (Actual pain)
b. Pot (Risk for Injury: falls)
c. Pot
d. Pot
e. Pos
f. A
g. Pos
h. Pot
i. A
j. Pos
k. A (She has signs and symptoms of pain.)
l. Pot (Her medical diagnosis and the signs of inflammation lead you to think she will develop pain if it is not already present. You might choose *possible*, but she really has no symptoms of pain.)
m. Pos (Limping is a sign of pain, but not enough for positive diagnosis, as it could be caused by weakness or joint stiffness.)

8. The nursing diagnoses are *b, c, d* and *e*.
a. This is a collaborative problem; the nurse cannot independently treat or prevent either arrhythmia or myocardial infarction.

In the nursing diagnoses, the parts you should have circled follow:
b. Low Self-Esteem and Perceived Sexual Inadequacy.
c. Risk for Skin Breakdown.
d. Perineal Rash and Excoriation, and perhaps Urinary Incontinence. Whether or not the nurse can intervene independently would depend upon the cause of the incontinence.
e. Confusion and Disorientation.

9.

Cluster 1
B/P 190/100
Hasn't been taking B/P pills because "don't make me feel any better."
Forgets to take B/P pills

Cluster 2
50 lb overweight
Eats fast food; snacks a lot
Sedentary job
No physical exercise
Eats out for fun

Cluster 3
B/P 190/100
Hasn't been taking B/P pills regularly
50 lb overweight
Sedentary job
No physical exercise
Eats fast food; snacks a lot

NANDA Pattern in Which Problem Occurs?

Choosing or Knowing

Exchanging (Nutrition) or Moving (Activity)

Exchanging (Regulation or Cardiac) or Exchanging (Nutrition), or Choosing, or Moving (Activity)

There seem to be three themes running through these cues: her failure to take pills, her obesity, and her hypertension. Because hypertension is a medical problem, the best way to handle it would be to use it as one of the cues in the "pills" and "obesity" group. Students often identify it as a problem, so it is included as a cue group (Cluster 3) here to show you how to deal with it if you have done that.

Step 1. In this step, determine which patterns seem to be involved. In Cluster 1 the cue *they don't make me feel any better* represents a lack of knowledge about the medication (Knowing)—antihypertensive medications usually don't improve the way a patient feels, since you can't feel high blood pressure. The cue *forgets* also represents Knowing. The cue *hasn't been taking B/P pills* represents the selection of alternatives (Choosing).

In Cluster 2, the cues *50 lb overweight, eats fast food, snacks a lot* and *eats out for fun* all relate to Exchanging (Nutrition). The cues *sedentary job* and *no physical exercise* relate to Moving (Activity).

In Cluster 3, some of the cues relate to Choosing, some to Moving, and some to Exchanging.

Step 2. In this step you must tentatively identify both the problem and the etiology to be able to determine in which pattern the problem resides (a preliminary to labeling the problem).

In Cluster 1 the problem is that she hasn't been taking the pills (Choosing). This is because she lacks knowledge about whether they are helping her and because she forgets (Knowing).

In Cluster 2 the best explanation is that she is overweight because she consumes too many calories and burns too few with exercise. The problem is obesity (Exchanging: Nutrition).

In Cluster 3 the best explanation is that she is hypertensive. The exact etiology of essential hypertension is unknown, but obesity, improper diet, lack of exercise, and failure to take her pills are all contributing factors. The problem is a medical one: hypertension (Exchanging). It is not clear whether you should use Exchanging (Regulation) or Exchanging (Cardiac), but most available information points to classifying this as an Exchanging

(Cardiac) problem. You can see how to classify this problem now, but you would not include it on your care plan, since it is a medical problem. For nurses, hypertension is merely a cue to other nursing diagnoses.

10. *Cluster 1*

Using your own terms you might have written something like "Failure to follow regimen for taking blood-pressure medications related to lack of knowledge about effects of the medication and forgetting."

Using NANDA labels you would write, "Noncompliance (blood-pressure medications) related to knowledge deficit (therapeutic effects) and forgetfulness."

Cluster 2

In your own words you might write, "Obesity related to improper eating habits and lack of exercise."
Using NANDA labels:
"Altered Nutrition: More than Body Requirements, related to improper eating habits and lack of exercise."

Cluster 3 is a medical diagnosis, hypertension.

11. a. Your explanations might be something like the following:

The client has a pressure sore on his sacrum because the paralysis keeps him from moving about in bed, and because his age causes his tissues to be fragile.

The client has broken skin on his sacrum because
1. he is old.
2. he is immobile secondary to being paralyzed on his left side.

You might have said, "Unable to move about in bed because of paralysis," but this is an incomplete explanation because it does not mention the broken skin.

b. Possible explanations:
Larry may become dehydrated because
1. he is losing fluids from diarrhea and vomiting, and
2. he cannot take in fluids because of the vomiting.

Possible fluid deficit because of excess fluid loss and inadequate fluid intake.

Insufficient fluids in body because of diarrhea and vomiting.

You might have said: "Losing fluids because of vomiting and diarrhea," but that is an incomplete explanation because it addresses only fluid loss and does not consider insufficient fluid intake nor the possible results of excess loss and inadequate intake (fluid deficit).

12. a. (3). The nurse might be generalizing from past experience; stereotypes are often based on very limited experience with members of a group. However, you cannot draw that conclusion because there is no information to indicate that.
b. (2).
c. (4) and (5). It could also be premature data collection—Susan could have asked, "Why is that?" It is not stereotyping, because stereotypes are based on *lack* of experience with a group.
d. (6). Actually, this case does not fully demonstrate that a diagnostic error was made. We are inferring that because the nurse was immobilized, she missed important diagnoses.

CHAPTER 5

1. a. Label   d. Qualifying term
   b. Risk factors   e. Related factors
   c. Label

2. a. 2   d. 3
   b. 1   e. 5
   c. 4

3. The correctly written diagnoses are *a, d, e, g, h*.
   b—Both parts of the statement mean the same thing.
   c—Elevated temperature is a symptom, not a combination of cues.
   f—Problem needs more specific descriptor; nurse cannot alter the problem or the etiology.
   i—Problem needs more specific descriptor; etiology is legally questionable.
   j—Crying is a symptom, not a problem.

4. Risk factors: possibility of going blind, post-op NPO
   Related factors: progressive loss of vision, effects of surgery, recent loss of job

5. a. Nonadherence to Medication Regimen r/t lack of understanding of effects of the medication and forgetting to take it. (This is not a NANDA label. See Nursing Diagnosis Guide, Noncompliance.)
   b. Impaired Skin Integrity: pressure sore on coccyx r/t inability to move about in bed (or r/t immobility)
   c. Altered Nutrition: More Than Body Requirements r/t irregular schedule, emotional eating pattern, and insufficient exercise
      or
      Altered Nutrition: More Than Body Requirements r/t excess calorie intake and inadequate exercise
   d. Potential Complication of Hysterectomy: Hemorrhage
   e. Risk for Infection Transmission r/t communicable nature of the disease
      or
      Possible Self-Esteem Disturbance r/t social implications of the disease
      or
      Risk for Altered Sexuality Patterns r/t pain, infectious nature of the disease, and implications for relationships

6. Altered Nutrition: More Than Body Requirements
   Diarrhea   Constipation
   Risk for Infection   Altered Protection
   Risk for Aspiration   Activity Intolerance
   Social Isolation

7. *a, c, d, e*

8. *Examples:*
   a—Activity Intolerance **(Level II)**
   c—Sensory-Perceptual Alteration **(Visual)**
   d—**Moderate** Chronic **Back** Pain
   e—Impaired Physical Mobility **(inability to sit up)**

9. a. Bowel Incontinence
   b. Diarrhea
   c. Ineffective Individual Coping
   d. High Risk for Aspiration
   e. Ineffective Airway Clearance

10. 1. *a*   4. *b*
    2. *c*   5. *e*
    3. *d*   6. *f*

11. a. Ineffective Denial
    b. Dressing/Grooming Self-Care Deficit +2
    c. Unilateral Neglect

d.   Stress Incontinence
e.   Urge Incontinence
f.   Altered Tissue Perfusion (Peripheral)
g.   Risk for Fluid Volume Deficit
h.   Parental Role Conflict
i.   Decisional Conflict (whether to have an abortion)
j.   Activity Intolerance

12. Long-term stress
Loss of belief in God
Prolonged activity restriction creating isolation

13. a.   Ms. Petrie
b.   Jill
c.   Mr. A.

14. a.   Perceived Constipation r/t impaired thought processes A.M.B. overuse of laxatives and suppositories, and expectation of a daily bowel movement
b.   Colonic Constipation r/t unknown etiology
c.   Colonic Constipation r/t inadequate fluid and fiber intake and inadequate physical activity 2° weakness from chronic lung disease
d.   Ineffective Individual Coping r/t complex etiology A.M.B. verbalizing inability to cope and observed inability to problem-solve
e.   Potential Complication of IV Therapy: phlebitis, infiltration, infection
f.   Possible Risk for Violence to Self, possibly r/t toxic reaction to medications
g.   Health-Seeking behaviors (exercise)

15. a.   Low   e.   High   i.   Medium
b.   Low   f.   Medium
c.   High   g.   Medium
d.   Medium   h.   Low

16. a.   4   d.   3   g.   1
b.   5   e.   1   h.   1
c.   1   f.   3   i.   3

CHAPTER 6

1. The measurable goals are

Eats fruit at least 3 times/day.	Rates pain as 3 on a 1–10 scale.
Skin warm and dry to touch.	States less anxious than before exercise.
Temp. will be < 100.1°.	Will not have foul-smelling lochia.
States he feels more confident.	Verbalizes understanding of home-care instructions.

2. Some suggested opposite, normal responses are given below. You may have thought of others that are slightly different; they should be similar, however.
b.   Absence of redness or swelling at site. Skin intact. Wound edges intact if healing by primary intention. Granulation tissue present if healing by secondary and tertiary intention.
c.   Temperature at least 98.0° F. Skin warm, dry, and pink. No shivering.
d.   Able to dress self. Able to dress self without assistance.
e.   Mucous membranes pink, moist, without lesions (intact). No bleeding.

3. Examples of expected outcomes using the opposite responses in Exercise 2:

	Subject	Verb Action	Special Conditions	Performance Criteria
a.	(Client)	will have	(none)	regular, soft, formed B. M.
b.	Skin	will be	(none)	without redness or swelling at site
	Skin	will be	(none)	intact.
	Wound edges	will be,	if healing by primary intention,	intact.
	Granulation tissue	will be,	if healing by secondary and tertiary intention	present.
c.	Temp.	will be	(none)	at least 98.0°F.
	Skin	will be	(none)	warm, dry, and pink.
	(Client)	will not	(none)	shiver.
d.	(Client)	will dress	(unassisted)	self.
e.	Mucous membranes	will be	(none)	pink, moist, without lesions or bleeding.

4. *Back Pain r/t incision of recent spinal fusion and muscle stiffness from decreased mobility.*
Good outcomes are individualized to fit the client. For instance, you would not say "VS—within normal limits," but would list the client's usual pulse, B/P, etc. Some ideas for outcome criteria follow:
a.   Experiences adequate pain relief, as evidenced by
(1)   Client will state pain is less than 3 on a 1–10 scale, within 20 minutes after receiving IM analgesic.
(2)   Will have no need for analgesics by day 7 postoperative.
(3)   After medication, will have no facial grimace or muscle tension; VS-WNL for client.
b.   Relief of muscle stiffness, as evidenced by
(1)   Client verbalizes he feels relaxed after being turned and repositioned.

5. Goals and nursing orders for Risk for Impaired Skin Integrity (Pressure Ulcers) r/t long periods of lying in bed follow.

Goals/Predicted Outcomes	Nursing Orders
1. Maintain skin integrity, as evidenced by a. No redness over bony prominences. b. Skin intact, good turgor.	1. Turn q2h around the clock. 2. Assess skin over bony prominences with @ turning. 3. Encourage balanced diet, with protein and Vit. C. 4. Use egg-crate mattress or foam-&-fatty-pad. 5. Keep sheets taut and wrinkle-free; check bed @ turning for foreign objects. 6. Don't use soap to bathe (skin is dry). Use lotion & light massage after bath.

6.

a.	O	d.	N	g,	O
b.	O	e.	N	h.	N
c.	N	f.	O	i.	N

j. O

7. The action verbs are *apply, demonstrate, verbalize.*

8.

a.	P	e.	A
b.	C	f.	P
c.	A	g.	C
d.	C	h.	P

9. The correctly written goals are *b, c, f, i, m, n,* and *o.*
Errors are as follows:

	Predicted Outcome	*Errors (Guideline Violated)*
a.	Client will develop adequate leg strength by 9/1.	*Develop* is not measurable; *adequate* is not observable/measurable. Should not write *client.*
b.	. . . VS-WNL, Hct and Hbg WNL.	"Within normal limits (WNL)" is not specific; but we do not know who the patient is so we cannot individualize the norms.
d.	Will feel better by morning.	*Feel better* is not specific, observable, or measurable.
e.	Improved appetite.	No verb; no special conditions or performance criteria; not observable/measurable.
g.	(On a 30-bed unit with only 2 wheelchairs) Will spend 4 hours each day in a wheelchair.	Not realistic.
h.	Client will discuss expectations of hospitalization and will relate the effects of a high carbohy-drate diet on blood-sugar levels with a basic knowledge of exchange diet for diabetes.	Should not write *client.* Too long and complex. Derived from more than one diagnosis (one relates to expectations of hospitalization, and one to diet).
j.	Injects self with insulin.	No performance criteria (e.g.,using sterile technique).
k.	Will state adequate pain relief from analgesics and will take at least 100 mL of p.o. fluids per hour.	Derived from more than one nursing diagnosis (pain & fluids).
l.	IV will remain patent and run at 125 mL/hr.	A nursing goal, not a statement of desired client response.

10. Independent: *a, b, e, f, g, h, i, j, k, l, m*
Dependent: *c, d*
Observation: *h, i; f* might be considered an observation order, since it states specifically *how* the observation is to be made.

Treatment:	Orders *a, b, e, g,* and *m* could be either treatment or prevention, depending on the problem (*m* is most likely health promotion). *c, d* are treatment only.
Prevention:	Orders *a, b, e, g,* and *m* could be either prevention or treatment (*m* is most likely health promotion). Orders *j, k, l* are prevention only. Order *f* is preventive in the sense that it would prevent injury to rectal mucosa.
Health promotion:	Order *b* might be considered health promotion, if Ms. Adkins's grief work is progressing normally, and she has no problem in that area. It would more likely be used to treat the etiology of some problem. Order *k* could be considered health promotion if done in a family of well clients. Order *m* is really the only nursing order that is clearly for health promotion.
Physical care:	*c, d, f, g, h, i, j,* possibly *e*
Teaching:	*a, k, m*
Counseling:	*b;* possibly *l* if persuasion or help with decision-making is needed.
Referral:	*l*
Environment management:	*e, g, j*

11. In order of priority: *b, e, c, a, d*

*b. <u>Chronic Pain</u> r/t inflammation of knees 2° rheumatoid arthritis

*d. <u>Risk for Noncompliance with NPO Order</u> r/t lack of understanding of its importance for anesthesia

a. <u>Risk for Low Situational Self-esteem</u> r/t unresolved feelings about inability to bear children after hysterectomy

c. <u>Altered Nutrition: More Than Body Requirements for Calories</u> r/t excess calorie intake from "emotional eating"

Rationale:
Diagnosis *b* has to take first priority. The pain will need to be under control in order to accomplish *e* (teaching about importance of NPO), since pain interferes with learning. Pain control is an immediate physical need.
Diagnosis *d* would be second because you would not want to teach about NPO after you had given pre-op medications, which depress the central nervous system.
Diagnosis *a* would probably come before *c* because (1) it may be more amenable to short-term intervention by the nurse, and (2) poor self-esteem might make the pattern of "emotional" eating worse. Teaching could be done for *d* while the client is in the hospital, but the problem does not seem to be caused by a lack of knowledge, so about all the nurse could do for this problem is make referrals.

12. See underlined nursing diagnoses in #11 above.

13. Examples of goals and nursing orders for the two top-priority nursing diagnoses follow. You may think of others that would be appropriate. (To save space, orders are not dated or signed.)

Nursing Diagnoses	Goals and Predicted Outcomes	Nursing Orders
b. Chronic Pain r/t inflammation of knees 2° rheumatoid arthritis	Will be able to carry out ADLs prior to surgery. Will state that pain is within acceptable limits prior to O.R., at all times.	1. Assess intensity of pain before & after meds. 2. Ask client what she usually does to manage/relieve pain. 3. Provide assistance with ADLs and ambulation prn 4. Obtain medical order for analgesics prn 5. WMP to knees, on 15 min., off 15 min. prn 6. Teach guided imagery or other pain-management techniques, day 2 post-op.
d. Risk for Noncompliance with NPO order r/t lack of understanding of its importance for anesthesia	Will remain NPO. After teaching, will relate side effects of anesthesia to need for NPO.	1. Assess client's knowledge of anesthesia and side effects, 3–11 today. 2. Teach rationale for NPO before anesthesia. 3. Remove water pitcher and glasses from room. 4. Put NPO sign above bed/note on Kardex.

14. Care Plan for Potential Complications of Intravenous Therapy.

(1) Signs and symptoms:

Inflammation: Localized diffuse redness of skin around insertion site; tender to touch; skin warm at area of redness. Possibly pus at insertion site.

Phlebitis: Hardness along vein, usually above insertion site; redness of vein and surrounding vein; warmth and tenderness at insertion site and along vein.

Infiltration: Swelling at site; painful to touch or to infusion of fluids; absence of blood return when bag lowered or tubing aspirated; skin around site hard, cold, pale; fluid not running well.

(2) Predicted outcomes and nursing orders for each complication:

Sign/Symptom	Outcomes	Nursing Orders
Inflammation	1. No redness, warmth or pus at insertion site. 2. States not tender 3. Temp. < 100°	1. Inspect site q4h for signs of inflammation. 2. Wash hands before IV care. 3. Teach pt. to avoid touching site. 4. Do not leave bottle hanging for > 8 hrs. 5. Change dressing & tubing q24h, on 3–11 shift. Use aseptic technique per agency procedure. 6. Do not disconnect tubing to change gown, etc. 7. If symptoms noted, DC IV and notify physician.
Phlebitis	1. No hardiness, redness or warmth along or around vein and site. 2. States not tender. 3. Pulse and temp. WNL.	1. Inspect site q4h for signs of phlebitis. 2. Check for tenderness. 3. Pulse and temp. q8h. Retake in 1 hr if elevated. 4. If symptoms occur, remove IV, restart at new site, and notify physician.
Infiltration	1. Skin not cool, pale, hard or swollen at insertion site. 2. States not tender to touch. 3. No c/o pain on infusion of fluid or meds. 4. Infusing at prescribed rate.	1. Inspect site hourly for signs of infiltration. 2. Check rate hourly. 3. If symptoms present, remove IV and restart at new site. 4. Teach pt. to call for help if any discomfort, if container nearly empty, or if flow changes.

CHAPTER 7

1. Dependent Nursing Actions

Definition: Any action that requires a medical order.
Examples: (a) Ibuprofen 500 mg p.o. $\bar{q}$ 3–4h prn pain (per medical order); (b) Obtain physician's order for analgesic if needed to relieve arthritis pain.

Independent Nursing Actions

Definition: Any action that does not require a physician's order.
Examples: (a) Offer client a backrub at HS. (b) Find out what time client usually goes to sleep. Offer milk or other protein at HS. (c) Do pre-op teaching and routines early so client will have time to relax before HS.

Interdependent Nursing Actions

Definition: Require collaboration with other health-care professionals, such as a dietitian, visiting nurse, or social worker.

Examples: (a) Refer client to Social Services Dept. if necessary for home help. (b) Refer client to home health agency if needed. (c) Interview client further to determine if there is a friend or someone who will be available to help her at home.

2. Ms. Atwell's privacy and dignity may be threatened by the enema, most obviously. However, the nurse should also respect her privacy when she takes the pHisohex shower. Ms. Atwell may be embarrassed that she has difficulty walking. She may be uncomfortable talking about her hysterectomy or loss of childbearing ability. She will have her hip exposed for the pre-op injection.

3. a. A possible collaborative nursing action might be to refer Ms. Atwell to a home health agency or a visiting nurse agency. Another possibility might be to arrange for outpatient physical therapy.

    b. A possible independent nursing action might be to talk with Ms. Atwell about alternative ways to manage household chores, such as sitting down to iron or not ironing at all.

4. She should look up pHisohex in the Hospital Formulary or call the pharmacist to ask what it is. She might also read the unit procedures for preoperative preparations. She should not instruct Ms. Atwell to take the shower until she knows what it is expected to accomplish and if there are any potential problems it could cause.

5. To prepare Ms. Atwell for implementation of the medical order, first assess whether she still needs a sleeping pill. If she is asleep, do not wake her to give her the pill. If she does need it, tell her what it is and what it is expected to do for her. Explain how she can make it more effective (e.g., by turning off the lights and staying in bed).

6. Therapeutic communication that might be needed by Ms. Atwell:

    You might talk with her to help her identify and relieve anxiety. She states she is not anxious about surgery, but she might have other anxieties (loss of childbearing function, how she will manage at home). Communication could help you identify whether she is grieving over loss of childbearing ability. You would need to communicate to assess her understanding of the importance of NPO and to do preoperative teaching.

7. a. *Determine that the action is appropriate. Assess for readiness.* The turning is postponed because one need takes priority over another, not because the action would be less successful if performed at this time. You might also have chosen *respects client dignity*—the client might not like to have her visitor see her in pain.

    b. *Be sure you know the rationale for the intervention. Question any actions that you do not understand. Improve your knowledge base.*

    c. *Provide for privacy and comfort.*
    Perform interventions according to professional standards. (The ANA Code of Ethics requires that you maintain client dignity.)

d. *Perform interventions according to professional standards of care and agency policies.* Most agencies have a policy that requires insulin dosage to be checked by two professional nurses. The nurse in this case does not lack knowledge of the intervention; she is simply guarding against error.

e. *Perform interventions according to professional standards* (which include safety).

f. *Determine that the action is still needed and appropriate.* The antihypertensive medication may not be needed if the client's blood pressure is now lower than normal.

8. *If nurse was unable to chart until 8 P.M.:*
    12/6/92, 8:00 P.M.
    D—Says his head hurts and light makes his eyes hurt. Eyes shut tightly.
    A—Cool cloth placed on head; door closed. Tylenol #3, tabs i, given p.o. at 6 P.M. (see medication record). Plan: Disturb as little as possible, keep room dark, notify Dr. King if headache unrelieved after second dose of Tylenol #3.
    R—At 7 P.M., stated head still hurts.————L. Nye, RN.

    Alternatively, if charting was done at 6 and 7 P.M.:
    12/6/92, 6:00 P.M.
    D—Says his head hurts and light makes his eyes hurt. Eyes shut tightly.————————
    A—Cool cloth placed on head; door closed. Tylenol #3, tabs i, given p.o. (see medication record).—L. Nye, RN.
    12/6/92, 7:00 P.M.
    R—States head still hurts.————————
    A—Disturb as little as possible, keep room dark, notify Dr. King if headache unrelieved after second dose of Tylenol #3.————————L. Nye, RN.
    (Did you remember to date, time, and sign your entry, and to draw lines through blank spaces?)

9. See Figure 7–8.

10. 12/9/92   #2—Risk for Noncompliance with Pre- and
    2100   Post-op Instructions r/t lack of knowledge.
              S—States she understands preoperative teaching, including need for NPO.
              O—Preoperative teaching done. Explained NPO after 2400, including rationale.————
              A—No knowledge deficit regarding pre-op procedures.————————
              P—Remove water pitcher at 2400 today.———— When awake, remind her not to drink or eat anything.————L. Nye, RN.
    (Did you remember to date, time, and sign your entry?)

CHAPTER 8

1. The specific, measurable or observable criteria are *b*, *c*, and *d*.

    a. "Safe" is not measurable. "Side rails up" would demonstrate this.

    e. "Adequate number" is not measurable. "Three w/c on each unit" is measurable.

    f. "Systematic" is not measurable. "A complete abdominal assessment is recorded in the client's chart once per shift" is measurable.

DATE 1-6-96	2300-0700	0700-1500	1500-2300
SIGNATURE			*L. Nye R.N.*

		2300-0700	0700-1500	1500-2300

EXERCISE/REST	Type of activity
	How far? How long?
	Repositioned
	ROM
	Aides (walker, cane, crutches, etc.)
	Sleep
		___Bedrest
		___Reposition
		   q 2 hrs
		___BRP/BSC
		___Chair/WC
		___Walk
		___Sleeping
		___Check q hr
		___Request SR down
		___Tx ___ hrs
		Patient Response
			___Bedrest
			___Reposition
			   q 2 hrs
			___BRP/BSC
			___Walk
			___Up ad lib
			___Tx ___ hrs
			Patient Response
				___Bedrest
				___Reposition
				   q 2 hrs
				___BRP/BSC
				___Walk
				_X_Up ad lib
				___Tx ___ hrs
				Patient Response *Walks erect. Steady gait.*

NUTRITION/ FLUID/ELEC	N/V Feeding assistance Tube feedings	___No Problems identified ___Not assessed/sleeping ___NPO	___No Problems identified ___Feed ___Assist Feed ___NPO	_X_No Problems Identified ___Feed ___Assist Feed ___NPO
ELIMINATION	Stool: freq/char Urine: freq/char Bowel sounds flatus, distention	___No Problems Identified ___Urine ___Abd. status ___Stool ___Incontinent	___No Problems Identified ___Urine ___Abd. status ___Stool ___Incontinent	___No Problems Identified ___Urine ___Abd. status 2100 Stool *S. S. enema, c̄ large unformed stool.* ___Incontinent

OXYGENATION	Breathing pattern
	Breath sounds
	Chest tubes
	Sputum
	O₂
	Tissue perfusion
		___Eupneic
		___Lungs clear to
		  auscultation
		___O₂
		___IS c assist
		___Cough/sputum
			___Eupneic
			___Lungs clear to
			  auscultation
			___O₂
			___IS c assist
			___Cough/sputum
				_X_Eupneic
				_X_Lungs clear to
				  auscultation
				___O₂
				___IS c assist
				___Cough/sputum

CIRCULATION	Pulse quality/presence
	Heart sounds
	Edema
		___No problems identified
		___Pedal pulses
		___Cap Refill
		___Numbness/tingling
		___Edema
		___TED Hose
		___R/L toes/fingers
		  pink/pale & warm/cool
			___No problems identified
			___Pedal pulses
			___Cap refill
			___Numbness/tingling
			___Edema
			___TED Hose
			___R/L toes/fingers
			  pink/pale & warm/cool
				___No problems identified
				_X_Pedal pulses = *bil.*
				___Cap refill
				___Numbness/tingling
				_X_Edema +1, (L) ankle
				___TED Hose
				___R/L toes/fingers
				  pink/pale & warm/cool

TEMP REGUL/ SKIN INTEGRITY	Skin assessment
	Wound/incision
	Rash
	Heparin Lock Site
		___Hep Lock
		___Dressing/incision
		  Normal
		___Warm/dry
		___Cast dry/intact
		___Brace/splint
		___Checked q 2 hr
		  for fit/position
			___Hep Lock
			___Dressing/incision
			  normal
			___Warm/dry
			___Cast dry/intact
			___Brace/splint
			___Checked q 2 hr
			  for fit/position
				___Hep Lock
				___Dressing/incision
				  Normal
				_X_Warm/dry
				___Cast/dry intact
				___Brace/splint
				___Checked q 2 hr
				  for fit/position

PATIENT DAILY ASSESSMENT SUMMARY FLOW SHEET
2 NORTH (PILOT)

Figure 7–8. Patient Daily Assessment Summary Flowsheet—Completed. Courtesy of Shawnee Mission Medical Center.

DATE	2300-0700	0700-1500	1500-2300
SIGNATURE			*L. Nye, R.N.*

		2300-0700	0700-1500	1500-2300
SENSORY/ NEURO	Visual/hearing aid Communication aid Perceptual ability Pain Neuro assessment Level of conscious.	__Alert/oriented __No c/o pain __C/o pain (Location) __See MAR __Dorsi/Plantar flex __Indicates pain relief	__Alert/oriented __No c/o pain __C/o pain (Location) __See MAR __Dorsi/Plantar flex __Indicates pain relief	X_Alert/oriented __No c/o pain X_C/o pain *abd cramps* (Location) X_See MAR __Dorsi/Plantar flex __Indicates pain relief
ENDOCRINE	Uterine/prostate status Menstrual/lactation Pregnancy Endocrine status	__NA __No s/s hypo/hyper glycemia __See Diabetic Record	__NA __No s/s hypo/hyper glycemia __See Diabetic Record	X_NA __No s/s hypo/hyper glycemia __See Diabetic Record
SELF CONCEPT/ INTERDEPENDENCE	Emotional status Coping mechanisms Role of S.O.	__Cooperative __Freq call lite use/ demands __Safety assessment min/mod/intense Posey/wrist restraints __Pt/family emotional support (Mod/intense	__Cooperative __Freq. call lite use/ demands __Safety assessment min/mod/intense Posey/wrist restraints __Pt/family emotional support (mod/intense	X_Cooperative __Freq call lite use/ demands __Safety assessment min/mod/intense Posey/wrist restraints __Pt/family emotional support (Mod/intense)
ROLE FUNCTION	Knowledge deficit Learning abilities Discharge planning Adaptive difficulty to new roles	__Nursing cares/ procedures explained __Special teaching: __Pt. indicates understanding	__Nursing cares/ procedures explained __Special teaching: __Pt. indicates understanding	X_Nursing cares/ procedures explained X_Special teaching: *pre-op. see No. Prog. notes* X_Pt. indicates understanding

NURSING PROGRESS NOTES

TIME	
1800	Sensori-Neuro- Ibuprofen given for c/o. abd cramping (see MAR.) *L. Nye, R.N.*
1900	Sensori-Neuro- States, "I feel better now." Role Function- Pre-op teaching done, including NPO at midnight & rationale for NPO. *L. Nye, R.N.*

Figure 7–8. Concluded.

2. 1. *b* and *c*

2. *a* (The data would come from the manual in structure evaluation. In process evaluation, one might note whether a nurse is following procedures, but the data itself would come from one's observation of the nurse's activities.)

3. *c* (possibly *b*—client might report whether nurse has done required teaching, etc.)

4. *c*
5. *b*
6. *a*
7. *b*
8. *a*

3.
1. *c*   5. *a*
2. *b*   6. *a* (possibly *b*)
3. *a*   7. *a*
4. *c*

4. a. Possible outcome criteria:
Oral mucosa pink, moist, intact
States no oral pain
No inflammation or ulcerations in oral cavity
Able to swallow without difficulty (when no longer NPO)

b. Examples of methods for obtaining data for the criteria:
Examine the patient's oral cavity.
Ask the client if his mouth is sore.
Examine the parient's oral cavity.
Observe the client swallowing, or ask him if he is having any difficulty.
(If you were performing a retrospective audit, you would look for this evidence in the chart— probably in the progress notes.

5. a. The following are examples; you may have thought of other cues. Verbal cues that would indicate achievement of the objective:
Ms. Atwell states, "I'm confident everything will go all right. I certainly don't have any experience with this kind of thing, but I know you will tell me what I need to know. I feel pretty relaxed, actually."

b. Nonverbal cues that would indicate achievement of the objective:
Client shows no facial tension.
Hands folded loosely in lap.
Sitting quietly; no fidgeting.

c. Verbal cues that would indicate the objective has not been achieved:
"I'd really rather not talk about it now."
"I'm still pretty scared."

d. Nonverbal cues that would indicate the objective has not been achieved:

Moving restlessly in bed	Tearful; pale
Perspiring heavily	Facial muscles tense
Not making eye contact	Wringing hands
Voice is shaky, tremulous	Pulse elevated

6. *Risk for Anxiety.* Goal met. Ct. verbalizes understanding of procedure and effects of surgery; exhibits no physical signs of anxiety. (Could also quote progress notes verbatim as evidence of goal achievement.)
Risk for Grief. Goal partially met. Client expressed feelings of relief at no longer having menses, but avoided discussion of inability to bear children. Will need to follow up after surgery.

Risk for Noncompliance with NPO. Goal partially met. Client verbalized reasons for NPO and verbalized intent to comply with restriction; however, she did drink some water at 0230, stating "I forgot."

7. *Risk for Anxiety* . . . You could discontinue this entire section of the plan: nursing diagnosis, goals, and nursing orders. The problem has been resolved.
Risk for Grief . . . This is still a potential problem. You should keep the diagnosis and goal.
Risk for Noncompliance . . . Because the goals are only partially met, you need to keep the diagnoses. You should mark off the first goal, because she has already done this.

8. b.   Even though the client does not have Actual Impaired Skin Integrity, Risk for Impaired Skin Integrity still exists. If the nursing interventions are discontinued, the client will undoubtedly develop Impaired Skin Integrity.

CHAPTER 9

1.

	Nursing Diagnosis	Predicted Outcomes	Nursing Orders
Verbally denies he is ill. Observed out of bed in spite of medical order for bedrest. Refused to take his 3 P.M. meds.	Noncompliance (Medical Treatment Plan) r/t denial of illness.	Pt will adhere to activity limitations. Pt will acknowledge consequences of not complying with treatment regimen. Pt will agree to follow plans for care (eg., meds, bedrest).	Encourage to express feelings & concerns about being hospitalized. Give positive reinforcement for compliance (e.g., staying in bed, taking meds). Develop a written contract with pt regarding bedrest and meds. Evaluate pt's support system and need for emotional support from staff.

2.   *Table 9.1 and Figure 9.9. Care Plan for Luisa Sanchez*

Guideline 1:   Does not apply. This care plan is for client nursing diagnoses only and is not intended to address the client's medical plan of care nor her routine basic needs. It does, however include some client-profile information (name, admitting date, and diagnosis and some medical orders).

Guideline 2:   Not met. Problems are dated but not signed.

Guideline 3:   Met. The problems are numbered in order of priority.

Guideline 4:   Probably met. The plan does not indicate that the nursing orders are listed in order of priority, but they appear to be.

Guideline 5:   Met, for the most part. Plan occasionally fails to abbreviate.

Guideline 6:   Met. Written legibly, typed (not in ink).

Guideline 7:   Met. Refers to other sources for detailed treatments (e.g., IV therapy).

Guideline 8: Partially met. Considers physiological and psychological (self-esteem) needs. Does not address spiritual needs. However, Mrs. Sanchez's data base does not indicate that she has any special needs in these areas.

Guideline 9: The problem list is individualized. There is not enough data about Mrs. Sanchez to adequately individualize her nursing orders. For instance, we do not know what kinds of fluids and fiber-foods she likes to eat.

Guideline 10: Some collaborative aspects are included e.g., IV Therapy, Heparin administration). Lab tests, X ray, and so forth would probably be in another section.

Guideline 11: This plan does not show any discharge planning. However, it may be included in the Standards of Care for Abdominal Hysterectomy or the Nursing Care Plan for Thrombophlebitis.

3. The care plan for Harvey Cain appears in the figures below and on the following page.

PROBLEM LIST FOR HARVEY CAIN		
Date and Initials	Nursing Diagnoses/Problems	Source for Goals and Nursing Orders
1-1-96 *JW*	Potential Complications of Bowel Obstructions	Refer to Standards of Care for Intestinal Obstruction.
1-1-96 *JW*	Risk for Altered Tissue Integrity (Pressure Ulcer) r/t decreased mobility, poor nutrition . . .	Nurse will develop goals and nursing orders.
1-1-96 *JW*	Abdominal Pain r/t abdominal distention	Refer to standardized care plan for Pain.
1-1-96 *JW*	Altered Oral Mucous Membranes r/t fluid loss from vomiting 2° intestinal obstruction	Refer to standardized care plan for altered Oral Mucous Membrane.
1-1-96 *JW*	Possible Fear or Anxiety r/t hospital environment, diagnostic tests, equipment, and procedures	Nurse will develop goals and nursing orders.
1-1-96 *JW*	Possible Fear of Dying r/t unknown outcome of illness and lack of information	Nurse will develop goals and nursing orders.
1-1-96 *JW*	Potential Complications of Upper GI: Perforations . . .	Nurse will develop goals and nursing orders.
1-1-96 *JW*	Potential Complications of IV Therapy . . .	See "Policies and Procedures for IV Therapy."
1-1-96 *JW*	Potential Complications of Nasoenteric Intubation: Ulceration —> Hemorrhage	See "Policies and Procedures for Nasoenteric Intubation and Suction."
1-1-96 *JW*	Potential Complications of Barium Enema	See "Protocol for Barium Enema."

Problem List for Harvey Cain

SHAWNEE MISSION MEDICAL CENTER

Date ord.	Radiology	Date Sch	DONE	Date ord.	Laboratory	Date Sch	DONE	Date ord.	Special Procedures	Date Sch	DONE
1-1	Upper GI	1/1		1-1	CBC, Lytes	1-1	✔				
1-1	Flat plate abd	1/1			SMA12						
									Daily Tests		
	Ancillary Consults										
									Daily Weight		

Diet: NPO

Food Allergies: none stated

Hold:

Feeding/Fluids NPO
- ☐ Self
- ☐ Assist
- ☐ Feeder
- ☐ Force
- ☐ Restrict

	meal	Ext	IV
7-3			
3-11			
11-7			

☒ I&O (hourly)
☒ IV D5LR 1250 c/hr
☐ Other_____

Safety Measures
- ☒ Siderails
- ☐ Restraints
- ☐ Other_____

Activities
- ☒ Bedrest
- ☐ BRP
- ☐ Dangle
- ☐ Chair
- ☐ Commode
- ☐ Up ad Lib
- ☒ Turn
- ☐ Ambulate

Transportation
per cart

Hygiene
- ☒ Bedbath
- ☐ Assist
- ☐ Self Bath
- ☐ Shower
- ☐ Tub
- ☐ Vanity
- ☐ Oral Care

Bowel/Bladder
- ☒ Foley   IN 1-1   OUT _____
- ☒ Cath care Bid
- ☐ Incontinent
- ☐ Colostomy
- ☐ Ileostomy
- ☐ Urostomy

Communication

1-1   Save any stools

Physical Therapy | **Date** | **Treatments**

1/1 Nasoenteric tube to Gomco

Cardio-Pulmonary

Drug Allergies: Codeine.

Isolation: In   Out

Emergency Instructions:
Relatives: Mildred Cain (wife)
Phone: 631-1098
Clergy: Fr. Wise 842-0097
Religion: Catholic
Religious Rites: No Special
Code Blue

Diagnosis: Intestinal Obstruction; Dehydration
Surgery & Dates:
Consults & Dates: Martin Botha, M.D.

Room	Name	Adm Date	Age	Physician
426	Cain, Harvey	1-1-96	78	ELTON HOBBS, M.D.

Kardex for Harvey Cain. Courtesy of Shawnee Mission Medical Center.

INDEX